Hypertensive Disease: Current Challenges, New Concepts, and Management

Guest Editor

EDWARD D. FROHLICH, MD, MACP, FACC

MEDICAL CLINICS OF NORTH AMERICA

www.medical.theclinics.com

May 2009 • Volume 93 • Number 3

SAUNDERS an imprint of ELSEVIER, Inc.

W.B. SAUNDERS COMPANY
A Division of Elsevier Inc.

1600 John F. Kennedy Boulevard • Suite 1800 • Philadelphia, Pennsylvania 19103-2899

http://www.theclinics.com

MEDICAL CLINICS OF NORTH AMERICA Volume 93, Number 3
May 2009 ISSN 0025-7125, ISBN-13: 978-1-4377-1004-5, ISBN-10: 1-4377-1004-2

Editor: Rachel Glover
Developmental Editor: Donald Mumford

Medical Clinics of North America (ISSN 0025-7125) is published bimonthly by W.B. Saunders, 360 Park Avenue South, New York, NY 10010-1710. Business and editorial offices: 1600 John F. Kennedy Boulevard, Suite 1800, Philadelphia, PA 19103-2899. Accounting and circulation offices: 6277 Sea Harbor Drive, Orlando, FL 32887-4800. Periodicals postage paid at New York, NY, and additional mailing offices. Subscription prices are USD 187 per year for US individuals, USD 334 per year for US institutions, USD 96 per year for US students, USD 238 per year for Canadian individuals, USD 434 per year for Canadian institutions, USD 151 per year for Canadian students, USD 288 per year for international individuals, USD 434 per year for international institutions and USD 151 per year for international students. To receive student/resident rate, orders must be accompanied by name of affiliated institution, date of term, and the *signature* of program/residency coordinator on institution letterhead. Orders will be billed at individual rate until proof of status is received. Foreign air speed delivery is included in all *Clinics* subscription prices. All prices are subject to change without notice. POSTMASTER: Send address changes to *Medical Clinics of North America*, Elsevier Periodicals Customer Service, 11830 Westline Industrial Drive, St. Louis, MO 63146. Customer Service (orders, claims, online, change of address): Elsevier Periodicals Customer Service, 11830 Westline Industrial Drive, St. Louis, MO 63146. Tel: 1-800-654-2452 (U.S. and Canada); 314-453-7041 (outside U.S. and Canada). Fax: 314-453-5170. E-mail: journalscustomerservice-usa@elsevier.com (for print support); journalsonlinesupport-usa@elsevier.com (for online support).

Reprints. For copies of 100 or more of articles in this publication, please contact the Commercial Reprints Department, Elsevier Inc., 360 Park Avenue South, New York, NY 10010-1710. Tel.: 212-633-3812; Fax: 212-462-1935; E-mail: reprints@elsevier.com.

Medical Clinics of North America is also published in Spanish by McGraw-Hill Interamericana Editores S. A., P.O. Box 5-237, 06500 Mexico, D.F., Mexico.

Medical Clinics of North America is covered in *MEDLINE/PubMed (Index Medicus), Current Contents, ASCA, Excerpta Medica, Science Citation Index, and ISI/BIOMED.*

Printed in the United States of America.

GOAL STATEMENT
The goal of *Medical Clinics of North America* is to keep practicing physicians up to date with current clinical practice by providing timely articles reviewing the state of the art in patient care.

ACCREDITATION
The *Medical Clinics of North America* is planned and implemented in accordance with the Essential Areas and Policies of the Accreditation Council for Continuing Medical Education (ACCME) through the joint sponsorship of the University of Virginia School of Medicine and Elsevier. The University of Virginia School of Medicine is accredited by the ACCME to provide continuing medical education for physicians.

The University of Virginia School of Medicine designates this educational activity for a maximum of 15 *AMA PRA Category 1 Credits*™ for each issue, 90 credits per year. Physicians should only claim credit commensurate with the extent of their participation in the activity.

The American Medical Association has determined that physicians not licensed in the US who participate in this CME activity are eligible for a maximum of 15 *AMA PRA Category 1 Credits*™ for each issue, 90 credits per year.

Credit can be earned by reading the text material, taking the CME examination online at http://www.theclinics.com/home/cme, and completing the evaluation. After taking the test, you will be required to review any and all incorrect answers. Following completion of the test and evaluation, your credit will be awarded and you may print your certificate.

FACULTY DISCLOSURE/CONFLICT OF INTEREST
The University of Virginia School of Medicine, as an ACCME accredited provider, endorses and strives to comply with the Accreditation Council for Continuing Medical Education (ACCME) Standards of Commercial Support, Commonwealth of Virginia statutes, University of Virginia policies and procedures, and associated federal and private regulations and guidelines on the need for disclosure and monitoring of proprietary and financial interests that may affect the scientific integrity and balance of content delivered in continuing medical education activities under our auspices.

The University of Virginia School of Medicine requires that all CME activities accredited through this institution be developed independently and be scientifically rigorous, balanced and objective in the presentation/discussion of its content, theories and practices.

All authors/editors participating in an accredited CME activity are expected to disclose to the readers relevant financial relationships with commercial entities occurring within the past 12 months (such as grants or research support, employee, consultant, stock holder, member of speakers bureau, etc.). The University of Virginia School of Medicine will employ appropriate mechanisms to resolve potential conflicts of interest to maintain the standards of fair and balanced education to the reader. Questions about specific strategies can be directed to the Office of Continuing Medical Education, University of Virginia School of Medicine, Charlottesville, Virginia.

The faculty and staff of the University of Virginia Office of Continuing Medical Education have no financial affiliations to disclose.

The authors/editors listed below have identified no professional or financial affiliations for themselves or their spouse/partner:
Rohit Amin, MD; Javier Díez, MD, PhD; Edward D. Frohlich, MD, MACP, FACC (Guest Editor); Krishna K. Gaddam, MD; Michael Gardner, MD; Rachel Glover (Acquisitions Editor); Maria Carolina Gongora, MD; David G. Harrison, MD; Tareq Islam, MPH; Avanelle V. Jack, MD; Rigas G. Kalaitzidis, MD; William B. Kannel, MD, MPH, FACC; Nitin Khosla, MD; Marie A. Krousel-Wood, MD, MSPH; Edward G. Lakatta, MD; Guido Lastra, MD; Camila Manrique, MD; Donald E. Morisky, ScD, MSPH; Paul Muntner, PhD; Brian P. Murphy, MBChB, MRCP; Samer S. Najjar, MD; Richard N. Re, MD, FACP; Michel E. Safar, MD; Scott D. Solomon, MD; Tony Stanton, PhD, MBChB, MRCP; Stephen C. Textor, MD; Mark Thompson, MD; Anil Verma, MD; Mingyi Wang, MD, PhD; Larry S. Webber, PhD; and Andrew Wolf, MD (Test Author).

The authors/editors listed below identified the following professional or financial affiliations for themselves or their spouse/partner:
George L. Bakris, MD serves as a consultant for Abbott, Takeda, Glaxo-Smith-Kline, Boerhinger-Ingelheim, Gileada, Novartis, and Merck, serves on the Speakers Bureau for Novartis and Forest, serves on the Advisory Board for Abbot, Boerhinger-Ingelheim, Forest, Merck, Novartis, Walgreens, Gilead, and Diachii-Sankyo, has received grants from NIH(NIDDK), Glaxo-Smith-Kline, Forest, and Juvenile Diabetes Foundation, and has received remuneration from Abbott, Boerhinger-Ingelheim, Forest, Glaxo-Smith-Kline, Merck, Novartis, Walgreens, Gileada, Daiichi/Sankyo, and Takeda.
Francis G. Dunn, MBChB, FRCP, FACC receives funding from BristolMeyresSquibb and Meck Sharpe and Dohme.
Efrain Reisin, MD is a consultant for Mission Pharmacal and is an industry funded research/investigator for Amgen, Shire, and Mitsubichi.
James R. Sowers, MD has received grants from Novartis and Forrest
Hector O. Ventura, MD serves on the Advisory Board GlaxoSmithKline, Astra Zenexa, and Scios

Disclosure of Discussion of Non-FDA Approved Uses for Pharmaceutical Products and/or Medical Devices.
The University of Virginia School of Medicine, as an ACCME provider, requires that all faculty presenters identify and disclose any off-label uses for pharmaceutical and medical device products. The University of Virginia School of Medicine recommends that each physician fully review all the available data on new products or procedures prior to clinical use.

TO ENROLL
To enroll in the Medical Clinics of North America Continuing Medical Education program, call customer service at 1-800-654-2452 or visit us online at http://www.theclinics.com/home/cme. The CME program is available to subscribers for an additional fee of USD 205.

FORTHCOMING ISSUES

July 2009
Care of the Cirrhotic Patient
David A. Sass, MD, *Guest Editor*

September 2009
Preoperative Medical Consultation
Lee Fleisher, MD, and
Stanley Rosenbaum, MD,
Guest Editors

November 2009
Cutaneous Manifestations of Internal Medicine
Neil Sadick, MD, *Guest Editor*

RECENT ISSUES

March 2009
Common Neurologic Disorders
Randolph W. Evans, MD,
Guest Editor

January 2009
Osteoarthritis
David J. Hunter, MBBS, MSc, PhD,
Guest Editor

November 2008
New and Emerging Infectious Diseases
Mary Elizabeth Wilson, MD, FACP, FIDSA,
Guest Editor

September 2008
Women's Health
Tony Ogburn, MD, and Carolyn Voss, MD,
Guest Editors

RELATED INTEREST

Clinics in Geriatric Medicine, May 2009 (Volume 25, Issue 2)
Hypertension in the Elderly
Mahboob Rahman, *Guest Editor*
www.geriatric.theclinics.com

THE CLINICS ARE NOW AVAILABLE ONLINE!

Access your subscription at:
www.theclinics.com

Contributors

GUEST EDITOR

EDWARD D. FROHLICH, MD, MACP, FACC
Alton Ochsner Distinguished Scientist, Ochsner Clinic Foundation; Professor of Medicine and Physiology, Louisiana State University School of Medicine; Clinical Professor of Medicine; Adjunct Professor of Pharmacology, Tulane University School of Medicine, New Orleans, Louisiana

AUTHORS

ROHIT AMIN, MD
Fellow, Cardiovascular Diseases, Ochsner Clinic Foundation, New Orleans, Louisiana

GEORGE L. BAKRIS, MD
Professor of Medicine; Director, Hypertensive Diseases Unit, University of Chicago-Pritzker School of Medicine, Chicago, Illinois

JAVIER DÍEZ, MD, PhD
Full Professor of Cardiovascular Medicine, School of Medicine; Director, Division of Cardiovascular Sciences, Centre for Applied Medical Research; Head of Molecular Cardiology, Department of Cardiology and Cardiovascular Surgery, University Clinic, University of Navarra, Pamplona, Spain

FRANCIS G. DUNN, MBChB, FRCP, FACC
Consultant Cardiologist, Cardiac Department, Stobhill Hospital, Glasgow, Scotland, United Kingdom

EDWARD D. FROHLICH, MD, MACP, FACC
Alton Ochsner Distinguished Scientist, Ochsner Clinic Foundation; Professor of Medicine and Physiology, Louisiana State University School of Medicine; Clinical Professor of Medicine; Adjunct Professor of Pharmacology, Tulane University School of Medicine, New Orleans, Louisiana

KRISHNA K. GADDAM, MD
Fellow, Cardiovascular Diseases, Ochsner Clinic Foundation, New Orleans, Louisiana

MICHAEL GARDNER, MD
Assistant Professor of Medicine, Department of Internal Medicine, Diabetes and Cardiovascular Center, University of Missouri, Columbia, Missouri

MARIA CAROLINA GONGORA, MD
Division of Cardiology, Department of Medicine, Emory University School of Medicine and the Atlanta Veterans Administration Hospital, Atlanta, Georgia

DAVID G. HARRISON, MD
Bernard Marcus Professor of Medicine, Division of Cardiology, Department of Medicine, Emory University School of Medicine and the Atlanta Veterans Administration Hospital, Atlanta, Georgia

TAREQ ISLAM, MPH
Biostatistician, Department of Epidemiology, Tulane University School of Public Health and Tropical Medicine, New Orleans, Louisiana

AVANELLE V. JACK, MD
Assistant Professor of Clinical Medicine; Fellowship Program Director, Section of Nephrology and Hypertension, Department of Medicine, Louisiana State University Health Sciences Center, New Orleans, Louisiana

RIGAS KALAITZIDIS, MD
Department of Medicine, Hypertensive Diseases Unit, Section of Endocrinology, Diabetes, and Metabolism, University of Chicago-Pritzker School of Medicine, Chicago, Illinois

WILLIAM B. KANNEL, MD, MPH, FACC
Professor Emeritus, Boston University School of Medicine/Framingham Heart Study, Framingham, Massachusetts

NITIN KHOSLA, MD
Department of Medicine, Section of Nephrology and Hypertension, University of California at San Diego, San Diego, California

MARIE A. KROUSEL-WOOD, MD, MSPH
Director, Center for Health Research, Ochsner Clinic Foundation; Clinical Professor, Department of Epidemiology, Tulane University School of Public Health and Tropical Medicine; Clinical Professor, Department of Family and Community Medicine, Tulane University School of Medicine, New Orleans, Louisiana

EDWARD G. LAKATTA, MD
Laboratory of Cardiovascular Science, Intramural Research Program, National Institute on Aging, National Institutes of Health, Baltimore, Maryland

GUIDO LASTRA, MD
Endocrinology Fellow, Department of Internal Medicine, Diabetes and Cardiovascular Center, University of Missouri, Columbia, Missouri

CAMILA MANRIQUE, MD
Endocrinology Fellow, Department of Internal Medicine, Diabetes and Cardiovascular Center, University of Missouri, Columbia, Missouri

DONALD E. MORISKY, ScD, MSPH
Professor, Department of Community Health Sciences, UCLA School of Public Health, Los Angeles, California

PAUL MUNTNER, PhD
Associate Professor, Department of Community and Preventive Medicine, Mount Sinai School of Medicine, New York, New York

BRIAN P. MURPHY, MBChB, MRCP
Specialist Registrar, Cardiac Department, Stobhill Hospital, Glasgow, Scotland, United Kingdom

SAMER S. NAJJAR, MD
Laboratory of Cardiovascular Science, Intramural Research Program, National Institute on Aging, National Institutes of Health, Baltimore, Maryland

RICHARD N. RE, MD, FACP
Scientific Director, Ochsner Clinic Foundation; Clinical Professor of Medicine; Adjunct Professor of Physiology, Tulane University School of Medicine, New Orleans, Louisiana

EFRAIN REISIN, MD
Professor of Medicine; Chief, Section of Nephrology and Hypertension, Department of Medicine, Louisiana State University Health Sciences Center, New Orleans, Louisiana

MICHEL E. SAFAR, MD
Professor of Therapeutics, Université Paris Descartes, Assistance Publique-Hôpitaux de Paris, Hôtel-Dieu, Centre de Diagnostic et de Thérapeutique, Paris, France

SCOTT D. SOLOMON, MD
Associate Professor of Medicine, Director of Non-Invasive Cardiology, Harvard Medical School, Brigham and Women's Hospital, Boston, Massachusetts

JAMES R. SOWERS, MD
Professor of Medicine and Physiology, Department of Internal Medicine, Diabetes and Cardiovascular Center, University of Missouri; Department of Physiology and Pharmacology, University of Missouri; Harry S. Truman VA Hospital, Columbia, Missouri

TONY STANTON, PhD, MBChB, MRCP
Specialist Registrar, Department of Medicine, University of Queensland, Princess Alexandra Hospital, Brisbane, Australia

STEPHEN C. TEXTOR, MD
Professor of Medicine; Vice-chair, Division of Nephrology and Hypertension, Mayo Clinic, Rochester, Minnesota

MARK THOMPSON, MD
Fellow, Cardiovascular Diseases, Ochsner Clinic Foundation, New Orleans, Louisiana

HECTOR VENTURA, MD
Director, Cardiovascular Fellowship Program, Ochsner Clinic Foundation, New Orleans, Louisiana

ANIL VERMA, MD
Fellow, Cardiovascular Diseases, Ochsner Clinic Foundation, New Orleans, Louisiana

MINGYI WANG, MD, PhD
Laboratory of Cardiovascular Science, Intramural Research Program, National Institute on Aging, National Institutes of Health, Baltimore, Maryland

LARRY S. WEBBER, PhD
Professor, Department of Biostatistics, Tulane University School of Public Health and Tropical Medicine, New Orleans, Louisiana

Contents

Preface   xv

Edward D. Frohlich

Current Challenges and Unresolved Problems in Hypertensive Disease   527

Edward D. Frohlich

> Over the past four or five decades, hypertension and cardiovascular
> medicine has experienced dramatic and innovative changes that have
> significantly reduced morbidity and mortality. A vast array of new antihy-
> pertensive compounds have been developed, which are able to inhibit
> many pathophysiologic mechanisms of the disease and prevent many of
> the outcomes in patients with hypertension. Much of this series of thera-
> peutic breakthroughs have been the result of active participation of clinical
> scientists with tremendous and remarkable knowledge of and experience
> with the fundamental mechanisms of disease. In more recent years, much
> new information has appeared concerning the basis genetic and biologic
> mechanisms involved in cardiovascular and renal diseases. What remains
> of utmost importance is for members of the academic community with
> a wide spectrum of experience and points of view to continue to work
> with the fundamental problems and mechanisms of the diseases.

Hypertension: Reflections on Risks and Prognostication   541

William B. Kannel

> Framingham Heart Study cardiovascular disease prospective population
> epidemiologic research has played an important role in the evolution of
> modern cohort study design and the advancement of preventive cardiol-
> ogy. To date no single essential factor has been identified; multiple inter-
> related factors are promoting increased risk for development of CHD.
> Elevated blood pressure has emerged as a prominent member of cardio-
> vascular risk factors. The study's documentation of a strong link of blood
> pressure to development of cardiovascular events stimulated the pharma-
> ceutical industry to develop medications for controlling blood pressure
> and, in turn, national campaigns to combat hypertension and its adverse
> vascular outlook.

New Insights into Target Organ Involvement in Hypertension   559

Richard N. Re

> Optimization of the care of the hypertensive patient will require not only
> attention to the regulation of arterial pressure but also to blunting the
> hypertension-related processes that lead to vascular disease. It is clear
> that the regulation of these processes is much more complex than
> previously understood. Here several new insights into the pathogenesis
> of hypertension-related vascular disease are explored with an emphasis
> on the role played by the renin-angiotensin systems.

The Renin Angiotensin Aldosterone System in Hypertension: Roles of Insulin Resistance and Oxidative Stress   569

Camila Manrique, Guido Lastra, Michael Gardner, and James R. Sowers

Hypertension (HTN) is a leading risk factor for cardiovascular disease (CVD) and chronic kidney disease (CKD)-related morbidity and mortality. Several abnormalities participate in the development of HTN. Inappropriately activated systemic and local tissue renin angiotensin aldosterone systems (RAAS) contribute to the hemodynamic and metabolic abnormalities that lead to endothelial dysfunction, HTN, CVD, and CKD. There is a growing body of evidence demonstrating a close relationship between RAAS activation, excessive production of reactive oxygen species, insulin resistance, and HTN. From a therapeutic standpoint, RAAS blockade results in improved insulin resistance, glucose homeostasis, and improved cardiovascular and renal outcomes. This article is focused on the role of RAAS-mediated insulin resistance and oxidative stress in the pathogenesis of HTN, CVD, and CKD.

Arterial Aging and Subclinical Arterial Disease are Fundamentally Intertwined at Macroscopic and Molecular Levels   583

Edward G. Lakatta, Mingyi Wang, and Samer S. Najjar

The structure and function of arteries change throughout a lifetime. Age is the dominant risk factor for hypertension, coronary heart disease, congestive heart failure, and stroke. The cellular/molecular proinflammatory alterations that underlie arterial aging are novel putative candidates to be targeted by interventions aimed at attenuating arterial aging as a major risk factor for cardiovascular diseases. This review provides a landscape of central arterial aging and age-disease interactions, integrating perspectives that range from humans to molecules, with the goal that future therapies for cardiovascular diseases, such as hypertension, also will target the prevention or amelioration of unsuccessful arterial aging.

Hypertension, Systolic Blood Pressure, and Large Arteries   605

Michel E. Safar

This article discusses the following: (1) factors modulating central and peripheral SBP and PP in hypertensive subjects; (2) mechanisms enhancing PP variations in this population; (3) Analysis of pulsatile arterial hemodynamics as predictors of CV risk; and (4) Pulsatile hemodynamics and strategies lowering CV risk in the treatment of hypertension.

Oxidative Stress and Hypertension   621

David G. Harrison and Maria Carolina Gongora

Reactive oxygen species (ROS) oxidize, reduce, or combine with other molecules in both physiologic and pathophysiologic ways. This article examines the role of ROS in hypertension, especially in certain tissues, such as the brain, the kidney, and the vasculature. A major clinical challenge is that the routinely used antioxidants are ineffective in preventing or treating cardiovascular disease and hypertension. This is likely because these drugs are either ineffective or act in a nontargeted fashion, such that they remove not only injurious ROS but also those involved in normal cell signaling. Inflammatory cells such as T cells may contribute to hypertension, and further investigation of how this occurs may lead to new therapies.

Towards a New Paradigm About Hypertensive Heart Disease   **637**

Javier Díez

A new paradigm is emerging related to the impact of chronic hypertension on the cardiac parenchyma. Whereas left ventricular hypertrophy may be detected early and accurately in hypertensive patients by electrocardiography and echocardiography, newer cardiac imaging methods and the monitoring of several circulating biomarkers holds promise as a noninvasive tool for the diagnosis of myocardial remodeling. A large number of clinical studies have shown that long-term antihypertensive treatment may be associated with regression of left ventricular hypertrophy, and this is associated with the decrease of the risk of cardiovascular morbidity and mortality. However, because the remaining risk is unacceptably high, new therapeutic strategies aimed not just to decrease left ventricular mass, but also to repair myocardial remodeling are necessary. All of these aspects are reviewed in brief in this article.

Diastolic Dysfunction as a Link Between Hypertension and Heart Failure   **647**

Anil Verma and Scott D. Solomon

Hypertension significantly contributes to cardiovascular morbidity and mortality by causing substantial structural and functional adaptations, including left ventricular diastolic dysfunction. Left ventricular diastolic dysfunction is characterized by abnormalities in left ventricular filling, including decreased diastolic distensibility and impaired relaxation, and it may represent an early measure of myocardial end-organ damage. Diastolic dysfunction may well precede development of left ventricular hypertrophy in hypertension and possibly is characteristic of an important pathophysiologic link between hypertension and heart failure with preserved ejection fraction. No specific therapeutic regimen has shown to benefit patients who have heart failure with preserved ejection fraction, and thus there is a need to understand the potential mechanisms primarily responsible for this clinical syndrome and its relationship to hypertension and diastolic dysfunction.

Hypertension and Cardiac Failure in its Various Forms   **665**

Krishna K. Gaddam, Anil Verma, Mark Thompson, Rohit Amin, and Hector Ventura

Aging population and poorly controlled hypertension contribute to an ever-increasing prevalence of heart failure. Two different phenotypes of heart failure, namely, heart failure with reduced ejection fraction and heart failure with preserved ejection fraction, are being increasingly recognized. However, they may not necessarily be separate processes and may actually represent a continuum. Nevertheless, either form of heart failure is associated with very high morbidity and mortality. Significant advances have been achieved in understanding the pathophysiology and treatment of patients who have heart failure with reduced ejection fraction. However, heart failure with preserved ejection fraction is less well understood and no convincing evidence-based treatment options are available in treating these patients. Given the poor prognosis with either form of heart failure, it is imperative to recognize and treat hypertension early.

Hypertension and Myocardial Ischemia   681

Brian P. Murphy, Tony Stanton, and Francis G. Dunn

There is an impressive evidence base for the presence of myocardial ischemia in patients who have hypertension. This relationship ranges from the obvious association with obstructive coronary artery disease to more subtle mechanisms related to hemodynamic, microcirculatory, and neuroendocrine abnormalities. All of these factors serve to destabilize the critical balance between myocardial oxygen supply and demand. We have at our disposal a range of sophisticated investigations that allow us to demonstrate the presence and extent of the ischemia and therefore to target specific therapies to reduce the risk to these patients. Achieving target blood pressure and managing all reversible components of the patient's cardiovascular risk status help to minimize the clinical sequelae of myocardial ischemia in this vulnerable population.

The Kidney, Hypertension, and Remaining Challenges   697

Nitin Khosla, Rigas Kalaitzidis, and George L. Bakris

There is an epidemic of chronic kidney disease in the Western world, with hypertension being the second most common cause. Blood pressure control rates, while improving, are still below 50% for the United States population. The following three challenges remain for the treatment of hypertension and associated prevention of end-stage kidney disease. First, a better understanding by the general medical community of how and in whom to use renin angiotensin aldosterone system blockers is needed. Second, the appropriate initiation of fixed-dose combination therapy to achieve blood-pressure goals needs to be clarified. Finally, the subgroup of patients with kidney disease needs more aggressive blood pressure lowering.

Current Approaches to Renovascular Hypertension   717

Stephen C. Textor

This article examines the status regarding prevalence, mechanisms, clinical manifestations and management of renovascular hypertension at this point in time. It should be viewed as a work in progress. As with most complex conditions, clinicians must integrate the results of published literature studies while considering each patient's specific features and comorbid disease risks. Beyond identifying renovascular disease as a cause of secondary hypertension, one must manage renal artery stenosis (RAS) itself as an atherosclerotic vascular complication. This disease warrants follow-up regarding progression and potential for ischemic tissue injury. These elements often determine the role and timing for revascularization. In this respect, atherosclerotic renal artery stenosis is analogous to progressive carotid or aortic aneurysmal disease.

Obesity and Hypertension: Mechanisms, Cardio-Renal Consequences, and Therapeutic Approaches   **733**

Efrain Reisin and Avanelle V. Jack

Obesity and its relationship to hypertension is growing worldwide and is considered today to be a pandemic. This article focuses on the impact of obesity and hypertension on the cardiovascular and renal systems. It also summarizes the nonpharmacological and pharmacological approaches used to control hypertension in the obese population.

Barriers to and Determinants of Medication Adherence in Hypertension Management: Perspective of the Cohort Study of Medication Adherence Among Older Adults   **753**

Marie A. Krousel-Wood, Paul Muntner, Tareq Islam, Donald E. Morisky, and Larry S. Webber

Low adherence to antihypertensive medication remains a public health challenge. Understanding barriers to, and determinants of, adherence to antihypertensive medication may help identify interventions to increase adherence and improve outcomes. The Cohort Study of Medication Adherence in Older Adults is designed to assess risk factors for low antihypertensive medication adherence, explore differences across age, gender, and race subgroups, and determine the relationship of adherence with blood pressure control and cardiovascular outcomes over time. This article discusses the relevance of this study in addressing the issue of barriers to anithypertensive medication adherence.

Index   **771**

Preface

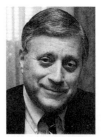

Edward D. Frohlich, MD, MACP, FACC
Guest Editor

Organizing this issue on hypertension every five (or so) years has been a truly satis-fying, stimulating, and tremendously rewarding experience for me. This educational exercise has permitted me to review the present state of the art about the pathophys-iological and clinical aspects of a remarkable and unusual field of medicine. On first reflection, I was compelled to look back upon an area of clinical medicine that was responsible for most of the hospital admissions at the time when I entered into medi-cine. These patients included those with cardiac failure, myocardial infarction, severe angina pectoris, dissecting aortic aneurysm, end-stage renal disease, malignant hypertension, hypertensive encephalopathy, and many other problems that we lump into the heterogeneous category we now term as "hypertensive emergencies." In fact, many of these latter problems have not been included in the hypertensive symposia of the *Medical Clinics of North America* for the past 20 years.

In its place, I believe a far more relevant sequence of discussions for this time now appears in our current overview. The discussions now include my personal reflections on some of the major clinical challenges concerning the pathophysiological aspects and clinical issues concerning the management of the hypertensive disease. One issue in particular concerns a subject that I had avoided in our pathophysiological studies until three or four decades ago; and that deals with the role of salt in hypertensive disease. (I was more concerned with the role of obesity in hypertension.) It was because of our experimental laboratory studies involving salt-loaded spontaneously hypertensive rats that I became convinced long-term salt-loading did much more than simply raising arterial pressure. We learned repeatedly in our studies that it also adversely affected the structure and function of the "target organs" of hypertensive diseases (ie, heart, kidneys, blood vessels). Through these experimental studies we have become convinced that conventional antihypertensive therapy can not only reverse but actually prevent these changes. This concept is particularly important at this juncture because one wonders why, despite the important (and frequently cited effects) of antihypertensive therapy to dramatically reduce cardiovascular morbidity and mortality, the important therapeutic trials and epidemiological reports failed to modify the adverse effects of hypertensive disease and its therapy on the increasing

Med Clin N Am 93 (2009) xv–xx
doi:10.1016/j.mcna.2009.02.016
0025-7125/09/$ – see front matter
medical.theclinics.com

rates of end-stage renal disease or of cardiac failure. My introductory discussion of this issue relates to this important subject and expands on this concept.

In the succeeding article, Dr. William B. Kannel, former director of the famous Framingham Heart Study, reflects on the risks inherent with untreated hypertension; and he also expands on some of his thoughts and prognostications. In this respect, it was Dr. Kannel who first coined the term "risk factors" in one of his earlier reports on identifying the first group of factors of risk responsible for the morbidity and mortality associated with coronary heart disease.

In recent years, much of our current thinking about the pathophysiological alterations associated with hypertension has been revitalized by new biological concepts that participate in the target organs of the disease. Perhaps much of this new information has been stimulated by a broadened concept of the role of the renin-angiotensin-aldosterone system (RAAS). We still consider the time-honored concept of this system in terms of its endocrine expression, thus, the enzyme renin is produced and released by the juxtaglomerular apparatus in the kidney and acts upon its substrate angiotensinogen produced in the liver. As a result of this action, the decapeptide angiotensin I is produced, which, in turn, is converted by the angiotensin-converting enzyme that cleaves off its terminal dipeptide to form angiotensin II. It is this octapeptide that acts upon vascular smooth muscle to promote vasoconstriction and on the adrenal cortex to release aldosterone, which is the most important steroid in regulating salt and water balance and metabolism. But, today, we have come to realize that there are local RAASs in heart, arteries, brain, adrenal, kidney, uterus, and additional organs that mediate other functions that are critically important in health and disease. Indeed, evidence is rapidly appearing that these local systems explain much of the mitogenic, inflammatory, oxidative stress, and other, heretofore unimagined actions that Irvine H. Page and Eduardo Braun-Menendez never conceived of when they and their colleagues first synthesized this octapeptide. These effects may be expressed through autocrine, paracrine, and, yes, even intracrine actions to explain many undreamed-of actions of this system. The concept of these local RAAS systems is cogently discussed by my colleague Dr. Richard N. Re of the Ochsner Clinic Foundation.

Many of us have been stimulated by new thinking about the multifactorial expressions of systemic hypertensive disease that we now term the "metabolic syndrome." However, this syndrome is not really new. Clear thinking by W. W. Herick in 1923 (shortly after Banting and Best's report of the production of insulin by the pancreas) was impressed by the frequency of the co-existence of hypertensive disease and hyperglycemia. Indeed, this astute clinician reported not only this observation in his published papers but also in a specific book detailing his large clinical experience at the Joslin Clinic in patients who have diabetes and hypertension. In that text, he was able to detail the prevalence of the co-existence of these two common diseases in over 50 percent of patients older than 50 years of age. Today, many recent reports express concern that the frequency of their co-existence is identical to that reported in 1923. And, in those early days, the definition of hypertension was usually greater than l60 mmHg systolic (not the 135 or 140 mmHg published in JNC-7)—particularly when co-existing with diabetes mellitus. What is new in the syndrome today is the close relationship between obesity and hyperlipidemia (the latter was not measurable in the 1920s); and the obvious association with aldosterone and insulin, the RAAs, and oxidative stress. These associations are discussed in detail by Dr. Camila Manrique and other associates of Dr. James R. Sowers at the University of Missouri in Columbia, Missouri, and the editor-in-chief of the new *Journal of Cardiometabolic Diseases*. No doubt these concepts will also be linked to the local RAASs and the problem of endothelial dysfunction, which is so commonly discussed in today's cardiovascular literature.

In recent years, much information has appeared in the literature that relates to the co-existence of the aging process and hypertension (primarily systolic hypertension in the elderly). The earlier literature, while not stating that these two areas of major cardiovascular interest are interdependent, suggested that this relationship was explainable by the frequent appearance of the atherosclerotic process as part of the aging process in the elderly patient as a natural occurrence. It is true that atherosclerosis frequently appears in aging individuals, but the pathogenesis of isolated systolic hypertension in the elderly is not necessarily associated with atherosclerosis for several reasons. First, not all patients with atherosclerosis develop hypertension, and, secondly, not all elderly patients with isolated systolic hypertension have atherosclerotic vascular disease.

Much of our current thinking about these problems has been stimulated by the appearance of the results from recent multicenter, double-blinded, and placebo-controlled trials that firmly established the concept that cardiovascular morbidity and mortality could be safely reduced; and that this problem is eminently treatable with conventional antihypertensive therapy. But, additional concurrent research contributions (well-known and published prior to these trials) primarily by two groups of investigators who demonstrated that both biological processes, aging and development of systolic hypertension, were independent of atherosclerosis. One group was led by Dr. Edward G. Lakatta of the Laboratory of Cardiovascular Science of the National Institute of Aging of the National Institutes of Health in Baltimore. Their carefully conducted clinical and laboratory studies demonstrated fundamental biological changes associated with aging. These studies, conducted at the macroscopic and molecular levels, are carefully detailed in their discussion in this issue of *Medical Clinics of North America*. One lesson from their studies is that much of the microcirculatory findings reported from epidemiological studies in aging patients do not necessarily reflect changes associated with the development of atherosclerotic vascular disease. Thus, impaired forearm flow in these studies does not necessarily reflect atherosclerosis but the aging process itself. The second group of investigators has been led by Dr. Michel E. Safar of the Universite Paris Descarte and the Centre de Diagnostic et de Therapeutique in Paris. It was his team's work (as well as studies conducted by the many workers trained by Safar) and the early fundamental clinical studies reported by Dr. Michael O'Rourke in Australia. Their findings were painstakingly elucidated in their hemodynamic laboratories that demonstrated the changes that take place in the large arteries of aging individuals. For years they stressed that the changes occurring with age (impaired distensibility and loss of elasticity of the large arteries) had vast clinical implications on their function as well as the left ventricle and on the microcirculation. The bottom line of their findings is the importance of measurable hemodynamic indices on ascertaining the changes associated with aging and the development of systolic hypertension in the elderly. The current thinking of Lakatta and Safar are detailed in this issue of the *Clinics*.

The most common cause of hospitalization in Medicare patients in the United States is cardiac failure and, perhaps, the earliest involvement of the heart in hypertension is that of left ventricular hypertrophy (LVH). Indeed, discussion still abounds relating to the most sensitive clinical means of detecting LVH, which is by echocardiography, although, clearly, the most practical and cost-effective approach is by electrocardiography. Hence, the latter technique is employed most frequently for the initial clinical evaluation of the patient with hypertension. It is true that LVH is the earliest means of detecting clinical cardiac involvement; but surrounding this simple yet practical concept is our understanding of the development and implication s of LVH. To be sure, in order for the heart to overcome the unrelenting increase in left ventricular afterload is the concurrent compensatory development of LVH. Moreover, for many years we have looked upon the presence of LVH as a major factor predisposing the patient with hypertension to increased risk of premature cardiovascular morbidity and mortality from coronary heart disease. Indeed, this was one of the first risk factors identified in their initial Framingham Heart Study on risk factors. But, if LVH is a normal adaptive phenomenon to the increased ventricular workload, what should be the underlying mechanism(s) predisposing the hypertensive patient to increased risk? In recent years, several pathophysiological epiphenomena have been identified that seem to explain that risk, and these include: ischemia of the ventricular muscle (either an absolute reduction in coronary blood flow or in coronary flow reserve, both of which are associated with increased coronary vascular resistance); fibrosis in the extracellular matrix as well as perivascular fibrosis within that wall; apoptosis of the ventricular myocyte, which reduces the number of contractile elements in the chamber, predisposing to cardiac failure; inflammatory changes within the ventricular chamber; and, most likely, other changes. It seems that these changes, in turn, are promoted, at least in part, through autocrine, paricrine, and intracrine mechanisms involving the local cardiac RAAS, and still others, no doubt, may account for production of these epiphenomena. This concept associated with specific approaches to treatment is discussed by Dr. Javier Díez, director of Cardiovascular Sciences and of the Centre for Applied Medical Research at the University of Navarra, Pamplona, Spain. His investigative group has contributed much exciting new information in recent years to our understanding of the development of a new paradigm related to hypertensive heart disease (HHD), also discussed herein.

Related to that subject is a series of discussions of the different aspects of cardiac failure and ischemia in this large group of patients. Perhaps the most common expression of cardiac failure in patients with HHD and, no doubt, the most frequent diagnosis is that of left ventricular diastolic dysfunction with preserved systolic function. This aspect of HHD is discussed by Drs. Anil Verma and Scott D. Solomon of the Ochsner Heart and Vascular Institute in New Orleans and the Brigham and Women's Hospital in Boston, respectively. Their vast experience in understanding the underlying clinical mechanisms associated with cardiac failure in patients with hypertension, as well as with occlusive ischemic cardiac disease in HHD, is widely perceived. Indeed, their personal experience concerning the well known contributions of the Brigham Group on the agents that inhibit the RAAS through controlled, double-blinded, multicenter trials. Their findings and those of others are detailed in their report that follows.

Cardiac failure is also manifest in other forms associated with hypertension. It may develop as a result of ischemic heart disease, following myocardial infarction complicated by other comorbid diseases (eg, diabetes mellitus, cardiac myopathy, etc.); and these common clinical experiences are detailed by Dr. Hector O. Ventura, director of the Cardiovascular Disease Training Program and section head of the Cardiomyopathy and Heart Transplant Program at the Ochsner Clinic Foundation in New Orleans. His and his colleagues' experiences with these patients are detailed in the following article.

The succeeding discussion on hypertension and myocardial ischemia in all its manifestations related to increased myocardial oxygen demand or by diminished myocardial oxygen supply is discussed by Dr. Francis G. Dunn and his colleagues of the Cardiac Department of the Stobhill Hospital, Glasgow, Scotland. Of great interest and importance is their discussion of the underlying mechanisms of ischemia—whether due to coronary atherosclerosis, microcirculatory dysfunction, structural dysfunctional changes, or by endothelial dysfunction and neurogenic factors—which are reviewed clinically, diagnostically, and, of course, therapeutically.

Several other aspects of comorbid diseases associated with hypertension are discussed in the following articles. Perhaps the co-existence of diabetes mellitus and renal vascular dysfunction is of increasing importance because of our appreciation for the frequency of this complicating factor of diabetic vascular disease systemically and intrarenally in patients with hypertension is ever-increasing. Many nephrologists have pointed to the finding of proteinuria (or microalbuminuria) in the patient with diabetic renal disease that predisposes that patient to increased cardiovascular risk. However, we must appreciate that the existence of diabetic renal disease is the intrinsic renal vascular disease itself, which is part of the overall cardiovascular risk in these patients. This problem is discussed in clear detail by Dr. George L. Bakris, director of the Hypertension Center at The University of Chicago, and his colleagues. They discuss these and other aspects of the co-existence of the two diseases, including the current thinking about the approach to therapy and the various therapeutic trials that have served as the basis for our present-day recommendations for treatment.

Another aspect of the kidney and hypertension relates to the one underlying diagnostic cause of hypertension and its associated renal disease; and this relates to the diagnosis of renal vascular hypertension. One of our major authorities in this area is Dr. Stephen Textor, vice chair, Division of Nephrology and Hypertension at the Mayo Clinic in Rochester, Minnesota. His great experience with the diagnosis and the still-present controversies concerning its approach to therapy (eg, medically, surgically, and by endovascular stenting) is frequently sought out personally and at many national and international meetings. Each of these aspects of renovascular hypertension is highlighted in his review.

Still another co-existing problem associated with hypertension is that of exogenous obesity. An authority who has contributed much to this area over many years is Dr. Efrain Reisin, chief of the Section of Nephrology and Hypertension at Louisiana State University School of Medicine, New Orleans. He and his associate, Dr. Avanelle V. Jack, discuss many of the aspects related to the co-existence of these two very increasingly common problems. In their discussion, they cover the underlying pathophysiological mechanisms, the rationale for the nondrug as well as pharmacological approaches to each of the various classes of antihypertensive drugs, and the rationale for their use.

We conclude this issue with one of the major unresolved clinical problems with respect to the treatment of hypertension. This problem relates to the appalling number of patients who are known to have hypertension although they remain untreated optimally. This problem was initially termed as a "lack of compliance" in years past, suggesting that the fault explaining its existence resides with the patient's refusal to be subservient to the managing physician. In response to this untenable argument, Dr. Harriet P. Dustan and myself suggested another term to the National High Blood Pressure Education Program years ago, one that relates to the lack of adherence, suggesting that both therapeutic partners are at fault. This term remains unsatisfactory, although many efforts toward its containment continue to frustrate. At the very best, these approaches remain incomplete. One committed and long-standing worker in this area is Dr. Marie Krousel-Wood, director of the Center for Health Research at the Ochsner Clinic Foundation and assistant provost, at Tulane University School of Medicine, New Orleans. Her epidemiological investigations on medication adherence (the Cohort Study of Medication Adherence among Older Adults) has been concerned with a number of heretofore unexplored mechanisms underlying the lack of compliance or adherence to medication in patients with hypertension immediately following Hurricanes Katrina and Rita in New Orleans. One of the issues (in addition to the usual explanations for non-adherence) is the frequency of depression among these patients. While the ready explanation may be attributed to the many problems that can easily be associated with these tragic disasters, it may also be explained by the compounding of problems of a chronic illness, such as hypertension, or yet other mechanisms. To my way of thinking, her study is providing a fresh approach to this important clinical problem.

Perhaps one of the most recent of the many pathophysiological mechanisms underlying hypertension is the development of oxidative stress in hypertension. I have indicated above that in past issues we focused in great depth on the existence of many fundamental mechanisms participating in the mosaic of hypertension (in terms of the overall pathophysiology of the disease), but this relatively new mechanism has been shown to inter-relate with many other less appreciated mechanisms, including the role of the immune system and the expression of reactive oxygen species in the target organs of the disease. There is no doubt at this point that angiotensin II and its receptors are important actors in the process of oxidative stress in the response of the target organs of hypertension, most likely, in part, through the NADPH oxidases. Furthermore, at the rate that new biological mechanisms appear in the clinical literature, there is no doubt that this subject is an imminent and important topic for the clinician. To this point, Dr. David G. Harrison and his colleague, Maria Carolina Gongora, of the Division of Cardiology in the Department of Medicine at Emory University in Atlanta provide a most exciting discussion for us.

Thus, once again, I am excited and honored to have been invited to organize this symposium or issue of the *Medical Clinics of North America*. Presented herein is a current approach by clinical investigators with a lifetime commitment to our understanding of one of the most common multifactorial diseases. The overall material is thoughtfully presented and details new and current thinking of an important disease having major health implications.

Before I close my expression of many personal thoughts about hypertension and its understanding and clinical management, there is one more thought I wish to share with you, our readers. Today, there is a dearth of clinically oriented physicians committed to a systematic study of the underlying pathophysiological and clinical aspects of hypertension. On behalf of the various contributors to this issue of the *Clinics*, we hope that some of you who are also interested in this subject—particularly those still in your training years or early in your medical careers—have become stimulated in a field that has enjoyed many years of leading contributors. Please, therefore, accept our joint invitation to join us in this field. There are many investigators with exciting preclinical credentials, but we are in desperate need for new and fresh clinical blood.

Edward D. Frohlich, MD, MACP, FACC
Ochsner Clinic Foundation
1514 Jefferson Highway
New Orleans, LA 70121

E-mail address:
efrohlich@ochsner.org (E.D. Frohlich)

Current Challenges and Unresolved Problems in Hypertensive Disease

Edward D. Frohlich, MD, MACP, FACC

KEYWORDS

- Hypertension • Pathophysiology • Heart • Kidney • Salt
- Management • Treatment

EARLIER CHALLENGES FOR REFLECTION

Organizing this issue of the *Clinics* on hypertension every 5 years or so has been a truly satisfying, stimulating, and a tremendously rewarding experience for me personally. This educational exercise has permitted me to review the present "State of the Art" by outstanding authorities of a remarkable and unusual area of medicine. On first reflection, I was compelled to look back upon an area of clinical medicine, which was responsible for most of the hospital admissions at the time when I entered medicine. These patients included those with cardiac failure, myocardial infarction, severe angina, dissecting aortic aneurysm, end-stage renal disease, malignant hypertension, hypertensive encephalopathy, and many other problems, which we now lump into a heterogeneous category of "hypertensive emergencies." In fact, many of these latter problems have not been included in the hypertension symposia of the *Clinics* for the past 20 years.

In its place, I believe a far more relevant sequence of discussions now appear in the current issue. They include risks related to hypertension by the person who coined the term "risk factors" and was the leader of the Framingham Heart Study; new concepts participating in the pathophysiology of hypertensive disease, involving its target organs from local hormonal and humeral systems to the role of oxidative metabolic stress; an enlightened discussion of the metabolic syndrome by the editor of the new journal dedicated to that problem; the role of aging and an important consideration of the significance of the large arteries in hypertensive disease; a current analysis of the problems associated with hypertensive heart disease (including ventricular hypertrophy, its underlying risks, and epiphenomena; systolic and diastolic failure, oxidative stress, the co-morbidity of atherosclerosis); end-stage renal and renovascular diseases, with current concepts of their treatment; obesity; and current major concerns about the continued intolerable problem of lack of adherence to therapy in hypertensive disease management. How different are these challenging aspects

Ochsner Clinic Foundation, 1514 Jefferson Highway, New Orleans, LA 70121, USA
E-mail address: efrohlich@ochsner.org

Med Clin N Am 93 (2009) 527–540
doi:10.1016/j.mcna.2009.02.004
0025-7125/09/$ – see front matter © 2009 Elsevier Inc. All rights reserved.

of the hypertensive disease today when compared with our treatment of this subject almost 30 years ago.

The reader's brief reflections on these foregoing topics, I am certain, are equally as mind-boggling as mine. So, if the reader will bear with me for a moment more, consider the major contributions by the clinicians and dedicated investigators on the underlying mechanisms of hypertensive disease over these many years. Bear in mind that the first multicenter, placebo-controlled, therapeutic studies were first introduced to the broad field of cardiovascular therapeutics by Edward D. Freis' landmark innovation of the Veterans Administration that demonstrated the feasibility, safety, and efficacy of hypertension treatment over four decades ago. Remember, please, the developments that ensued in the succeeding generation of cardiovascular therapeutics, including the introduction of vasodilators for heart failure, cardiovascular remodeling, and reversing and preventing ischemia, fibrosis, apoptosis, and inflammation of heart, vessels, and kidney. And, during these years, we have witnessed over 70% and 50% reductions in deaths from stroke and coronary heart disease, respectively. Consider further the introduction of the discipline of clinical pharmacology to medicine by our early hypertension investigators. Furthermore, please also consider the impact of antihypertensive drugs on other areas of cardiovascular, renal, and endocrine diseases, and the remarkably not-yet conceived endocrine roles of the heart, vessels, kidney, brain, and adipose tissue by cardiovascular investigators of hypertension. Finally, consider the tremendous impact of these innovative approaches to hypertension and their consequences on the dramatic reduction of cardiovascular, renal, neurologic morbidity and mortality over these years. With these considerations now fresh in your mind, I am delighted to introduce this issue for your study and reflection, with some of our current challenges. I have no doubt that the material presented will provide many new practical concepts and insights for many medical clinics, not only in North America but certainly, worldwide.

CURRENT CONSIDERATIONS

From the foregoing introductory remarks, one might come to the conclusion that the problems related to hypertensive diseases have been resolved. But, now that we have achieved many therapeutic challenges, other major issues have emerged for greater pathophysiologic understanding and more specific means of treatment. Thus, once again, I am delighted to share with you several extremely exciting areas for elucidation and study. Therefore, although we now understand many of the underlying pathophysiologic processes associated with cardiac, vascular, and renal involvement of the disease, we must now look into others that have emerged, as well as new concerns and more specific means of unresolved problems.

Genetic Concepts

To my way of thinking, individual genes underlying hypertensive disease are not usually related to specific, causative biologic mechanisms of what we currently term "essential hypertensive disease." It is true that there are some forms of hypertension for which specific genes have and probably will continue to be identified. But for the tremendous numbers of patients with essential hypertensive disease, for whom an even greater number of their parents and their forbearers had hypertension, the likelihood of identifying the multiplicity of genes involved is far too great a challenge to envision at this time. Although this may eventually come to pass with improved sophistication of understanding the mechanisms of polygenetic diseases, this concept does not seem immediately probable. However, what seems more likely is that clinical investigators working at the bedside and in the laboratory may identify specific underlying biologic processes and their respective participating genetic mechanisms that will eventually provide new areas not only for diagnosis, but also for more specific forms of treatment. Indeed, they will provide new thinking and insights into these processes, as they relate to the target organ involvements of hypertensive disease. Personally, I believe that these newer findings will also explain how certain environmental stimuli interact with specific biologic processes that will help elucidate new mechanisms as to how and why target organ involvement develops under the extrinsic influence. These possibilities shall be discussed below, using as an example how dietary salt excess may operate to exacerbate hypertensive disease in the target organs (eg, heart, blood, vessels, kidney, brain). Therefore, it is not necessary to concentrate our intellectual resources on a search for a specific genetic cause of what appears to be a polygenetic disease at the present time. Rather, we should focus much of our efforts onto more enlightened searches for identifying biologic processes that have been closely identified with hypertensive disease (eg, salt or alcohol excess, obesity, and other issues) that interact with the myriad of specific mechanisms accounting for the many metabolic and other biologic alterations associated with hypertensive disease. Currently, many investigators are focusing on racial, gender, and other issues that have emerged as major biologic factors in our ongoing search for the potential causes of hypertension and other diseases.

TARGET ORGAN CONCERNS
Heart

Almost four decades ago, investigators initiated a series of studies directed to identifying the clinical correlates of hypertensive heart disease and, thereby, the potential mechanisms underlying the intrinsic risk associated with left ventricular hypertrophy (LVH). At the time, earlier ECG indices associated with the progression of LVH were identified.[1] It was shown that even before overt LVH could be recognized, evidence of left atrial enlargement could presage development of eventual cardiac dysrhythmias that are associated with LV structural and functional changes related to LVH.[2] Subsequently, the first echocardiographic (echo) study relating structural and functional changes to the progression of hypertensive heart disease was reported.[3] Thus, the ECG changes of atrial abnormality were associated with LV structural changes (ie, increased wall thicknesses and mass) that indicated early LVH. It was further demonstrated that with obvious LVH, there were more specific structural and functional ventricular alterations. Soon, these observations were related to the increased risk of LVH identified earlier by the team of investigators from the Framingham Heart Study,[4] and subsequently, it was reported that all antihypertensive agents and other therapeutic interventions that decreased arterial pressure reduced LV mass.[5]

Many investigators have confirmed these findings and related the therapeutically promoted decrease in LVH (by ECG or echo) to the efficacy of certain classes of these agents to "reversing hypertrophy." At this point, we only know clinically that this treatment reduced LV mass, although actual reversed hypertrophy of the cardiac myocytes was not demonstrated. It was also learned that associated with the therapeutically reduced LV mass, certain agents decreased ventricular collagen content, whereas other agents actually increased the collagen.[6,7] Investigators soon became concerned that certain antihypertensive therapy might convert the LV into a fibrous chamber, thereby predisposing the patient to early cardiac failure when that therapy was withdrawn.[8] Studies have demonstrated that most of the currently used agents were able to maintain LV function, and efforts were then directed to the underlying mechanisms associated with the risk of LVH.[9–17] Our studies, and those of others whose work is detailed elsewhere in this edition of the *Clinics*, demonstrated that the risk of LVH was not a result of the hypertrophied myocytes, but of the associated epiphenomena of ischemia, fibrosis, apoptosis, and inflammatory changes related to the LVH.[18] Our conclusion and present clinical and experimental efforts therefore, is not to demonstrate "reversed hypertrophy or mass" but to prevent or reverse those fundamental underlying mechanisms that promote the foregoing processes of ischemia, fibrosis, apoptosis, inflammation, and whatever other comorbid processes that occur in the heart with LVH.

Indeed, there is abundant and important recent laboratory and clinical evidence that clearly indicated that the therapeutic classes in current use accomplish much of these goals (see the article "Current thinking about hypertensive heart disease" by Diez, in this issue). Thus, to direct current costly efforts to simply demonstrate reduction in size of the LV without ascertaining whether the associated pathophysiologic alterations are also affected, only defers the need to consider a new paradigm for the understanding of LVH and its treatment (ie, to reduce the underlying mechanisms of risk). For current evidence of this effort, the reader is referred to the cited references in this and other articles in this issue. Furthermore, we also refer the reader to the articles concerning hypertensive heart disease, cardiac failure (systolic and diastolic), and to the associated comorbid disease of hypertensive heart disease coexisting with atherosclerotic epicardial cardiovascular disease, elsewhere in this issue (see articles by Solomon and Verma, Ventura and colleagues, and Dunn and colleagues).

The Large Arteries

As our knowledge concerning the pathophysiologic development of LVH was revealed, so did our concepts concerning the changes that occur in the aorta and other large arteries. Our diagnostic and instrumental sophistication concerning the assessment of the structure and function of the large arteries has improved greatly. Much of this information has been stimulated by the works of Michel Safar, in France, and Michael O'Rourke, in Australia.[19] The reader is referred to the article "Hypertension, systolic blood pressure and large arteries," by Safar in this issue of the *Clinics* and to a remarkable series of symposia, published approximately every 3 or 4 years in *Hypertension*, organized by Safar and his colleagues. Essentially, the thesis, which has been elaborated, demonstrated that with aging there is an impaired distensibility and loss of elasticity of the large vessels, which results in structural and functional changes as well as impairment of the recoil ability (ie, the "Windkessel" phenomenon) of the aorta. Much of these functional effects are translated into the increasing systolic pressure and pulse pressure that occurs with the aging process, and with the associated increasing prevalence of systolic hypertension in the elderly. A more detailed discussion of this important subject is presented in the related articles of this issue on hypertension, systolic pressure, and large arteries, and that of aging and hypertension. (See the article "Aging versus hypertension" by Lakata in this issue.) These discussions are of vital importance, as we face the need to approach this increasingly prevalent problem that has been shown to be eminently treatable and can reduce the associated cardiovascular morbidity and mortality.

Kidney

For many years, the problem of progressive decrease in renal structure and excretory function in hypertension had been only perfunctorily addressed in textbooks of hypertension and nephrology, and referred to as "benign nephrosclerosis." We now are acutely aware of the fact that there is nothing benign about these problems. Indeed, there was a notable absence of information until very recently, and what was published related to changes in renal function and microscopic studies of the kidney that severely affected the patients' overall health and the increased problem of end-stage renal disease. Much of the information that was available concerned the consequences of aging and the effects of diabetes mellitus. However, soon after the development of those therapeutic agents that inhibited the renin-angiotensin system, much valuable information became available and was initially focused on diabetes. I became concerned, however, that much physiologic and pathophysiologic data were extrapolated from experimental models that were in no way identical with that which could be attributed to essential hypertension with developing end-stage renal disease or in patients with diabetes mellitus. Early efforts were by Gomez,[20] who employed formulae to ascertain the progression of glomerular and arteriolar functional changes in patients with essential hypertension. These measurements were discounted by those who were focusing on the changes that could be ascertained experimentally by the technique of renal micropuncture. Of course, this latter methodology technique is not feasible for use in the patient with hypertension with structural and functional impairment.

Notwithstanding, the renal hemodynamic and glomerular dynamic effects of disease and their response to antihypertensive agents were studied, and there is general agreement on the renal involvement in patients with essential hypertension and nephrosclerosis, as well as in experimental models and treatment of hypertensive renal disease. We have devoted much time and effort to the spontaneously hypertensive rat (SHR), whose naturally developing hypertensive disease is exacerbated by the endothelial nitric oxide inhibitor L-NAME.[21] In brief, as renal involvement progresses, renal blood flow and glomerular filtration rate and the filtration fraction decline, while renal vascular resistance increases. Furthermore, in our micropuncture laboratory, single nephron renal flow, glomerular filtration rate, filtration fraction decrease as afferent, and efferent glomerular arteriolar resistance, as well as the glomerular hydrostatic pressure, increase; these changes are associated with adverse glomerular and arteriolar injury scores.[21-23] Furthermore, we showed that the angiotensin converting enzyme (ACE) inhibitors, angiotensin II (type I) receptor blockers (ARBs), and calcium antagonists (including those that bind with L-, N-, and T-type calcium channel receptors) will prevent, and to some extent, reverse these changes.[22-31] The aldosterone receptor inhibiting agent eplerinone will prevent the inflammatory damage, but provides far less dramatic hemodynamic effects.[32] These findings are in accordance with the renal hemodynamic and functional effects of these agents (although some controversy remains with the calcium antagonists) in patients with essential hypertension and diabetes mellitus. Thus, at the present time, there is strong advocacy for the use of the ACE inhibitors and ARBs in these patients.[33,34]

Furthermore, we found that the diuretic agent, hydrochlorothiazide, will aggravate the renal hemodynamic and glomerular dynamic involvement, and these changes are associated with further glomerular and arteriolar damage.[35] However, when the diuretic is combined with an ACE inhibitor or with an ARB (or both), these adverse effects of the diuretic when used alone were prevented.[36]

CONCERNS ABOUT LIFESTYLES
Smoking and Obesity

Much concern has been and continues to be focused on three major lifestyles that impact adversely on the outcomes of hypertension and its morbidity and mortality: tobacco smoking, exogenous obesity, and dietary salt excess.[33] Clearly, important inroads have been made in recent years to minimize the effects of smoking but, unfortunately, much more must be done. These changes have been accomplished by changes in social, political, and economic behavior, and this discussion will not elaborate further on this issue except for three important points. First, we still must make an impact on the continued increase in the smoking rates of women and young people. Second, while restrictions on places to smoke have been instituted, the effects of secondary smoking (so-called "side-stream" smoking) still must be emphasized. And, third, while the cigarette sales have been reduced selectively by certain vendors, it makes no sense at all to permit cigarette sales to take place in stores whose products are devoted to promote health (eg, food stores and pharmacies).

The second lifestyle concern relates to the widespread and increasing problem of obesity; this problem is only beginning to be addressed socially and economically. Our early studies have been directed to the hemodynamic effects of obesity and subsequent weight reduction, but these changes are not uniformly observed by all patients with obesity and hypertension.[37] It is important, at this juncture, to recognize the more recent efforts addressed by our colleagues, dealing more biologically with the major problem of obesity in children as well as adults. These studies are now focusing on the biologic role of the adipocyte and are discussed separately in this issue (see the article "Hypertension and the metabolic syndrome" by Sowers.) There is no doubt that much new and exciting information will soon appear with pertinence for this important and vital concern as it relates to hypertensive disease. There is much valuable information that will relate to hypertension, diabetes mellitus, the hyperlipidemias, and other metabolic problems; however, caution is urged for all of us to assimilate this information without exerting proper attention to making precipitous conclusions related to a single pathophysiologic entity. Let us remember that clear-thinking internists made the association of hypertension and diabetes over 80 years ago.[38] Moreover, in reports documenting their experiences with large numbers of patients with both diseases, the prevalence of diabetes mellitus in elderly patients with hypertension was no greater at that time as it is today.[39] Furthermore, their definition of hypertension began at much higher arterial pressure levels that we employ today. The lesson is clear: all answers to present concerns of disease are not presently available, especially with respect to an area of study that is experiencing vastly new concepts and exploding biologic information.

Salt

Perhaps one of the more perplexing problems that has confronted those of us in the area of hypertension has been the role of salt as a major concern.[40] Until the last century, mankind had only been concerned with salt in economic, social, political, and other nonmedical areas.[41] Then, astute clinicians became concerned with the role of salt in diseases.[42] At first this interest was related to hypertension; more recently, there has been a major interest in its role in other cardiovascular, renal, and neurologic diseases. One existing problem is the lack of an adequate explanation for the remarkably high correlation of salt to the underlying mechanisms that explain the epidemiologic morbidity and mortality data related to salt excess. Perhaps this is because the term "salt sensitivity" eluded a more primary cause-effect relationship than simply the provocation of an elevation of arterial pressure with intravenous or other means of excessive salt challenges. This relationship remains a major enigma because, if there is such a highly significant correlation between the daily intake of salt in large populations and risk of hypertension, one should wonder why the prevalence of salt sensitivity clinically with salt challenge should be as low as approximately

30%, when salt loads are administered to individual patients with essential hypertension.[43]

One of the problems with finding an explanation is in arriving at a testable definition of just what is meant by the term "salt sensitivity." This term has been used clinically over many years to refer to the response of arterial pressure to salt-loading in either short-term clinical studies or in epidemiologic investigations; it has not been used generally for application by the clinician. Thus, it seems inappropriate to relate this term simply to the response of arterial pressure to salt overload. Rather, it seems wiser to demonstrate the response of salt-loading not only to the response of arterial pressure, but also the structural and functional responses of the target organs of hypertensive disease (ie, heart, aorta, vessels, kidney, and brain). This can be related to measurable sodium intake (ie, by 24-hour urinary sodium collections). I have arrived at this concept because the traditional relationship between arterial pressure and salt-loading has been highly correlated statistically in epidemiologic studies, a less frequent relationship tested epidemiologically rather than clinically with individual patients. Thus, over the past three decades our experimental studies have related chronic salt-loading in the SHR, a genetic form of hypertension,[44] to the responses of not only arterial pressure, but to the structural and functional responses of the target organs of hypertensive disease. It has been most satisfying to see recent clinical studies concerned with target organ involvement by hypertensive disease (*vide infra*).

Our initial studies involved chronic dietary salt excess to increased cardiac mass even before arterial pressure and total peripheral resistance increased.[44,45] In contrast, their normotensive control Wistar-Kyoto rats did not increase arterial pressure, but they responded by an increased cardiac output,[44] suggesting that salt-loading exerts nonhemodynamic actions independent upon the response of arterial pressure. Our subsequent studies in the SHR demonstrated development of increased left and right ventricular mass associated with diminished coronary blood flow and flow reserve, increased fibrosis of the ventricular extracellular matrix and perivascularly, as well as impaired ventricular diastolic function, all important responses of the heart to aging.[45–48] With respect to the age factor, all older adult SHRs and 75% of the younger adult SHRs demonstrated diastolic dysfunction with preserved systolic function, very similar to cardiac failure in adult patients with essential hypertension without conclusive atherosclerotic coronary disease. The remaining 25% of the younger adult SHRs demonstrated impaired systolic function with overt cardiac failure.[47,48] Thus, with respect to the experimental laboratory cardiac responses to salt overload, there was a small but significant increase in arterial pressure; in addition, there was a more profound increase in ventricular fibrosis, bilateral ventricular ischemia, and impaired diastolic function.

More recently, clinical studies have confirmed our findings, providing credence to the highly common occurrence of cardiac failure (even without atherosclerotic coronary arterial disease).[33,49] Subsequently, we extended these findings by treating older adult SHRs with an angiotensin II (type 1) receptor blocking agent (ARB) and prevented the development of ventricular fibrosis and ventricular diastolic dysfunction, which was remarkably unassociated with any reduction in arterial pressure.[50] Additionally, in these studies we demonstrated that the cardiac alterations observed with salt overload was accompanied by impaired aortic distensibility, massive proteinuria, and severe renal dysfunction, which were also prevented by the ARB.[50–52]

These foregoing findings supported our conviction that prolonged dietary salt-loading promoted structural and function derangements of the target organs of hypertensive disease independent of its pressor action. We continued with our experimental studies on the kidney, using either 4%, 6%, or 8% chronic dietary salt loads. Each group developed severe proteinuria (and microalbuminuria), even before arterial pressure increased slightly (but significantly), within 2 weeks before arterial pressure increased further over the entire 8 weeks of study, the same time employed without cardiac studies.[51] Although it was not possible to perform renal micropuncture studies in those SHRs receiving the 8% salt overload, we did demonstrate diminished renal blood flow, glomerular filtration rate, and renal filtration fraction in these rats, as well as severe glomerular and arteriolar damage. However, in those SHRs receiving either the 4% or 6% salt overload, their renal micropuncture data demonstrated decreased single-nephron renal plasma flow and glomerular filtration rate, with increased filtration fraction, afferent and efferent glomerular arteriolar resistance, and glomerular hydrostatic pressure in proportion to the extent of the salt overload. In addition, microscopically, their kidneys demonstrated progressively more involved renal glomerular and arteriolar injury in proportion to the magnitude of the dietary sodium intake. More recently, using one of two different ARBs (including the agent used in our earlier cardiac study), the renal function and structural derangements were reversed without any pressure reduction.[51]

These data have continued to support our initial hypothesis that the role of salt excess in hypertensive disease is far more complex than that which had been concluded from earlier epidemiologic studies (ie, that salt or sodium excess simply raises arterial pressure). We are therefore convinced that chronic salt excess produces and exacerbates the adverse structural and functional derangements in the target organs of hypertensive disease, and that this may be totally independent of its pressure-elevating action.[40]

Recently, the Trial of Hypertension Prevention studies (TOPH I and II), involving 2,382 prehypertensive participants, reported that dietary sodium restriction (which had been previously shown to lower blood pressure) demonstrated highly significant cardiovascular risk reduction (by 25%–35%) than those individuals not receiving such a diet.[53] The highly significant primary outcomes (ie, composite of stroke, myocardial infarction, coronary artery bypass graft, percutaneous transluminal angioplasty, cardiovascular death—even when those patients who had bypass grafts and angioplasty—were excluded) were demonstrated in the large group of prehypertensive subjects whose diet was not restricted in sodium intake. Thus, these findings provided further support for those earlier more controversial epidemiologic reports in which a single determination of urinary sodium excretion was used to demonstrate diminished risk of stroke and coronary heart disease.[54,55] In addition, a number of clinical studies have been reported that demonstrated the structural and functional alterations associated with salt-loading and, taken together with the foregoing observation, strongly suggest that salt excess over a prolonged time produced not only an elevated arterial pressure in patients, but many of the long-term clinical derangements seen in patients, including progressive chronic diastolic cardiac failure with and without systolic dysfunction, increased prevalence of end-stage renal disease, and isolated systolic as well as systolic-diastolic hypertension.[40] Furthermore, our experimental findings suggest that angiotensin II receptor blockade may prevent (or, at least, ameliorate) these severe target organ findings.

We have therefore postulated that the pathophysiologic changes that we have demonstrated experimentally may be mediated through local cardiac, vascular, and renal mechanisms that involve local renin-angiotensin and, perhaps also, aldosterone-(RAAS) mediated actions.[40,56] In recent, years much evidence has accumulated supporting the existence of local RAAS systems in the heart, vessels, kidney, and in other organs.[49,57,58] Thus, despite the abundant evidence that renin release from the juxtaglomerular apparatus is suppressed with sodium overload, while renal and cardiac fibrosis occurs, we have documented that the use of small or large doses of ARBs produces impressive reversal of the structural and functional changes induced by sodium excess. Thus, a vast body of clinical information has accumulated over the years that have demonstrated the importance of inhibition of the RAAS in preventing cardiac, vascular, and renal endpoints of the disease.

We therefore propose that dietary salt excess does not simply raise arterial pressure, but that it also promotes severe structural and functional alterations that promote cardiac and renal failure. We further postulate that dietary sodium restriction will prevent cardiovascular and renal outcomes through structural and functional pathophysiologic changes induced by sodium that are independent of the RAAS, and will further diminish that risk by reversing those structural and functional derangements. In further support of this concept, we must be aware that cardiac failure is the most common cause of hospitalization in Medicare patients in this country in hypertensive and normotensive patients, and end-stage renal disease continues to increase in these patients at an alarming rate.[33]

CONCERNS REQUIRING FURTHER THOUGHT
Prolonged Diuretic Use Without Cardiovascular-Renal Protection

Over the years, successive national and international guidelines dealing with the evaluation, diagnosis, and treatment of hypertension have documented the increasing prevalence of cardiac failure and end-stage renal disease, despite the continued decrease in the morbidity and mortality resulting from stroke and coronary heart disease.[33,34] Why this enigmatic occurrence takes place, despite the continued use of antihypertensive therapy, remains to be explained. Perhaps some of our thinking about this major concern may be offered from our experiences with salt excess experimentally and in clinical studies.

In many patients with hypertension, long-term use of diuretics promotes increased plasma renin activity. It is believed that this is promoted through local and systemic RAAS in heart, vessels, and kidney.[40] These changes, in turn, may produce effects similar to the alterations that have been observed with prolonged dietary overloading with sodium excess. Furthermore, findings from experimental studies with prolonged treatment with hydrochlorothiazide that were produced by stimulation of the RAAS have been reported.[35] Moreover, these data suggested that local RAAS stimulation may be prevented with cotreatment with either an ACE or an ARB agent.[36] Others have also speculated on this occurrence and recent experience with salt excess and its effects on the target organs of hypertension.

ISSUES THAT YET REQUIRE CLEARER UNDERSTANDING
Meta-Analyses

Do studies involving meta-analysis have the full credibility of undeniable truths? One issue of concern is the acceptance of a metaanalytic report without some intellectual question. For example, a number of reports have been published in recent years that suggest that when one lumps all statistically acceptable articles into a statistically meaningful conclusion, that concludes that a specific approach to treatment is or is not acceptable. This has been raised in the area of at least two classes of antihypertensive agents in recent years: the calcium antagonists and the beta-adrenergic receptor-inhibiting drugs. The concerns about former agents have dissipated, for the most part. But excitement and controversy about the latter agents are more recent, and they threaten the well being of those individuals who have been the undeniable beneficiaries of their value. First, there are patients with hypertension who have been taking beta-blockers for control of arterial pressure and cardiovascular symptoms, as well as for the secondary prevention of a recurrent myocardial infarction. These patients have been frightened by reports in the lay media of the lack of value of the beta-blockers (if not injury), just as other patients were concerned earlier about the calcium antagonists. As a result, they have pressured their physicians to discontinue the beta-blocker drug. Second, there are some patients with hypertension (for example, the younger patient with a hyperdynamic circulation) who have had excellent control of their blood pressure, with remission of their cardiovascular symptoms. Although these individuals may be less in number than other patients receiving this treatment, their consideration has been ignored in the sweeping conclusion of the almighty meta-analysis. Trialists supporting these reports have disregarded these relatively fewer patients in the sweeping conclusion made in their "evidence-based" reports. These remarks do not invalidate the concept of evidence-based medicine. Rather, one should remember the caution once made in jocularity at the height of the calcium antagonist controversy: "analysis is to meta-analysis as physics is to metaphysics." Let us remember not to throw out the entire concept and rationale for the use of one form of therapy with the therapeutic bathwaters!

The Quest of the Holy Grail in Terms of "Biomarkers"

In recent years we have been captivated by the general acceptance of specific (or nonspecific) biomarkers. One such cardiovascular biomarker has been the C-reactive protein. There is much merit for using this index of pathophysiologic changes relating to the generation of specific inflammation or immunologic entities that suggest great diagnostic and therapeutic significance underlying an impending cardiovascular event. This biomarker is currently under intense study and has prompted the inquiry for introduction of other biomarkers of pathologic changes in other organs and diseases. Let us permit the scrutiny of the myriad of agents under study. Let us also remember the present day value of the erythrocyte sedimentation rate. It still is of value under certain circumstances, but should this measurement be done in all patients on hospital admissions, as has done until relatively recently? In this respect, we have recently witnessed the withdrawal of measurement of certain phase reactants for the patient with acute coronary syndrome following the abrupt decision by one respected institution. And what will be the ultimate fate of the brain natriuretic peptide measurement? Biomarkers are vitally important and have value, but should we rely on their value as an absolute index without great study and scrutiny?

What about Other Diagnostic and Therapeutic Issues?

At the present time we are awaiting judgment about the value for carotid and renal arterial stenting. At present there are several multicenter studies funded by the National Heart, Lung, and Blood Institute to provide recommendations from well-controlled studies. Let us not make premature decisions until the answers from these trials provide the appropriate rationale. And, in this relative lull in the introduction of new therapeutic classes for the treatment, let us once again await the recommendations from appropriate trials without precipitously initiating new forms of diagnosis or therapy without valid studies.

CONCLUDING THOUGHTS

Over the past four or five decades hypertension and cardiovascular medicine has experienced dramatic and innovative changes that have significantly reduced morbidity and mortality. A vast array of new antihypertensive compounds have been developed that are able to affect the outcomes of many pathophysiologic mechanisms in patients with hypertension. The result has become a remarkably bright outcome for our patients with hypertensive disease. Many of these therapeutic breakthroughs have been the result of active participation of clinical scientists, with tremendous and remarkable knowledge of and experience with the fundamental mechanisms of disease. In more recent years, much new information has appeared concerning the basis genetic and biologic mechanisms involved in cardiovascular and renal diseases. New information, both fundamental and clinical, has appeared, and these advances have provided new means to develop and conduct new approaches to evaluate disease mechanisms and therapeutic actions. No doubt, much more will appear and enthrall us. In addition, innovative approaches to drug evaluation will become elucidated through individual studies into disease and drug mechanisms. These advances have been accompanied by mind-boggling multicenter controlled trials involving thousands of patient volunteers. Still more amazing is the realization and pride that many of these remarkable changes have emanated from the hypertension academic community. What remains of utmost importance is for members of the academic community with a wide spectrum of experience and points of view to continue to work intimately with industry. These associations are mutually beneficial and should include academicians with a wide spectrum of experience and points of view whose relationships must never be tainted, and who must always be open and known to practicing physicians, medical scientists, and to the general public.

REFERENCES

1. Frohlich ED, Tarazi RC, Dustan HP. Clinical-physiological correlations in the development of hypertensive heart disease. Circulation 1971;44:446–55.
2. Tarazi RC, Miller A, Frohlich ED, et al. Electrocardiographic changes reflecting left atrial abnormality in hypertension. Circulation 1966;34:818–22.
3. Dunn FG, Chandraratna P, de Carvalho JGR, et al. Pathophysiologic assessment of hypertensive heart disease with echocardiography. Am J Cardiol 1977;39: 789–95.
4. Kannel WB, Dawber TR, Kagen A, et al. Factors of risk in the development of coronary heart disease: six year follow-up experience. The Framingham Study. Ann Intern Med 1961;55:33–56.
5. Frohlich ED, Apstein C, Chobanaian AV, et al. The heart in hypertension. N Engl J Med 1992;327:998–1008.
6. Frohlich ED, Tarazi RC. Is arterial pressure the sole factor responsible for hypertensive cardiac hypertrophy? Am J Cardiol 1979;44:959–63.
7. Frohlich ED. Hemodynamics and other determinants in development of left ventricular hypertrophy: conflicting factors in its regression. Fed Proc 1983;42: 2709–15.
8. Frohlich ED. Clinical conference: hypertensive cardiovascular disease: a pathophysiological assessment. Hypertension 1984;6:934–9.
9. Frohlich ED. State of the art. The heart in hypertension: unresolved conceptual challenges. Hypertension 1988;11:19–24.
10. Frohlich ED. (State of the Art): the first Irvine H. Page lecture: the mosaic of hypertension: Past, present, and future. J Hypertens 1988;6:S2–11.
11. Sasaki O, Kardon MB, Pegram BL, et al. Aortic distensibility and left ventricular pumping ability after methyldopa in Wistar-Kyoto and spontaneously hypertensive rats. J Vascular Med Biol 1989;1:59–66.

12. Natsume T, Kardon MB, Pegram BL, et al. Ventricular performance in spontaneously hypertensive rats with reduced cardiac mass. Cardiovasc Drugs Ther 1989; 3:433–9.
13. Frohlich ED. Overview of hemodynamic and non-hemodynamic factors associated with LVH. J Mol Cell Cardiol 1989;21(Suppl V):3–10.
14. Frohlich ED, Sasaki O. Dissociation of changes in cardiovascular mass and performance with angiotensin converting enzyme inhibitors in Wistar-Kyoto and spontaneously hypertensive rats. J Am Coll Cardiol 1990;16:1492–9.
15. Frohlich ED. Regression of cardiac hypertrophy and left ventricular pumping ability post-regression. J Cardiovasc Pharmacol 1991;17:81–6.
16. Frohlich ED, Horinaka S. Cardiac and aortic effects of angiotensin converting enzyme inhibitors. Hypertension 1991;18:2–7.
17. Frohlich ED, Sasaki O, Chien Y, et al. Changes in cardiovascular mass, left ventricular pumping ability, and aortic distensibility after calcium antagonist in Wistar-Kyoto and spontaneously hypertensive rats. J Hypertens 1992;10: 1369–78.
18. Frohlich ED. Risk mechanisms in hypertensive heart disease. Hypertension 1999; 34:782–9.
19. Safar ME, O'Roarke MF (editors): Arterial stiffness in hypertension, Volume 23 of Handbook of Hypertensioin (Series Editors: Birkenhäger WH and Ried JL). Amsterdam: Elsevier BV; 2006.
20. Gomez DM. Evaluation of renal resistances with special reference to changes in essential hypertension. J Clin Invest 1951;30:1143–55.
21. Ono H, Ono Y, Frohlich ED. Nitric oxide synthase inhibition in spontaneously hypertensive rats: systemic, renal, and glomerular hemodynamics. Hypertension 1995;26:249–55.
22. Ono H, Ono Y, Frohlich ED. ACE inhibition prevents and reverses L-NAME exacerbated nephrosclerosis in spontaneously hypertensive rats. Hypertension 1996; 27:176–83.
23. Frohlich ED. Arthur C. Corcoran memorial lecture: influence of nitric oxide and angiotensin II on renal involvement in hypertension. Hypertension 1997;29: 519–24.
24. Francischetti A, Ono H, Frohlich ED. Renoprotective effects of felodipine and/or enalapril in spontaneously hypertensive rats with or without L-NAME. Hypertension 1998;31:795–801.
25. Susic D, Frohlich ED. Nephroprotective effects of antihypertensive drugs in essential hypertension. J Hypertens 1998;16:555–67.
26. Ono H, Ono Y, Frohlich ED. L-Arginine reverses severer nephrosclerosis in aged spontaneously hypertensive rats. J Hypertens 1999;17:121–8.
27. Nakamura Y, Oho H, Frohlich ED. Differential effects of T- and L-type calcium antagonists on glomerular dynamics in spontaneously hypertensive rats. Hypertension 1999;34:273–8.
28. Nakamura Y, Ono H, Zhou X, et al. Angiotensin type 1 receptor antagonism and ACE inhibition produce similar renoptotection in L-NAME/SHR rats. Hypertension 2001;37:1262–7.
29. Zhou X, Frohlich ED. Functional and structural involvement of afferent and efferent glomerular arterioles in hypertension. Am J Kidney Dis 2001;37:1092–7.
30. Ono H, Ono Y, Takanohashi A, et al. Apoptosis and glomerular injury after prolonged nitric oxide synthase inhibition in SHR. Hypertension 2001;38:1300–6.
31. Zhou X, Ono H, Ono Y, et al. N- and L-type calcium channel antagonistic improves glomerular dynamics, reverses severe nephrosclerosis and inhibits

apoptosis and proliferation in an L-NAME/SHR model. J Hypertens 2002;20: 993–1000.

32. Frohlich ED. Clinical management of the obese hypertensive patient. Cardiol Rev 2002;10:127–38.

33. Chobanian AV, Bakris GL, Black HR, et al, and the National High Blood Pressure Education Program Coordinating Committee (2003) The seventh report of the Joint National Committee on Prevention, Detection, Evaluation, and Treatment of High Blood Pressure. Hypertension 2003;42:1206–52.

34. International Society of Hypertension Writing Group. International Society of Hypertension (ISH): statement on blood pressure lowering and stroke prevention. J Hypertens 2003;21:651–63.

35. Ono Y, Ono H, Frohlich ED. Hydrochlorothiazide exacerbates nitric oxide-blockade nephrosclerosis with glomerular hypertension in spontaneously hypertensive rats. J Hypertens 1996;14:823–8.

36. Zhou X, Matavelli LC, Ono H, et al. Superiority of combination of thiazide with angiotensin-converting enzyme inhibitor or AT_1-receptor blocker over thiazide alone on renoprotection in L-NAME/SHR. Am J Physiol Renal Physiol 2005;289:F871–9.

37. Reisin E, Frohlich ED, Messerli FH, et al. Cardiovascular changes after weight reduction in obesity hypertension. Ann Intern Med 1983;98:315–9.

38. Frohlich ED. The metabolic syndrome: there's little that's new under the sun. J Cardiometab Syndr 2006;1(5):293–4.

39. Herrick WW. Early reports on frequency of diabetes in patients with hypertension. In: Joslin EP, editor. The treatment of diabetes mellitus: the experience of the Joslin clinic in patients under and over 50 years of age. 3rd edition. Philadelphia: Lea & Febiger; 1923.

40. Frohlich ED. The salt conundrum: a hypothesis. Hypertension 2007;50:161–6.

41. Kurlansky M. Salt: a World history. New York: Penguin Books; 2003.

42. Ambard L, Beaujard E. Causes de l'hypertension arterialle. Arch Med Gen Trop 1904;1:520–33.

43. Weinberger MH, Miller JZ, Luft FC, et al. Definitions and characteristics of sodium sensitivity and blood pressure resistance. Hypertension 1986;8(Suppl II):127–34.

44. Chrysant SG, Walsh GM, Kem DC, et al. Hemodynamic and metabolic evidence of salt sensitivity in spontaneously hypertensive rats. Kidney Int 1979;15:33–7.

45. MacPhee AA, Blakeslley HL, Graci KA, et al. Altered cardiac beta-adrenergic receptors in SHR rats receiving salt excess. Clin Sci 1980;59(Suppl VI):169–70.

46. Frohlich ED, Chien Y, Sosoko S, et al. Relationships between dietary sodium intake, hemodynamic and cardiac mass in spontaneously hypertensive and normotensive Wistar-Kyoto rats. Am J Physiol 1993;264:R30–4.

47. Ahn J, Varagic J, Slama M, et al. Cardiac structural and functional responses to salt loading in SHR. Am J Physiol Heart Circ Physiol 2004;287:H767–72.

48. Varagic J, Frohlich ED, Diez J, et al. Myocardial fibrosis, impaired coronary hemodynamics, and biventricular dysfunction in salt-loaded SHR. Am J Physiol Heart Circ Physiol 2006;290:H1503–9.

49. Williams JS, Solomon SD, Crivaro M, et al. Dietary sodium intake modulates myocardium relaxation responsiveness to angiotensin II. Transgenic Res 2006;48:49–54.

50. Varagic J, Frohlich ED, Susic D, et al. AT-1 receptor antagonism attenuates target organ effects of salt excess in SHRs without affecting pressure. Am J Physiol Heart Circ Physiol 2008;294:H853–68.

51. Matavelli LC, Zhou X, Varagic J, et al. Salt loading produces severe renal hemodynamic dysfunction independent of arterial pressure in spontaneously hypertensive rats. Am J Physiol Heart Circ Physiol 2007;292:H814–9.

52. Susic D, Zhou X, Frohlich ED. Angiotensin blockade prevents salt-induced injury of the renal circulation in spontaneously hypertensive rats. Am J Nephrol 2009;29: 639–45.

53. Cook NR, Cutler JA, Obazanek E, et al. Long term effects of dietary sodium reduction on cardiovascular disease outcomes: observational follow-up of the trials of hypertension prevention (TOHP). BMJ 2007;334:885–94.

54. Tunstall-Pedoe H, Woodward M, Tavendale R, et al. Comparison of the prediction by 27 different factors of coronary heart disease and death in men and women of the Scottish Heart Health Study. BMJ 1997;351:722–9.

55. Toumilehto J, Iousilahti P, Restenyte D, et al. Urinary sodium excretion and cardio-vascular mortality in Finland: a prospective study. Lancet 2001;357:848–51.

56. Frohlich ED. The role of salt in hypertension: the complexity seems to become clearer. Nat Clin Pract Cardiovasc Med 2008;5:2–3.

57. Partovian C, Benetos A, Pommies JP, et al. Effects of a chronic high-salt diet on large artery structure: role of endogenous bradykinin. Am J Physiol 1998;274: H1423–8.

58. Du Cailar G, Ribstein J, Mimran A. Dietary sodium and target organ damage in essential hypertension. Am J Hypertens 2002;15:222–9.

Hypertension: Reflections on Risks and Prognostication

William B. Kannel, MD, MPH, FACC

KEYWORDS

• Hypertension • Risk stratification • Cardiovascular hazards

Framingham Heart Study cardiovascular disease (CVD) prospective population epidemiologic research has played an important role in the evolution of modern cohort study design and the advancement of preventive cardiology. Epidemiologic research on coronary heart disease (CHD) from the Framingham Study evolved the risk factor concept in 1961, indicating that multiple interrelated factors are promoting increased risk for development of CHD.[1] To date no single essential factor has been identified. Epidemiologists subsequently were induced to conceptualize vascular disease as an outcome of multiple forces, now a critical tenet of modern epidemiology. Such thinking has had clinical, public health, preventive, and therapeutic applications. The "risk factor" has become a prime feature of the current epidemiologic model and elevated blood pressure has emerged as a prominent member of the major cardiovascular risk factors.

Framingham Study population research has demonstrated the importance of distinguishing between usual (average) and optimal risk factor levels as normal and acceptable. It determined the influence of hypertension on the full clinical spectrum of CVD, including sudden death, silent and overt myocardial infarction, heart failure, and clinical and silent strokes. The study determined population CVD incidence attributable to hypertension at a time when only mortality statistics were available and, most recently, the lifetime risk for developing it and its vascular consequences. The study also provided some valuable insights on mechanisms of hypertension-induced CVD. Furthermore, the study's documentation of a strong linkage of blood pressure to development of cardiovascular events stimulated the pharmaceutical industry to develop medications for controlling blood pressure and to conduct trials indicating their efficacy for reducing elevated blood pressure and its adverse cardiovascular

From the National Heart, Lung and Blood Institute's Framingham Heart Study, National Institutes of Health. Framingham Heart Study research is supported by NIH/NHLBI Contract No. N01-HC-25195 and the Visiting Scientist Program, which is supported by Servier Amerique and Astra Zeneca.
Boston University School of Medicine/Framingham Heart Study, 73 Mt. Wayte Avenue, Framingham, MA 01702-5827, USA
E-mail address: billkannel@yahoo.com

consequences. National campaigns to combat hypertension and its adverse vascular outlook by the American Heart Association, American College of Cardiology, American Society of Hypertension, and the National Heart, Lung, and Blood Institute in turn were stimulated.

MISCONCEPTIONS CORRECTED

Control of hypertension and its cardiovascular consequences required the correction of many clinical misconceptions about hypertensive vascular disease, such as the significance of left ventricular hypertrophy (LVH), importance of small amounts of proteinuria, and the role of obesity and weight gain.[2] Of major importance was the Framingham Study investigation dispelling the concept of "benign essential hypertension" and belief in the greater importance of controlling the diastolic than systolic blood pressure. The cardiovascular hazard of hypertension was believed to derive chiefly from the diastolic pressure component and it was held that the disproportionate rise in systolic blood pressure with age was an innocuous accompaniment of arterial stiffening. It was believed that treatment of isolated systolic hypertension would be not only fruitless but also intolerable and dangerous. The tenaciously held belief in the prime importance of the diastolic pressure was convincingly refuted by Framingham Study data and later confirmed by other prospectively obtained data, demonstrating that the impact of systolic pressure is greater than the diastolic component and that even isolated systolic hypertension is dangerous.[3,4]

Women were believed to tolerate elevated blood pressure well, and it was held that there were age-related critical cardiovascular risk thresholds for blood pressure so that normal blood pressures in both genders should be designated at substantially higher levels in the elderly than in the middle aged. There was a recent attempt to resurrect this faulty concept.[5] Framingham Study data soundly refuted this assertion, however, indicating that although the hypertensive risk ratios for all the major atherosclerotic CVD events are larger for those under than over age 65, the absolute incidence of disease in hypertensive persons was greater in the elderly. Systolic blood pressures formerly regarded as normal for the elderly (100 plus age mm Hg) were shown to impose a substantial excess cardiovascular risk. Also, although the absolute incidence of all events except stroke in the elderly are lower in women than men, the risk ratios in women are similar to those in men. Thus, neither the elderly nor women tolerated hypertension well.[6]

Because of the concept of benign essential hypertension and a lack of effective and tolerable means for lowering blood pressure, emphasis in the past was placed on diagnosing and treating causes of secondary hypertension. As result of population research in the Framingham Study and elsewhere, routine testing to identify specific underlying causes of hypertension no longer is recommended unless there is history or physical findings that suggest secondary hypertension or that blood pressure cannot be controlled. Identifiable underlying causes were responsible for only a small percentage of the hypertension encountered in clinical practice.

In the past, initiation of antihypertensive treatment often was delayed until there was evidence of target organ involvement. Framingham Study data indicated that this practice was imprudent because 40% to 50% of hypertensive persons developed overt cardiovascular events before evidence of target organ damage, such as proteinuria, cardiomegaly, or electrocardiograph (ECG) abnormalities.

The perception of the hazard of hypertension was preoccupied with the diastolic blood pressure component since the beginning of the twentieth century and even today, there seems to be lingering uncertainty about the CVD impact of the various components of the blood pressure. Influenced by Framingham Study findings, the focus has shifted to the systolic blood pressure and, most recently, to the pulse pressure.[7,8] An increased pulse pressure in advanced age previously was considered an innocuous feature of progressive arterial rigidity. Assessment of the implications of blood pressure components by the Framingham Study, however, indicated that increments of pulse pressure at any systolic pressure are associated with increased CHD incidence. With increasing age there is a shift in importance of risk for CHD from diastolic to systolic and finally to pulse pressure.[7]

Framingham Study data have altered the concept of an acceptable blood pressure from what is usual in the population to what is optimal for avoiding hypertension-related CVD. Epidemiologic data showed that at all ages and in both genders, CVD risk increases incrementally with the blood pressure even within what was perceived as the normal range. Similar continuous graded relationships of blood pressure level to CHD and all-cause mortality also have been reported in other cohorts.[8,9] There is no threshold for blood pressure cardiovascular risk, as some claim, and in the Framingham Study cohort 45% of the CVD events in men occurred at a systolic blood pressure less than 140 mm Hg, the value recently claimed to be the threshold of risk.[5] Huge data sets are available that enable precise estimation of CVD incidence trends in the low blood pressure range. The Multiple Risk Factor Intervention Trial (MRFIT) data on more than 350,000 men screened and followed for CVD mortality and the Prospective Studies Collaboration involving almost 1 million participants and 56,000 vascular deaths found no indication of a threshold of blood pressure risk down to 115/75 mm Hg.[10,11] Persons aged 40 to 69 years had a doubling of stroke or CHD mortality with every 20/10–mm Hg increment of blood pressure throughout its entire range. A recent analysis of the relation of "nonhypertensive" blood pressure to the rate of development of CVD in the Framingham Study confirmed a significant graded influence of blood pressure from optimal (<120/80 mm Hg) to normal (120–129/80–84 mm Hg) to high-normal (130–139/85–89 mm Hg) among untreated men and women.[9] Compared with optimal pressure, high-normal blood pressure conferred a 1.6- to 2.5-fold age- and risk factor–adjusted risk for a CVD event (**Table 1**). Based on these findings, the Seventh Report of the Joint National Committee on Prevention, Detection, Evaluation, and Treatment of High Blood Pressure (JNC 7) guidelines have defined a "prehypertensive" blood pressure category.[8]

COMMENTARY ON PREHYPERTENSION

Recently, Liszka and colleagues[12] examined the CVD outlook for the JNC 7 promulgated prehypertension risk category, confirming that it carries an excess risk in a larger

Table 1
Relation of non–high blood pressure to cardiovascular disease

Blood Pressure (mm Hg)	Ten-Year Cumulative Incidence				
	Women		Men		
	Age-Adjusted Rate (%)	HR	Age-Adjusted Rate (%)	HR	
<120/80	1.9	1.0	5.8	1.0	
120–129/80–84	2.8	1.5	7.6	1.3	
130–139/85–89	4.4	2.5	10.1	1.6	
	P<.001		P<.001		

Framingham Study subjects, ages 35–90 years.
Abbreviation: HR, hazard ratio adjusted for age, BMI, cholesterol, diabetes, and smoking.
Data from Vasan R, Larson MG, Leip EP, et al. Impact of high normal blood pressure on the risk of cardiovascular disease. N Engl J Med 2001;345:1291–7.

and more generalizable population sample than the Framingham Study. The incremental blood pressure risk noted within the prehypertensive range reflects the continuous graded influence of blood pressure without critical values delineating normal from "hypertension." In the Framingham Study, 80% to 90% of the prehypertensive population sample had at least one additional cardiovascular risk factor. A weight gain–driven tendency for other risk factors to cluster with elevated blood pressure has been well documented by the Framingham Study.[13] CVD risk in the prehypertensive blood pressure range, although significantly increased compared with lower blood pressures, still is modest. The CVD risk in this prehypertensve blood pressure range increases with the number of associated risk factors present. Hence, persons in this category require global risk assessment to select those in need of changes of diet, weight control, and amount of exercise. For some who have multiple risk factors predicting a high multivariable risk, antihypertensive monotherapy along with control of the other risk factors can be justified. Only by using multivariable risk assessment is it possible to avoid needlessly alarming or falsely reassuring these prehypertensve patients and subjecting them to therapy they do not require.

THE J-CURVE CONTROVERSY

It has been alleged that there is an increased CVD risk at low and at high diastolic blood pressure (a so-called J-curve) generating fear of lowering the diastolic blood pressure too much.[14,15] The Framingham Study tested prospectively the hypothesis that the upturn in CVD incidence at low diastolic blood pressure largely is confined to persons who have increased systolic pressure, hence reflecting risk from an increased pulse pressure.[14] The10-year risk associated with 951 nonfatal CVD events and 205 CVD deaths was estimated at diastolic pressures of less than 80, 80 to 90, and greater than or equal to 90 mm Hg, according to concomitant systolic blood pressure. An increasing tendency for a J-curve relation of CVD incidence to diastolic blood pressure was observed with successive increments in accompanying systolic blood pressure (**Fig. 1**). In both genders, a statistically significant excess of CVD events was observed at diastolic blood pressures less than 80 mm Hg only when accompanied by a systolic pressure greater than 140 mm Hg, and this persisted after adjustment for age and associated CVD risk factors.[14] This finding is corroborated in the large MRFIT data set.[11,16] Persons who have this condition of isolated systolic hypertension have been shown in the large Systolic Hypertension in the Elderly Program

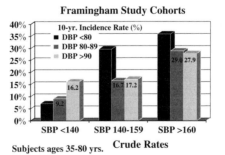

Fig. 1. CVD incidence by diastolic blood pressure according to systolic blood pressure Framingham Study cohorts. (*From* Kannel WB, Wilson PW, Nam BH, et al. A likely explanation for the J-curve blood pressure cardiovascular risk. Am J Cardiol 2004;94:380–4; with permission.)

(SHEP) and Systolic Hypertension in Europe (Syst-Eur) trials to safely benefit from anti-hypertensive treatment.[17,18]

LEFT VENTRICULAR HYPERTROPHY

The Framingham Study has for a long time advocated use of ECG data for CVD risk assessment. Unfortunately the ECG now often is looked on as an anachronism (compared with the echocardiogram) when it comes to assessing ominous LVH. The original Framingham Study multivariable CVD risk profiles included ECG-LVH until the guideline committees decided it was too insensitive, too low in prevalence, and too poorly defined for clinicians to use. The ECG, however, is more available, less labor intensive, and less costly than the more elegant echocardiogram. When present, ECG abnormalities, such as LVH, nonspecific abnormality, intraventricular block, and unrecognized myocardial infarction, are important contributors to cardiovascular risk assessment. LVH originally was considered compensatory, helping the heart deal with a blood pressure overload. LVH was shown by the Framingham Study to be an ominous harbinger of CVD rather than an incidental compensatory response to hypertension, CHD, and heart valve deformity. The Framingham Study showed that LVH is an ominous feature of hypertension that independently escalates the risk for future CVD, equivalent to that of persons who already have overt atherosclerotic CVD.[19,20] Increases in voltage and repolarization were associated with further escalation of cardiovascular risk and decreases with reduction in the adverse consequences.[21]

ELECTROCARDIOGRAPHIC ABNORMALITIES

Hypertension, particularly when associated with LVH, promotes ventricular premature beats. The Framingham Study evaluated the prevalence and prognostic significance of asymptomatic complex or frequent ventricular premature beats detected during ambulatory ECG monitoring of surviving participants of the Framingham Study cohort and offspring of the original cohort.[22] Those men who do not have CHD with such premature beats on 1-hour ambulatory ECG, after adjusting for age and traditional risk factors for CHD, were at significantly increased risk for all-cause mortality (relative risk 2.30) and the occurrence of myocardial infarction or death from CHD (relative risk 2.12). Curiously, in men who had CHD and in women who had and who did not have CHD, complex or frequent arrhythmias were not associated with an increased risk for either outcome.

The age-adjusted prevalence of complex or frequent arrhythmia (more than 30 ventricular premature complexes per hour or multiform premature complexes, ventricular couplets, ventricular tachycardia, or R-on-T ventricular premature complexes) was as high as 12% in the 2425 men who did not have clinically evident CHD and 33% in the 302 men who had CHD. The corresponding values in women (3064 who did not have disease and 242 who had disease) were 12% and 26%.

Thus, in men who did not have clinically overt CHD, the incidental detection of ventricular ectopy was associated with a twofold increase in the risk for all-cause mortality and myocardial infarction or death resulting from CHD. The preventive and therapeutic implications of these findings await further investigation.[22]

The risk for developing overt CHD also was examined in relation to occurrence of nonspecific ECG ST and T-wave abnormalities in the Framingham Study.[23] In the course of follow-up, 14% of the 5127 men and women participating in the Framingham Study had or developed nonspecific ECG abnormalities without clinically apparent intervening CHD. During 30 years of surveillance, 760 men and 578 women developed a first overt clinical manifestation of CHD. Nonspecific ECG abnormality seemed to be a hallmark of a compromised coronary circulation predicting the occurrence of every clinical manifestation of CHD independently of known risk factors, including hypertension, its chief determinant. Coronary morbidity and mortality was increased twofold in each gender. The more common T-wave abnormality alone carried a significant increased risk, although the combination of ST and T waves seemed most hazardous.[23]

Many studies have shown positive associations between heart rate and both all-cause and cardiovascular mortality. These relationships, however, were not investigated in persons who had hypertension until the Framingham Study did so using 36-year follow-up data evaluated from 4530 subjects, aged 35 to 74, whose blood pressures were greater than or equal to 140 mm Hg systolic or greater than or equal to 90 mm Hg diastolic and who were not on antihypertensive medication. On pooled logistic regression analysis it was found that for each of 40 beats/min heart rate increment (adjusted for age and systolic blood pressure), all-cause mortality increased 2.2-fold for men and twofold for women. Cardiovascular mortality increased 1.7-fold in men and women. Exclusion of outcomes in the first 2 or 4 years after measurement of heart rate did not change the results materially, suggesting that rapid heart is not merely an indicator of pre-existing illness. Consequently, heart rate on ECG examination is a useful independent risk factor for cardiovascular mortality in persons who have hypertension.[24]

The clinical implications of newly acquired left bundle branch block (LBBB) were investigated prospectively in the Framingham Study population.[25] During 18 years of observation, 55 subjects developed LBBB. The mean age at the onset was 62, the LBBB occurring largely in participants who had antecedent hypertension, cardiac enlargement, CHD, or a combination of these. Coincident with or subsequent to the onset of LBBB, 48% developed clinical coronary disease or congestive failure for the first time. Throughout the entire period of observation, only 11% who had this intraventricular conduction abnormality remained free of clinically overt cardiovascular events. Within 10 years of the onset of LBBB, 50% died from CVDs. In men, the ECG evidence of LBBB contributed independently to an increased risk for CVD mortality.[25] Comparison with age- and gender-matched control subjects free from LBBB confirmed that in the general adult population, newly acquired LBBB most often is a hallmark of advanced hypertensive or ischemic heart disease or both.

Consequently, it is no surprise to learn that recent Women's Health Initiative data support the usefulness of the ECG for CV risk assessment.[26] Abnormalities in the ECGs of 14,749 healthy women predicted increased risk for cardiovascular events and mortality. Women who had minor abnormalities had a 55% increased risk for an event, and those who had major abnormalities had a threefold increase in risk.

UNRECOGNIZED MYOCARDIAL INFARCTION

Hypertension is a powerful risk factor for the occurrence of a myocardial infarction. An investigation of the occurrence of unrecognized infarctions by blood pressure status was undertaken by the Framingham Study. This counterintuitively found that the proportion of infarctions that were unrecognized was substantially greater in hypertensive than normotensive persons. As many as 35% of infarctions in hypertensive men and 50% of such infarctions in women of the Framingham Study went unrecognized.[27] The high proportion of unrecognized infarctions among hypertensive persons persisted on adjustment for antihypertensive treatment, diabetes, and ECG-LVH (**Table 2**). This important finding seems to have escaped the notice of guideline crafters and prevention-minded physicians. Risk for all clinical manifestations of

Table 2						
Myocardial infarctions unrecognized by hypertensive status						
	Percent Unrecognized					
	Excluding Diabetics		**Excluding Anti–High Blood Pressure Prescription**		**Excluding Electrocardiogram–Left Ventricular Hypertrophy**	
High Blood Pressure Status	**Men**	**Women**	**Men**	**Women**	**Men**	**Women**
Normal	18	30	18	27	20	29
Mild	28	36	30	36	30	35
Definite	33	48	35	49	33	51

Framingham Study cohort, age adjusted.
From Kannel WB, Dannenberg AL, Abbott RD. Unrecognized myocardial infarction and hypertension in the Framingham study. Am Heart J 1985;109:581–5; with permission.

coronary disease is increased in hypertensive persons, in particular unrecognized myocardial infarctions, necessitating periodic ECG surveillance to detect them.

CARDIOVASCULAR HAZARDS

Hypertension (140/90 mm Hg) increases atherosclerotic CVD incidence, on average, two- to threefold. The chief hazard of hypertension often is believed a stroke. The Framingham Study established that although its risk ratio is smaller than for stroke or heart failure, coronary disease is the most common hazard for hypertensive patients of all ages.[2] Hypertension predisposes to all clinical manifestations of CHD, including myocardial infarction, angina pectoris, and sudden death; imposing a two- to threefold increased risk. For hypertension-induced strokes, the risk ratio for intracerebral hemorrhage was believed greater than for an atherothrombotic brain infarction. This proved incorrect; hypertension was as strong a risk for atherothrombotic brain infarction as intracerebral hemorrhage.[28] It also was widely believed that mild hypertension promotes brain infarctions whereas severe hypertension induces intracerebral hemorrhage. Framingham Study investigation indicated that the preponderance of hypertension-related strokes were atherothrombotic brain infarctions whether or not the hypertension was severe (70%) or mild (56%). The proportion of strokes resulting from hemorrhage in mild hypertension (5%) was virtually identical to that for severe hypertension.[28]

RISK STRATIFICATION OF HYPERTENSION

There is a need for greater use of risk stratification of hypertension to determine the type and intensity of treatment that are most appropriate. Hypertension per se can directly induce encephalopathy, renal insufficiency, and acute heart failure whereas its promotion of accelerated atherogenesis is more complex, involving lipid atherogenesis, thrombogenesis, insulin resistance and endothelial dysfunction, all of which are influenced by the blood pressure and its accompanying established cardiovascular risk factors. Evaluation of the hypertensive hazard for development of atherosclerotic CVD requires consideration of other metabolically linked risk factors. Hypertensive persons often have increased triglycerides, small dense low-density lipoprotein cholesterol, reduced high-density lipoprotein (HDL) cholesterol, elevated blood glucose, and visceral adiposity, the combination of which has been characterized as a metabolic syndrome. This cluster of risk factors derived from insulin resistance induced by weight gain and visceral adiposity greatly augments the cardiovascular hazard of elevated blood pressure. These other risk factors should be routinely sought in all patients who have elevated blood pressure because of the tendency for clustering and the great influence that these coexistent risk factors have on the CVD hazard imposed by an elevated blood pressure.

Hypertension occurs in isolation of the aforementioned metabolically linked risk factors in only approximately 20% of patients. The size of the cluster of accompanying risk factors mirrors weight gain and loss.[29] High-risk hypertension is that accompanied by one or more of the following: dyslipidemia, glucose intolerance, LVH, visceral adiposity, proteinuria, cardiomegaly, sinus tachycardia, or insulin resistance. The urgency for and choice of treatment should take into account these associated risk factors and the character and severity of the blood pressure elevation.

Because moderate blood pressure elevations are much more prevalent than severe elevations, a large fraction of the CVD attributable to hypertension derives from seemingly trivial elevations of blood pressure. Despite the 1.5- to 20-fold increased risk associated with moderate degrees of hypertension, the absolute hazard is modest, and many persons in this category need to be treated to prevent one case of CVD. Efficient selection of mildly hypertensive persons for aggressive treatment with medication requires multivariable global risk assessment of their level of risk. Also, the goal of therapy should be to improve the global risk profile and the blood pressure. Targeted therapy, based on a composite risk profile, improves the cost-benefit ratio of antihypertensive therapy.

Hypertension occurred in isolation of other standard risk factors in only 20% of patients. Clusters of three or more additional risk factors occur at 4 times the rate expected by chance.[30] Hypertension often is a consequence of decreased arterial compliance and an insulin resistance metabolic syndrome characterized by abdominal obesity, hypertension, glucose intolerance, and dyslipidemia. Abdominal obesity also imposes a natriuretic penalty that may increase sensitivity to salt intake promoting a rise in blood pressure[31] (**Table 3**). Risk for CVD in persons who have hypertension was shown by the Framingham Study to vary widely depending on the size of the associated burden of other risk factors.[30]

Table 3
Influence of obesity on odds of low plasma natriuretic peptides

	Risk Factor–Adjusted Odds Ratios			
	Low BNP		Low N-ANP	
BMI	Men	Women	Men	Women
Normal (<25)	1.00	1.00	1.00	1.00
Overweight (25–29)	1.64*	1.43**	3.47***	1.89***
Obese (≥30)	2.51***	1.84***	4.81***	2.85***

Odds ratios adjusted for age, prior myocardial infarction, atrial fibrillation, diabetes, smoking, blood pressure, serum creatinine, left atrial size, left ventricular systolic function, left ventricular mass.

Low BNP = 4 pg/mL; low N-ANP = <195 pmol/L.

* $P<.01$.

** $P<.05$.

*** $P<.001$.

Data from Wang TJ, Larson MG, Levy D, et al. Impact of obesity on plasma natriuretic peptide levels. Circulation 2004;109:594–6000.

Substantial risk in hypertensive persons who have mild to moderate hypertension was concentrated in those who had coexistent dyslipidemia, diabetes, and LVH. For stroke, the most feared hazard of hypertension in the elderly, risk varied over a wide range, reaching substantial proportions when accompanied by diabetes, LVH, atrial fibrillation, and coronary disease or heart failure. Hypertensive elderly commonly already had target organ damage, such as impaired renal function, silent myocardial infarction, strokes, transient ischemic attacks, retinopathy, or peripheral artery disease. At least 60% of older men and 50% of elderly women who had hypertension in the Framingham Study had one or more of these conditions.

Instruments for the global assessment of multivariable risk for coronary disease, stroke, peripheral artery disease, and heart failure have been crafted using Framingham Study data.[32–37] Recently a global risk assessment instrument for predicting total CVD has been produced.[38] This makes it convenient to estimate the global risk for hypertensive patients using ordinary office procedures and standard laboratory tests.

GUIDELINES VERSUS GLOBAL RISK ASSESSMENT FOR ANTIHYPERTENSIVE THERAPY

Various guidelines and many updates of guidelines have been promulgated to refine the definition of hypertension and improve treatment and prevention of the cardiovascular consequences hypertension promotes.[8,39–41] In response to clinical trials showing efficacy of treating milder degrees of hypertension, increasingly lower blood pressure goals have been set. Recent guidelines also have factored in the coexistence of associated conditions and compelling indications into therapeutic decisions for more aggressive blood pressure lowering and individualized antihypertensive therapy for diabetes, chronic renal disease, post–myocardial infarction, and recurrent stroke prevention.[8]

Despite advocacy of these revised guidelines by prestigious organizations, it seems that the recommendations are not being implemented acceptably in clinical practice. A Framingham Study assessment of control of systolic and diastolic blood pressure by the physicians of participants in that cohort found that 50% of hypertensive persons referred for treatment do not have blood pressure levels at the recommended systolic blood pressure goals.[42] Also, diastolic pressures were controlled better than systolic pressures. A survey of self-reported hypertension rates from National Health and Nutrition Examination Survey (NHANES) data over the past decade suggests an increase in hypertension prevalence with only 31% achieving target goals of adequate control.[43] A survey of hypertension management of veterans who had diabetes found that more aggressive therapy for blood pressure is needed because 73% had blood pressures above 140/90 mm Hg. Persons who had diabetes received less intensive therapy than those who did not have diabetes and this was not attributed to distraction by the need to treat the diabetes itself.[44] Compliance with guidelines for treatment of dyslipidemia with hypertension also is suboptimal.[45]

It is uncertain why there is such a high failure rate in achieving adequate blood pressure control. One possibility is physician inertia, disenchanted by multiple complex sets of guidelines, each targeting a specific risk factor. It seems that multiple iterations of guidelines may be too difficult for an average primary care physician to keep up with, let alone remember and implement. Understandingly, guidelines may be unable to take into consideration all the diverse problems clinicians encounter in practice, such as patients under treatment who have medications for a variety of coexisting medical conditions. The JNC 7 hypertension guideline modifications recommends reclassification of blood pressure categorizing prehypertension as stage 1 hypertension, renaming current stage 1 and stage 2 hypertension categories to stages 2 and 3, respectively, and introducing further complexity into the guidelines by using ill-defined "early disease markers," "target organ disease," and "vascular damage" to develop a risk algorithm for therapy.[8] Practicing clinicians may have difficulty in applying and adhering to such guidelines.

It now is evident that it is the degree of blood pressure elevation that promotes CVD and not arbitrarily defined hypertension stages. Cardiovascular risk increases incrementally with the blood pressure with no critical blood pressure values defining risk stages. Furthermore, blood pressure is best regarded as one component of a multivariable cardiovascular risk profile because at any level of blood pressure the CVD risk varies widely in relation to the number accompanying risk factors.[30] It is advantageous, therefore, to link the aggressiveness of blood pressure–lowering therapy to the level of multivariable CVD risk. This policy has become critical because near-average levels of blood pressure now are recommended for treatment of high-risk persons.[8] Because the number needed to treat to prevent one cardiovascular event is inversely proportional to the level of absolute CVD risk, only in this way is it possible to efficiently target the population segment with moderate blood pressure elevation for treatment. Trials specifically testing the efficacy of multivariable risk-linked therapy (compared with therapy disregarding absolute cardiovascular risk) are lacking; nevertheless, it seems eminently likely that such an approach would prove more cost effective and efficacious. Many clinical trials have tested the hypothesis that treatment of hypertension is most effective in patients who have multiple risk factors and higher risk for CVD events. For example, using the American Heart Association multiple risk factor equation on data from SHEP, a global CVD risk score was calculated for 4189 participants free of cardiovascular events and in 264 participants who had CVD at baseline. Cardiovascular event rates in the placebo group were progressively higher in relation to higher quartiles of predicted cardiovascular risk. The protection afforded by treatment was similar across quartiles of risk, but the number needed to treat to prevent one cardiovascular event decreased progressively at higher predicted CVD risk quartiles.[46]

The absolute long-term benefit associated with a 12–mm Hg reduction in blood pressure over 10 years was estimated by Ogden and colleagues according to the JNC VI risk stratification system using data from the NHANES follow-up study. As expected, the number needed to treat to prevent a CVD event/death was reduced in relation to increasing levels of blood pressure in each of the risk strata; furthermore, the number needed to treat was much smaller in persons who had one or more additional major cardiovascular risk factors compared with those who did not have additional risk factors. This analysis demonstrates that the absolute benefit of antihypertensive therapy depends not only on the level of blood pressure but also on the presence or absence of additional risk factors.[47] It also is virtually certain that a subgroup analysis of existing trials of antihypertensive therapy using competing drugs would show that the therapy was more effective in those who have dyslipidemia or impaired glucose tolerance (which most hypertensive patients have) compared with those who do not have these conditions.

The Adult Treatment Panel III lipid guidelines have linked the treatment of dyslipidemia to the Framingham Study CHD multivariable risk algorithm, thereby simplifying the process of risk assessment.[48] It is likely that such a multivariable assessment applied to hypertension will result in better risk assessment and control of hypertension and more appropriate targeting of antihypertensive therapy.

Framingham Study multivariable risk evaluation tools exist for evaluating hypertensive hazards for developing coronary disease, stroke, heart failure, peripheral artery disease, and, most recently, total CVD.[32–38] The Framingham Study recently crafted a global total CVD risk assessment instrument[38] that enables risk assessment in hypertensive persons based on the standard major risk factors, which tend to cluster with hypertension (**Table 4**). This profile was a robust predictor of each of its components. Furthermore, a simplified version substituting body mass index (BMI) for the laboratory components also was produced, which can be used to target high-risk CVD candidates for the more complete profile (**Table 5**).

Framingham Study investigation of the major risk factors, including hypertension, has long contended that each risk factor needs to be dealt with as an ingredient of a multivariable cardiovascular risk profile because each often is accompanied by a cluster of other metabolically linked risk factors that markedly influence their cardiovascular risk. Guidelines for all these individual risk factors need to be coalesced to reflect the goal of reducing global cardiovascular risk rather than correction of an individual risk factor. Because all the risk factors for which guidelines are being formulated are contained in the multivariable CVD risk formulations (eg, blood pressure, dyslipdemia, and diabetes) the time has come to consider abandoning multiple complex guidelines, each targeting individual risk factors, shifting instead to multivariable cardiovascular formulations for risk assessment and goals for therapy. This provides a less complex means for hypertensive risk assessment than the current guidelines.

Table 4
Framingham Heart Study cardiovascular disease risk profile for men

Points	Age	HDL Cholesterol	Total Cholesteral	Systolic Blood Pressure	Systolic Blood Pressure RX'd	Smoker	Diabetic
−2	—	60+	—	<120	—	—	—
−1	—	50–59	—	—	—	—	—
0	<35	40–49	<160	120–120	<120	No	No
1	—	35–44	160–199	130–139	—	—	—
2	35–39	<35	200–239	140–159	120–129	—	—
3	—	—	240–279	160+	130–139	—	Yes
4	—	—	280+	—	140–159	Yes	—
5	40–44	—	—	—	160+	—	—
6	45–49	—	—	—	—	—	—
7	—	—	—	—	—	—	—
8	50–54	—	—	—	—	—	—
9	—	—	—	—	—	—	—
10	—	—	—	—	—	—	—

Points	Risk (%)	Points	Risk (%)	Points	Risk (%)	Points	Risk (%)	Points	Risk (%)
≤3	<1	2	2.4	7	5.9	12	13.9	17	>30
−2	1.2	3	2.9	8	7.0	13	16.4	—	—
−1	1.4	4	3.5	9	8.3	14	19.2	—	—
0	1.7	5	4.1	10	9.9	15	22.6	—	—
1	2.0	6	4.9	11	11.7	16	26.4	—	—

Data from D'Agostino RB, Vasan RS, MJ Pencina, et al. General cardiovascular risk profile for use in primary care. Circulation 2008;117:743–53.

Table 5
Framingham Heart Study simplified cardiovascular disease risk profile for men

Risk Factor	Points									
	1	2	3	4	5	6	7	8	9	10
Age (y)	30–34	35–39	40–44	45–49	50–54	55–59	60–64	65–69	70–74	75+
Systolic blood pressure (untreated)	—	130–139	140–159	160+	—	—	—	—	—	—
Systolic blood pressure (treated)	—	—	120–129	130–139	140–149	160+	—	—	—	—
BMI	—	—	25–30	>30	—	—	—	—	—	—
Smoker	—	—	—	—	Yes	—	—	—	—	—
Diabetes	—	—	Yes	—	—	—	—	—	—	—

Points	Risk (%)	Points	Risk (%)	Points vasc.	Age	Points vasc.	Age
1	2.8	9	11.2	1	35	9	55
2	3.3	10	13.3	2	37	10	58
3	4.0	11	15.7	3	39	11	62
4	4.7	12	18.5	4	41	12	65
5	5.6	13	21.7	5	44	13	69
6	6.7	14	25.4	6	46	14	73
7	8.0	15	29.6	7	49	15	78
8	9.5	16+	>30	8	52	16	>80

Data from D'Agostino RB, Vasan RS, MJ Pencina, et al. General cardiovascular risk profile for use in primary care. Circulation 2008;117:743–53.

RISK FACTORS PREDISPOSING TO HYPERTENSION

An assessment of the frequency of progression to hypertension in participants in the Framingham Study cohort who did not have hypertension was undertaken to establish the best frequency of blood pressure screening by assessing the rates and determinants of progression to hypertension.[13] Patients who had optimum (<120/80 mm Hg), normal (120–129/80–84 mm Hg), and high normal (130–139/85–89 mm Hg) blood pressure commonly progress to "hypertension" (>140/90 mm Hg). In subjects below age 65, a stepwise increase in hypertension incidence occurred across three nonhypertensive blood pressure categories: 5.3% of participants who had optimum blood pressure, 17.6% who had normal blood pressure, and 37.3% who had high normal blood pressure progressed to hypertension over 4 years. Corresponding 4-year rates of progression to hypertension for subjects 65 years and older were 16.0%, 25.5%, and 49.5%, respectively (**Table 6**). Obesity and weight gain greatly contributed to progression; a 5% weight gain on follow-up was associated with 20% to 30% increased odds of developing hypertension. The finding that high normal and normal blood pressure frequently progress to hypertension over a short period (4 years), especially in older adults, supports recommendations for yearly monitoring of persons who have high normal blood pressure and monitoring those who have normal blood pressure every 2 years. The data also indicate the importance of blood pressure

Table 6
Development of hypertension by nonhypertensive blood pressure status

Baseline Blood Pressure (mm Hg)	High Blood Pressure Rate (%)	Odds Ratio
Optimum (<120/80)	16	Referent
Normal (120–129/80–84)	25.5	2.0 (1.4–2.7)
High-normal (130–139/85–89)	49.5	5.5 (4.0–7.4)

Four-year high blood pressure rate adjusted for age, gender, BMI, and systolic and diastolic blood pressure. Framingham Study subjects were ages 65–94 years.

Data from Vasan RS, Larson MG, Leip EP, et al. Assessment of frequency of progression to hypertension in non-hypertensive subjects in the Framingham Heart Study. Lancet 2001;358:1682–6.

monitoring in the obese and emphasize the importance of weight control for primary prevention of hypertension.

Several population determinants of hypertension have been documented. A high-normal systolic blood pressure is 2 to 3 times more likely to progress to "hypertension." A 5% increase in obesity and weight gain is associated with 20% to 30% increase in odds of developing hypertension. Arterial stiffness disproportionately increases systolic pressure causing increased pulse pressure and isolated systolic hypertension. High intake of salt promotes hypertension in salt-sensitive persons. Low circulating natriuretic peptides associated with increased activation of the sympathetic renin-angiotensin system results in hypertension. Elevated aldosterone causes excessive renal sodium retention, potassium wasting, and blood volume expansion, resulting in hypertension.

The Framingham Study has crafted a risk assessment instrument for predicting likelihood of developing hypertension from the following ingredients: gender, parental history of hypertension, BMI, smoking, and systolic and diastolic blood pressure in the normotensive range (**Table 7**). In multivariable analysis, each of theses variables was a significant predictor of hypertension. According to the risk score derived from these predisposing factors, the 4-year incidence of hypertension was deemed low (<5%) in 34% of participants, medium (5%–10%) in 19%, and high (>10%) in 47%. The risk score needs to be validated in other cohorts and is based on single measurements of risk factor and blood pressure. Such a risk factor scoring instrument can be used, however, to refine management of prehypertensive persons.[49]

Addition of natriuretic peptides and aldosterone to this hypertension risk algorithm could further enhance its predictive value. The prevalence of hypertension is strongly related to the degree of obesity. Risk for developing hypertension in overweight or obese subjects of the Framingham Study offspring cohort was increased threefold. As much as 59% of the hypertension developing in men and 42% in women ages 20 to 49 years was attributable to overweight and obesity. As people gain weight their blood pressure rises, and as they lose weight it falls. Obesity seems to impose a natriuretic handicap because brain natriuretic peptide and N-terminal pro-atrial natriuretic peptide decline with increase in weight leaving overweight and grossly obese persons with low natriuretic peptide levels. This imposed natriuretic handicap could contribute to the susceptibility of obese persons to hypertension and its cardiovascular sequelae.[31]

PREVENTIVE IMPLICATIONS

Because modifiable risk factors predisposing to hypertension have been identified and hypertension risk assessment algorithms developed, there now is an opportunity

Table 7
Framingham Heart Study risk score predicting high blood pressure

Systolic Blood Pressure (mm Hg)	Points		Gender	Points		Smoking		Points
<110	-4		Men	1		No		0
110–114	0		Women	0		Yes		1
115–119	2		Parental High Blood Pressure	Points		BMI		Points
120–124	4		None	0		<25		0
125–129	6		One	1		25-29		1
130–134	8		Both	2		>30		3
135–139	10		Points	4-Year Risk %	Points	4-Year Risk %	Points	4-Year Risk %

Points	4-Year Risk %	Points	4-Year Risk %	Points	4-Year Risk %
<0	<1.0	8	5.2	17	23.8
0	1.2	9	6.3	18	27.4
1	1.4	10	7.5	19	31.4
2	1.7	11	9.0	20	35.7
3	2.1	12	10.7	21	40.3
4	2.5	13	12.6	22	45.0
5	3.0	14	14.9	23	49.7
6	3.6	15	17.5	24	54.5
7	4.4	16	20.5	25	59.3

Diastolic Blood Pressure (mm Hg) Points					
AGE	<70	70-74	75-79	80-84	85-89
20–29	-7	-2	0	3	5
30–39	-4	0	2	4	6
40–49	-1	2	4	6	7
50–59	2	5	6	7	8
60–69	5	7	8	8	9
70–79	9	9	9	10	10

Data from Parikh NI, Pencina MJ, Wang TJ, et al. A risk score for predicting near term hypertension. Ann Intern Med 2008;148:102–10.

to prevent much of hypertension itself and its cardiovascular consequences.[49] This opportunity should be acted on.

Moderate blood pressure elevations are more prevalent than severe elevations, so that a large fraction of the CVD in the population is attributable to seemingly trivial elevations of blood pressure. Because the absolute hazard associated with moderate degrees of hypertension is modest, and many persons in this category need to be treated to prevent one CVD event, efficient selection of mildly hypertensive persons for treatment with medication requires multivariable global risk assessment. The goal of therapy should be more to improve the global risk profile than the blood pressure level per se. Targeting therapy based on a composite risk profile should be used to improve the cost-benefit ratio of antihypertensive therapy for prehypertensive patients.

Despite that it is now firmly established that systolic blood pressure exerts a greater influence on CVD incidence than diastolic blood pressure (particularly in the elderly) control of systolic pressure still lags behind diastolic blood pressure control.[42] Why physicians still regard diastolic blood pressure as the chief culprit in hypertension needs to be investigated. There also is unjustified fear of aggressive treatment of systolic hypertension because of an apparent excess CVD risk at low diastolic blood pressure (the J-curve). This apprehension is unfounded because the excess of CVD observed at low diastolic blood pressure is confined to those who have a high pulse pressure, incriminating the pulse pressure. The SHEP and Syst-Eur trials have shown that treatment of elderly patients who have isolated systolic hypertension and, therefore, a disproportionately low diastolic pressure and increased pulse pressure are benefited by treatment without penalty of feared intolerable side effects.[17,18] Isolated systolic hypertension and a widened pulse pressure auger ill and need to be treated at all ages. Such antihypertensive therapy is safe, well tolerated, and efficacious for CVD without any penalty of overall mortality.

Hypertension, dyslipidemia, and diabetes are best regarded as ingredients of a CVD multivariable risk profile comprised of metabolically linked risk factors because the hazard of each varies widely, contingent on the associated burden of other risk factors. Maximum CVD risk reduction in hypertensive persons is best achieved by concomitant control of the accompanying burden of risk factors. Evaluation and treatment of the dyslipidemia that often accompanies hypertension is important and can be guided by the total/HDL cholesterol lipid ratio and the aggressiveness of therapy for hypertension and dyslipidemia linked to the global CVD risk.

Physicians treating hypertension also can seek out more aggressive therapy for those who have preclinical atherosclerotic disease signified by an abnormal ankle brachial index, arterial vascular bruits, coronary artery calcification, LVH, other ECG abnormalities, a low ejection fraction, silent myocardial infarction, or proteinuria, among other risk factors.

High-risk hypertensive candidates for CVD who have an ominous multivariable risk profile indicating a 10-year risk for a CVD event exceeding, for example, 20% require more aggressive risk factor modification. The goal of therapy for hypertension should be linked to the global level of CVD risk. Because CVD risk factors usually cluster with hypertension, and the risk imposed by it varies widely in relation to this, such multivariable CVD risk assessment is a necessity, especially now that near-average blood pressure levels are recommended for treatment. Measures taken to prevent any particular CVD hypertensive outcome also can be expected to benefit the other adverse CVD events. Novel risk factors deserve attention, but the standard CVD risk factors seem to account for as much as 85% of CVD arising within the population.

Just as the cardiovascular risk factors identified by the Framingham Study have been found to apply universally, the Framingham Study multivariable risk functions have been validated and found to have transportability with calibration in culturally diverse populations around the world.[27] The risk profiles have been shown accurate even in low-risk areas, such as in Chinese and Spanish populations.[50,51]

Health care providers might be encouraged to undertake multivariable risk assessment whenever patients are evaluated or treated for hypertension if laboratories being sent blood samples for testing of blood sugar or blood lipids could be encouraged to request the other ingredients of the CVD risk profile, including blood pressure and cigarette smoking, and provide a multivariable estimate of risk along with the requested lipid or glucose determination. Serial assessment of global CVD risk can be used to monitor progress of patients on treatment of hypertension. Demonstrating improvement in their multivariable risk score can be used to motivate patients to comply better with the recommended preventive management of their hypertension.

The hypertension-induced CVD epidemic cannot be conquered solely by cardiologists caring for referred patients. Multiple elements of the health care system have to be mobilized. Unfortunately, the health care system rewards doing procedures more than preventive services. Despite means available to identify high-risk hypertensive candidates for CVD and proof of the efficacy of controlling their blood pressure and associated risk factors, goals for prevention of CVD are not often met. There is an unmet need to more aggressively implement established guideline goals for management of hypertensive, dyslipidemic, and diabetic patients at risk for atherosclerotic CVD.

REFERENCES

1. Kannel WB, Dawber TR, Kagan A, et al. Factors of risk in the development of coronary heart disease—six-year follow-up experience. The Framingham Study. Ann Intern Med 1961;55:33–50.
2. Kannel WB. Framingham study insights into hypertensive risk of cardiovascular disease. Hypertens Res 1995;18:181–96.
3. Kannel WB, Gordon T, Schwartz MJ. Systolic versus diastolic blood pressure and risk of coronary heart disease: the Framingham Study. Am J Cardiol 1971;27:335–45.
4. Kannel WB, Dawber TR, McGee DL, et al. Perspectives on systolic hypertension: the Framingham Study. Circulation 1980;61:1179–82.
5. Port S, Demer L, Jennrich R, et al. Systolic blood pressure and mortality. Lancet 2000;355:175–80.
6. Kannel WB, Vasan RS, Levy D. Is the relation of systolic blood pressure to risk of cardiovascular disease continuous and graded, or are there critical values? Hypertension 2003;42: 453–6.
7. Franklin SS, Kahn SA, Wong NA, et al. Is pulse pressure useful in predicting risk for coronary heart disease? The Framingham Study. Circulation 1999;100:354–60.
8. Chobanian AV, Bakris GL, Black HR, et al. Joint National Committee on Prevention, Detection, Evaluation, and Treatment of High Blood Pressure. National Heart Lung and Blood Institute; National High Blood Pressure Education Program Coordinating Committee. Seventh report of the Joint National Committee on prevention, detection, evaluation and treatment of high blood pressure. Hypertension 2003;42:1206–52.
9. Vasan R, Larson MG. Impact of high normal blood pressure on the risk of cardiovascular disease. N Engl J Med 2001;345:1291–7.
10. Lewington S, Clarke R, Qizilbash N, et al. Age-specific relevance of usual blood pressure to vascular mortality: a meta-analysis of individual data for one million adults in 61 prospective studies. Prospective Studies Collaboration. Lancet 2002;360:1903–13.
11. Neaton JD, Wentworth D. Serum cholesterol, blood pressure, cigarette smoking, and death from coronary heart disease. Overall findings and differences by age for 316,099 white men. Multiple Risk Factor Intervention Trial Research Group. Arch Intern Med 1992;152:56–64.
12. Liszka HA, Mainous AG, King DE, et al. Prehypertension and cardiovascular morbidity. Ann Fam Med 2005;3:294–9.
13. Vasan RS, Larson MG, Leip EP, et al. Assessment of frequency of progression to hypertension in non-hypertensive subjects in the Framingham Heart Study. Lancet 2001;358:1682–6.
14. Kannel WB, Wilson PW, Nam BH, et al. A likely explanation for the J-curve blood pressure cardiovascular risk. Am J Cardiol 2004;94:380–4.
15. Cruickshank JM, Thorp JM, Zacharias FJ. Benefits and potential harm of lowering high blood pressure. Lancet 1987;1:581–4.
16. Neaton JD, Kuller L, Stamler J, et al. Impact of systolic and diastolic blood pressure on cardiovascular mortality. In: Laragh JH, Brenner BM, editors. Hypertension: pathophysiology, diagnosis and management. 2nd edition. New York: NY Raven Press Ltd; 1995. p. 127–44.
17. SHEP Cooperative Research Group. Prevention of stroke by antihypertensive drug treatment in older persons with isolated systolic hypertension. JAMA 1991;265:3255–64.

18. Stassen JA, Fagard R, Thijs L, et al. Randomized double blind comparison of placebo and active treatment for older patients with isolated systolic hypertension. Lancet 1997;350:757–64.
19. Kannel WB, Dannenberg AL, Levy D. Population implications of left ventricular hypertrophy. Am J Cardiol 1987;60:851–931.
20. Kannel WB. Left ventricular hypertrophy as a risk factor in hypertension. Eur Heart J 1992;13:82–8.
21. Levy D, Salomon M, D'Agostino RB, et al. Prognostic implications of baseline electrocardiographic features and their serial changes in subjects with left ventricular hypertrophy. Circulation 1994;90:1786–93.
22. Bikkina M, Larson MG, Levy D. Prognostic implications of asymptomatic ventricular arrhythmias: the Framingham Heart Study. Ann Intern Med 1992;117(12):990–6.
23. Kannel WB, Anderson K, McGee DL, et al. Nonspecific electrocardiographic abnormality as a predictor of coronary heart disease: the Framingham Study. Am Heart J 1987;113:370–6.
24. Gillman MW, Kannel WB, Belanger A, et al. Influence of heart rate on mortality among persons with hypertension: the Framingham Study. Am Heart J 1993;125:1148–54.
25. Schneider JF, Thomas HE Jr, Kreger BE, et al. Newly acquired left bundle-branch block: the Framingham study. Ann Intern Med 1979;90:303–10.
26. Denes P, Larson JC, Lloyd-Jones DM, et al. Major and minor ECG abnormalities in asymptomatic women and risk of cardiovascular events and mortality. JAMA 2007;297:978–85.
27. Kannel WB, Dannenberg AL, Abbott RD. Unrecognized myocardial infarction and hypertension in the Framingham study. Am Heart J 1985;109:581–5.
28. Kannel WB. Fifty years of Framingham study contributions to understanding hypertension. J Hum Hypertens 2000;14:83–90.
29. Wilson PWF, Kannel WB. Clustering of risk factors, obesity and syndrome X. Nutr Clin Care 1999;1:44–50.
30. Kannel WB. Risk stratification of hypertension; new insights from the Framingham Study. Am J Hypertens 2000;13:3S–10S.
31. Wang TJ, Larson MG, Levy D, et al. Impact of obesity on plasma natriuretic peptide levels. Circulation 2004;109:594–600.
32. Kannel WB, D'Agostino RB, Silbershatz H, et al. Profile for estimating risk of heart failure. Arch Intern Med 1999;159:1197–204.
33. Wolf PA, D'Agostino RB, Belanger AJ, et al. Probability of stroke: a risk profile from the Framingham study. Stroke 1991;3:312–8.
34. Murabito JM, D'Agostino RB, Silberschatz H, et al. Intermittent claudication: a risk profile from the Framingham Heart Study. Circulation 1997;96:44–9.
35. Kannel WB, McGee D, Gordon T. A general cardiovascular risk profile: the Framingham study. Am J Cariol 1976;38:46–51.
36. Anderson KM, Wilson PWF, Odell PM, et al. An updated coronary risk profile: a statement for health professionals. Circulation 1991;83:357–63.
37. Wilson PWF, D'Agostino RB, Levy D, et al. Prediction of coronary heart disease using risk factor categories. Circulation 1998;97:1837–47.
38. D'Agostino RB, Vasan RS, Pencina MJ, et al. General cardiovascular risk profile for use in primary care. Circulation 2008;117:743–53.
39. Guidelines Committee. 2003 European Society of Hypertension–European Society of Cardiology guidelines for the management of arterial hypertension. J Hypertens 2003;21:1011–53.

40. Mancia G. Guidelines Committee. 2003 European Society of Hypertension—European Society of Cardiology guidelines for the management of arterial hypertension. J Hypertens 2003;21;1011–53.

41. Joint National Committee. The sixth report of the Joint National Committee on prevention, detection, evaluation and treatment of high blood pressure. Arch Intern Med 1997;157:2314–446.

42. Lloyd-Jones DM, Evans JC, Larson MG, et al. Differential control of systolic and diastolic blood pressure: factors associated with lack of blood pressure control in the community. Hypertension 2000;36:504–50.

43. Hajjar T, Kotchen TA. Trends in prevalence awareness, treatment and control of hypertension in the U.S. 1988–2000. JAMA 2003;290:199–206.

44. Berlowitz DR, Ash AS, Hickey EC, et al. Hypertension management in patients with diabetes. The need for more aggressive therapy. Diabetes Care 2005;26:355–9.

45. Fonarow GC, French WJ, Parsons LS, et al. Use of lipid-lowering medications at discharge in patients with acute myocardial infarction data from the National Registry of Myocardial Infarction 3. Circulation 2001;103:38–44.

46. Ferrucci L, Furberg CD, Penninx WJH, et al. Treatment of isolated systolic hypertension is most effective in older patients with high-risk profile. Circulation 2001;104:1923–6.

47. Ogden LG, He J, Lydick E, et al. Long-term absolute benefit of lowering blood pressure in hypertensive patients according to JNC VI risk stratification. Hypertension 2000;35:539–43.

48. Expert Panel on Detection, Evaluation and Treatment of High Blood Cholesterol in Adults. Executive Summary of the Third Report of the NCEP Expert Panel. Adult Treatment Panel III. JAMA 2001;285:2486–97.

49. Parich NI, Pencina MJ, Wang TJ, et al. A risk score for predicting near term hypertension: the Framingham Heart Study. Ann Intern Med 2008;148:102–10.

50. Marrugat J, D'Agostino RB, Sullivan L, et al. An adaptation of the Framingham coronary heart disease risk function to European Mediterranean Areas. J Epidemiol Community Health 2003;57:634–8.

51. Liu J, Hong Y, D'Agostino RB, et al. Predictive value for the Chinese of the Framingham CHD risk assessment tool compared with the Chinese Multi-Provincial Cohort Study. JAMA 2004;291:2591–9.

New Insights into Target Organ Involvement in Hypertension

Richard N. Re, MD, FACP

KEYWORDS

- Hypertension • Renin angiotensin system • Prorenin
- Vascular disease • Intracrine

The therapy of hypertension is in large measure directed to the prevention of target organ disease in the brain, kidney, heart, and vasculature. It is noteworthy that some of the factors that participate in the raising of arterial pressure also participate in the pathogenesis of hypertension-related target organ disease. Foremost among these factors is the renin-angiotensin system (RAS), which is both a powerful regulator of intravascular volume and arterial pressure as well as a mediator of tissue damage. Over recent years new knowledge has been developed regarding the participation of the RAS in the development of target organ damage and these insights in turn suggest improved methods of therapy.[1–8]

THE RENIN-ANGIOTENSIN SYSTEM AND VASCULAR DISEASE

It has been shown that infusion of angiotensin II, the major effector peptide of the RAS, can lead to hypertension accompanied by cardiac fibrosis, vascular remodeling, vascular hyalinization, and fibrinoid necrosis in various animal models.[4–9] Thus, many of the major findings in acute severe hypertension can be reproduced by angiotensin-induced hypertension. At the same time, atherosclerosis, a longer term potential sequela of high blood pressure, has come to be seen as a complex process involving the genesis of fatty streaks, vascular inflammation, plaque formation, and at times plaque rupture. Angiotensin II participates in many phases of this process. Recent work in a primate model of atherogenesis demonstrates that blockade of the AT-1 angiotensin II receptor results in marked diminution in fatty streak formation in large arteries. Monocyte adherence to the vessel walls of these animals is reduced and in fact remains reduced for some weeks after cessation of AT-1 blocker therapy suggesting an effect of angiotensin II blockade on the differentiation of monocyte precursors.[10,11] Similarly, angiotensin has been shown to be proinflammatory, through

Ochsner Clinic Foundation, 1514 Jefferson Highway, New Orleans, LA 70121, USA
E-mail address: rre@ochsner.org

Med Clin N Am 93 (2009) 559–567
doi:10.1016/j.mcna.2009.02.009
0025-7125/09/$ – see front matter © 2009 Elsevier Inc. All rights reserved.

medical.theclinics.com

the production of oxidative stress as well as the up-regulation of inflammatory mediators such as transforming growth factor (TGF)-beta.[4,12] In cell culture and other models, angiotensin can either stimulate cellular proliferation or hypertrophy depending on cell type and culture conditions.[13–16] In this regard it is interesting to note that converting enzyme inhibition or AT-1 blockade when administered to hypertensive subjects can be shown to improve hypertension-induced vascular remodeling in arterioles studied at biopsy. Beta blockers do not produce a similar effect even when blood pressure is equally controlled.[17] Angiotensin-converting enzyme is up-regulated in the shoulders of arterial plaques and this makes it reasonable to suppose that increased angiotensin II production at these sites could lead to a proinflammatory environment, an up-regulation of matrix metalloproteinases, and ultimately to plaque rupture.[18,19]

Thus considerable evidence points to the participation of the RAS in the development of the sequelae of hypertension. Recent findings further extend this participation.

THE (PRO)RENIN RECEPTOR

One of the most exciting findings of recent years has been the discovery and initial characterization of the (pro)renin receptor.[20,21] It has for some time been known that glycosylated renin could be taken into cells via the mannose/insulin-like growth factor II cell surface receptor. Renin binding to this receptor leads to receptor signaling but the internalized renin does not act within the cell and appears to be destroyed.[22,23] That is, this appears to be a clearance receptor without significant implications for local angiotensin II generation. More recently, a second receptor has been characterized. Termed the (pro)renin receptor, this molecule is a portion of the vacuolar ATPase-associated protein, a near ubiquitously expressed intracellular protein. On the cell surface, however, this receptor binds both prorenin and renin with the generation of second messengers and the up-regulation of among other factors, plasminogen activator inhibitor-1. These cell surface receptors have been reported on vascular smooth muscle cells, mesangial cells of the kidney, and other cell types. Also, upon prorenin binding to the receptor, the pro segment of prorenin is moved away from the enzymatic active site and surface-bound prorenin becomes non-enzymatically activated. That is to say, the pro segment is not cleaved from the protein but, nonetheless, the enzyme on the cell surface can generate angiotensin I from angiotensinogen. The availability of angiotensin-converting enzyme on cell surface in proximity to angiotensin AT-1 receptors on targets cells makes local generation of angiotensin II by cell surface bound prorenin of considerable physiologic importance. Moreover, as already noted, the receptor binds renin whereupon bound renin becomes more enzymatically active than when in an unbound state, a situation that again leads to the generation of large amounts of angiotensin II in close proximity to the cell's AT-1 receptors.[20,21,24] Recently, small decoy peptides designed to bind to the so-called handle region of the (pro)renin receptor have been synthesized. Because the handle region is responsible for displacing the pro segment from the prorenin active site and thereby activating the enzyme, it was assumed that these small peptides would interfere with the activation of prorenin at the receptor. When these peptides were administered to diabetic rodents, diabetic nephropathy was almost entirely prevented—an effect more robust than was seen with traditional AT-1 blockers. Moreover, this beneficial effect was seen in AT-1 knockout mice suggesting a novel mode of producing pharmacologic benefit. These results are controversial in part because they have not yet been reproduced and in part because it is unclear why the decoy peptides provided benefit when renin was presumably left free to bind to the receptor.[24-26] Nonetheless, these are promising observations suggesting the existence of previously unsuspected ways of mitigating vascular disease in the glomerulus.

Irrespective of the efficacy of decoy peptides, the (pro)renin receptor has important implications for the pathogenesis of disease. It has long been know that circulating prorenin concentration can be very high in diabetic patients. Prorenin concentrations are also high in eyes of diabetic patients and, in fact, prorenin can be synthesized in situ in the retina.[27,28] In the 1970s it was reported that elevations of circulating prorenin concentration in type I diabetic patients presage microvascular complications such as retinopathy and nephropathy.[27] Until the discovery of the prorenin receptor these findings were inexplicable. The only known site of prorenin activation was the kidney. Thus, any circulating prorenin would be expected to be inert. However, the existence of the (pro)renin receptor means that high concentrations of prorenin can be activated at local sites and lead to local generation of angiotensin II. In this way, the (pro)renin receptor greatly expands the complexity of the local renin angiotensin system. Moreover, direct signaling by high concentrations of prorenin at the (pro)renin receptor could also have physiologic implications. Aliskiren is a recently available renin inhibitor.[27-29] It can block the enzymatic activity of prorenin and renin bound to the (pro)renin receptor and therefore should be beneficial in cases of high local angiotensin generation. An interesting question is whether aliskiren can prevent the direct activation of receptor signaling by either prorenin or renin; cell culture studies suggest that it cannot.[30] Receptor signaling is not impaired by aliskiren but nonetheless the drug likely will produce considerable benefit through the inhibition of local angiotensin II formation. Another facet of aliskiren action should be touched on. Aliskiren is associated with marked reactive up-regulation of renin.[27-29] Circulating renin concentrations are much higher after aliskiren therapy than after AT-1 blocker therapy. Although this was initially felt to be the result of more complete blockade of the renin angiotensin system, it seems more likely a result of the measurement of renin concentration in the blood being artifactually elevated because of bound inhibitor. Also, the clearance of renin may be reduced once it is bound to aliskiren, another possible cause for artifactually high concentrations of renin.[27-29] Nonetheless, renin concentration rises after aliskiren as it does after AT-1 blocker therapy or after the administration of converting enzyme inhibition. Even though circulating renin in the case of aliskiren is not enzymatically active, could it be detrimental by virtue of direct stimulation of the (pro)renin receptor? A recent cell culture study suggests that there is a mitigating process that would lessen any such deleterious effects. The binding of renin to the (pro)renin receptor activates a rapid down-regulation of the receptor gene, thereby presumably down-regulating receptor number at the cell surface and dampening any effects of high circulating renin.[31] The lack of any obvious deleterious effects of the hyperreninemia associated with AT-1 blocker or converting enzyme inhibitor therapy is consistent with this view.

THE AT-1 RECEPTOR

The effects of angiotensin II at the cell surface are mediated by two G-protein coupled receptors termed the AT-1 and AT-2 receptors. Although the AT-2 receptors are abundantly expressed in the fetus, their number declines in adults with the result that the AT-1 receptor becomes the predominant receptor in most tissues. The most well-known actions of angiotensin II, such as vasoconstriction, as well as stimulation of hypertrophy, hyperplasia and fibrosis, stimulation of aldosterone secretion, and augmentation of renal tubular sodium re-absorption, are mediated by the AT-1 receptor. Angiotensin II binding to the AT-2 receptor for the most part appears to have actions opposite to angiotensin II binding at the AT-1 receptor so that the AT-2 receptor in part mitigates the stimulation of the AT-1 receptor.[4,5,32] AT-2 receptor stimulation up-regulates bradykinin and eventually nitric oxide synthesis thereby producing a vasodilating effect. AT-2 stimulation also plays a role in enhancing natriuresis and in the blunting of cell proliferation.

It has recently become apparent that the AT-1 receptor participates in cross-talk with the epidermal growth factor (EGF) receptor such that activation of the AT-1 by angiotensin II leads to the cleavage of bound EGF from the cell surface with subsequent stimulation of cell-surface EGF receptors.[33] This provides a link between the proliferative effects of angiotensin II and EGF such that stimulation of target cells can produce enhanced actions via the stimulation of EGF receptors and therefore the actions of both hormones become involved in generating tissue pathology. Also of note, it is now clear that the AT-1 receptor can physically interact at the cell surface with the bradykinin B2 receptor with the result that AT-1 signaling in the presence of angiotensin II is enhanced.[34,35] This receptor interaction has the effect of sensitizing target cells to angiotensin II with likely pathologic results. Indeed, there is evidence to indicate that AT-1 B 2 interaction plays a role in the genesis of the hypertension and vascular pathology seen in preeclampsia.

Yet other recent findings point to an interaction between the pathogenic effects of hyperlipidemia and hypertension—two potent risk factors for atherosclerosis. Oxidized low-density lipoprotein—an established risk factor for atherogenesis—can be oxidized whereupon it can bind to the so-called lectin-like oxidized low density lipoprotein (LDL) receptor, LOX-1. Angiotensin II increases the synthesis of oxidized LDL in the arterial wall through the production of oxidative stress with the result that increased amounts of oxidized LDL are taken up by macrophages through a scavenger pathway leading to enhanced macrophage synthesis of cholesterol. However, angiotensin II also produces pro-atherogenic effects on endothelial cells including the stimulation of apoptosis and these effects are mediated by LOX-1. It has recently been shown that angiotensin II up-regulates LOX-1 expression, whereas oxidized LDL up-regulates AT-1 expression.[36,37] This suggests that AT-1 and LOX-1 act synergistically in the production of vascular inflammation and pathology.

A homolog of angiotensin-converting enzyme (ACE) has been identified, so-called ACE2. This enzyme does not generate angiotensin II from angiotensin I but rather cleaves angiotensin I to angiotensin, (1-9) which in some circumstances may be cleaved to angiotensin (1-7) by ACE. But more important, it also cleaves angiotensin (1-7) directly from angiotensin II.[38–40] Angiotensin (1-7) is an important mediator of angiotensin action, likely operating through the Mas receptor.[41] Angiotensin (1-7) is antiproliferative and vasodilating. Thus, it tends to offset the pathogenic actions of angiotensin II. The balance between angiotensin II and angiotensin (1-7) is an important determinant of vascular health and the ratio of these factors in large part determined by the availability and regulation of ACE2.[38–41]

TRANSFORMING GROWTH FACTOR

An exciting, although still preliminary, new field of investigation involves the role of TGF in the vascular pathology of Marfan's syndrome. Patients with Marfan's syndrome suffer from a variety of abnormalities, most notably from aortic aneurysm and dissection. The defect in Marfan's syndrome involves the gene for fibrillin, a structural protein in the vascular wall. Conventional thinking assumed that abnormalities of a connective tissue protein such as fibrillin resulted in abnormal connective tissue strength in large vessels leading to lessened tissue integrity and eventual aneurysm formation.

Treatment consisted in lowering blood pressure and pulse pressure so as to reduce stress on the aortic wall and this therapy has provided significant benefit by slowing the progression of aortic distension.[42]

However, recent studies have revealed that the fibrillin molecule contains multiple binding sites for TGF and that the protein serves as a reservoir for this protein, binding it in tissue in an inactive state. Defects in the fibrillin gene are associated with a reduction in TGF binding sites. These observations and studies in transgenic animal models of the disease led to the hypothesis that a major lesion in Marfan's syndrome was the absence of a tissue sink for TGF leading to enhanced TGF activity in the tissue, the stimulation thereby of metalloproteinases, and the degradation of vascular connective tissue. Because angiotensin II up-regulates TGF, it was hypothesized that AT-1 blockade could blunt the progression of vascular pathology in Marfan's syndrome. Studies in the transgenic model of the disease, and more recently a preliminary study in humans, bear this out. AT-1 blockade results in a slowing of the progression of aortic root dilatation.[39,43,44] This suggests that the possibility that similar benefit can be obtained in patients with non-Marfan's vascular dilatation should be explored.

INTRACRINE RENIN-ANGIOTENSIN

Considerable evidence has been developed over recent years to indicate that a variety of peptide factors, including hormones, growth factors, DNA binding proteins, enzymes, and others, can serve both as extracellular signaling molecules and also function in the intracellular space either after retention in the cells that synthesized them or after internalization by target cells.[45–52] Early on we termed these factors *intracrines* and developed hypotheses regarding their biologic origins and the principles that regulate their function.[45,46] These ideas are reviewed in detail elsewhere.[45–52] Important for the present discussion is the realization that angiotensin II was one of the earliest identified intracrine hormones and recent evidence strongly suggests that renin, angiotensinogen, and even angiotensin-converting enzyme can act as intracrines in their own right.

Recent studies using either an angiotensinogen construct lacking the signal sequence for secretion and therefore destined to be retained in the cell, or using a construct expressing an angiotensin II molecule that must be retained in the intracellular space demonstrated that up-regulation of intracellular angiotensin II is associated with proliferation in several cell types.[53–55] These observations were followed by the demonstration that the transfection of cultured cardiac myocytes with a construct expressing a nonsecreted angiotensin II moiety resulted in marked cellular hypertrophy within 48 to 96 hours. Moreover, when the intracellular angiotensin construct was incorporated in a plasmid under the regulation of the alpha myosin heavy chain promoter and the plasmid injected into the left ventricles of rodents, marked cardiac hypertrophy again occurred within 96 hours.[56,57] Collectively, these results point to the possibility that the intracrine angiotensin system could play an important role in cardiac hypertrophy. Still more recent studies indicate that both in cell culture and in vivo hyperglycemia up-regulates intracellular cardiac myocyte angiotensinogen and renin, leading to apoptosis. These findings support earlier reports of increased angiotensin II and apoptosis in human diabetic heart disease.[58]

Other studies have demonstrated that intracellular angiotensin II can have important effects on intracellular calcium currents and on junctional conductance.[59–64] Moreover, intracellular angiotensin as opposed to extracellular hormone causes cell volume to decrease.[64–66] All these effects suggest a role for the intracellular renin angiotensin system in the regulation of cardiac rhythm and in the genesis of pathologic arrhythmia.

SUMMARY

Hypertension and its sequelae are complex processes. Optimization of the care of the hypertensive patient requires not only attention to the regulation of arterial pressure but also attention to blunting the hypertension-related processes that lead to vascular disease. It is clear that the regulation of these processes is much more complex than previously understood. Here several new insights into the pathogenesis of hypertension-related vascular disease have been explored. While this review is not exhaustive, it does serve to point out the varied nature of the biologic processes that must be taken into account and it points to new avenues for the development of therapeutic agents.

REFERENCES

1. Prisant LM. Management of hypertension in patients with cardiac disease: use of renin-angiotensin blocking agents. Am J Med 2008;121(8 Suppl):S8–15.
2. Pedelty L, Gorelick PB. Management of hypertension and cerebrovascular disease in the elderly. Am J Med 2008;121(8 Suppl):S23–31.
3. Palmer BF. Management of hypertension in patients with chronic kidney disease and diabetes mellitus. Am J Med 2008;121(8 Suppl):S16–22.
4. Re RN. The renin-angiotensin systems. Med Clin North Am 1987;71:877–95.
5. Re RN. Tissue renin angiotensin systems. Med Clin North Am 2004;88:19–38.
6. Re RN. The clinical implication of tissue renin angiotensin systems. Curr Opin Cardiol 2001;16:317–27.
7. Wolf G. Novel aspects of the renin-angiotensin-aldosterone-system. Front Biosci 2008;13:4993–5005.
8. Burchfiel CM, Tracy RE, Chyou PH, et al. Cardiovascular risk factors and hyalinization of renal arterioles at autopsy. The Honolulu Heart Program. Arterioscler Thromb Vasc Biol 1997;17:760–8.
9. Johnson RJ, Alpers CE, Yoshimura A, et al. Renal injury from angiotensin II-mediated hypertension. Hypertension 1992;19:464–74.
10. Strawn WB, Richmond RS, Ann Tallant E, et al. Renin-angiotensin system expression in rat bone marrow haematopoietic and stromal cells. Br J Haematol 2004; 126:120–6.
11. Strawn WB, Ferrario CM. Angiotensin II AT1 receptor blockade normalizes CD11b+ monocyte production in bone marrow of hypercholesterolemic monkeys. Atherosclerosis 2008;196:624–32 [Epub 2007 Aug 9].
12. Re RN. Cellular biology of the renin-angiotensin systems. Arch Intern Med 1984; 144:2037–41.
13. Geisterfer AA, Peach MJ, Owens GK. Angiotensin II induces hypertrophy, not hyperplasia, of cultured rat aortic smooth muscle cells. Circ Res 1988;62:749–56.
14. Campbell-Boswell M, Robertson AL Jr. Effects of angiotensin II and vasopressin on human smooth muscle cells in vitro. Exp Mol Pathol 1981;35:265–76.
15. Re RN, Chen L. Growth factors and cardiovascular structure. Implications for calcium antagonist therapy. Am J Hypertens 1991;4(7 Pt 2):460S–5S.
16. Schlüter KD, Wenzel S. Angiotensin II: a hormone involved in and contributing to pro-hypertrophic cardiac networks and target of anti-hypertrophic cross-talks. Pharmacol Ther 2008;119:311–25.
17. Schiffrin EL. Vascular remodeling and endothelial function in hypertensive patients: effects of antihypertensive therapy. Scand Cardiovasc J Suppl 1998; 47:15–21.

18. Ribichini F, Pugno F, Ferrero V, et al. Cellular immunostaining of angiotensin-converting enzyme in human coronary atherosclerotic plaques. J Am Coll Cardiol 2006;47:1143–9 [Epub 2006 Feb 23].
19. Diet F, Pratt RE, Berry GJ, et al. Increased accumulation of tissue ACE in human atherosclerotic coronary disease. Circulation 1996;94:2756–67.
20. Nguyen G, Delarue F, Burckle C, et al. Pivotal role of the renin/prorenin receptor in angiotensin II production and cellular responses to renin. J Clin Invest 1996;109:1417–27.
21. Nguyen G, Delarue F, Berrou J, et al. Specific receptor binding of renin on human mesangial cells in culture increases plasminogen activator inhibitor-1 antigen. Kidney Int 1996;50:1897–903.
22. Saris JJ, Derkx FH, Lamers JM, et al. Cardiomyocytes bind and activate native prorenin: role of soluble mannose 6-phosphate receptors. Hypertension 2001;37:710–5.
23. Saris JJ, van den Eijnden MM, Lamers JM, et al. Prorenin-induced myocyte proliferation: no role for intracellular angiotensin II. Hypertension 2002;39(2 Pt 2):573–7.
24. Campbell DJ. Critical review of prorenin and (pro)renin receptor research. Hypertension 2008;51:1259–64 [Epub 2008 Mar 17].
25. Nguyen G, Contrepas A. Physiology and pharmacology of the (pro)renin receptor. Curr Opin Pharmacol 2008;8:127–32 [Epub 2008 Feb 19].
26. Muller DN, Klanke B, Feldt S, et al. (Pro)renin receptor peptide inhibitor "handle-region" peptide does not affect hypertensive nephrosclerosis in Goldblatt rats. Hypertension 2008;51:676–81 [Epub 2008 Jan 22].
27. Wilson DM, Luetscher JA. Plasma prorenin activity and complications in children with insulin-dependent diabetes mellitus. N Engl J Med 1990;323:1101–6.
28. Kida T, Ikeda T, Nishimura M, et al. Renin-angiotensin system in proliferative diabetic retinopathy and its gene expression in cultured human Muller cells. Jpn J Ophthalmol 2003;47:36–41.
29. Re RN, Messerli FH. Renin excess after renin inhibition: malefactor or innocent bystander? Int J Clin Pract 2007;61:1427–9.
30. Messerli FH, Re RN. Do we need yet another blocker of the renin-angiotensin system? J Am Coll Cardiol 2007;49:1164–5 [Epub 2007 Mar 6].
31. Batenburg WW, de Bruin RJ, van Gool JM, et al. Aliskiren-binding increases the half life of renin and prorenin in rat aortic vascular smooth muscle cells. Arterioscler Thromb Vasc Biol 2008;28:1151–7 [Epub 2008 Ap].
32. Schefe JH, Neumann C, Goebel M, et al. Prorenin engages the (pro)renin receptor like renin and both ligand activities are unopposed by aliskiren. J Hypertens 2008;26:1787–94.
33. Schefe JH, Unger T, Funke-Kaiser H. PLZF and the (pro)renin receptor. J Mol Med 2008;86:623–7 [Epub 2008 Mar 12].
34. Jones ES, Vinh A, McCarthy CA, et al. AT(2) receptors: functional relevance in cardiovascular disease. Pharmacol Ther 2008;120:292–316.
35. Tang H, Nishishita T, Fitzgerald T, et al. Inhibition of AT1 receptor internalization by concanavalin A blocks angiotensin II-induced ERK activation in vascular smooth muscle cells. Involvement of epidermal growth factor receptor proteolysis but not AT1 receptor internalization. J Biol Chem 2000;275:13420–6.
36. AdbAlla S, Abdel-tawab AM, Quitterer U. The angiotensin II AT2 receptor is an AT1 receptor antagonist. J Biol Chem 2001;276:39721–6.
37. AbdAlla S, Lother H, el Massiery A, et al. Increased AT(1) receptor heterodimers in preeclampsia medicate enhanced angiotensin II responsiveness. Nat Med 2001;7:1003–9.

38. Singh BM, Mehta JL. Interactions between the renin-angiotensin system and dyslipidemia: relevance in the therapy of hypertension and coronary heart disease. Arch Intern Med 2003;163:1296–304.

39. Hu C, Dandapat A, Sun L, et al. Modulation of angiotensin II-mediated hypertension and cardiac remodeling by lectin-like oxidized low-density lipoprotein receptor-1 deletion. Hypertension 2008;52:556–62 [Epub 2008 Jul 21].

40. Crackower MA, Sarao R, Oudit GY, et al. Angiotensin-converting enzyme 2 is an essential regulator of heart function. Nature 2002;417:799–802.

41. Brosnihan KB, Li P, Tallant EA, et al. Angiotensin-(1-7): a novel vasodilator of the coronary circulation. Biol Res 1998;31:227–34.

42. Chappell MC, Allred AJ, Ferrario CM. Pathways of angiotensin (1-7) metabolism in the kidney. Nephrol Dial Transplant 2001;16(Suppl I):22–6.

43. Pearson GD, Devereux R, Loeys B, et al. National Heart, Lung, and Blood Institute and National Marfan Foundation Working Group. Report of the National Heart, Lung, and Blood Institute and National Marfan Foundation Working Group on research in Marfan syndrome and related disorders. Circulation 2008;118: 785–91.

44. Brooke BS, Habashi JP, Judge DP, et al. Angiotensin II blockade and aortic-root dilation in Marfan's syndrome. N Engl J Med 2008;358:2787–95.

45. Habashi JP, Judge DP, Holm TM, et al. Losartan, an AT1 antagonist, prevents aortic aneurysm in a mouse model of Marfan syndrome. Science 2006;312: 117–21.

46. Zhou Y, Poczatek MH, Berecek KH, et al. Thrombospondin 1 mediates angiotensin II induction of TGF-beta activation by cardiac and renal cells under both high and low glucose conditions. Biochem Biophys Res Commun 2006;339: 633–41 [Epub 2005 Nov 18].

47. Re RN, Bryan SE. Functional intracellular renin-angiotensin systems may exist in multiple tissues. Clin Exp Hypertens Theory Practice 1984;A6(10–11):1739–42.

48. Re RN. The cellular biology of angiotensin: paracrine, autocrine and intracrine actions in cardiovascular tissues. J Mol Cell Cardiol 1989;21(Suppl V):63–9.

49. Re R. The nature of intracrine peptide hormone action. Hypertension 1999;34: 534–8.

50. Re RN. The origins of intracrine hormone action. Am J Med Sci 2002;323:43–8.

51. Re RN. Toward a theory of intracrine hormone action. Regul Pept 2002;106:1–6.

52. Re RN. The intracrine hypothesis and intracellular peptide hormone action. Bioessays 2003;25:401–9.

53. Re RN, Cook JL. The intracrine hypothesis: an update. Regul Pept 2005;133:1–9 [Oct 12, e-published ahead of print].

54. Re RN. The implications of intracrine hormone action for physiology and medicine. Am J Physiol Heart Circ Physiol 2003;284:H751–7.

55. Cook JL, Zhang Z, Re RN. In vitro evidence for an intracellular site of angiotensin action. Circ Res 2001;89:1138–46.

56. Cook JL, Mills SJ, Naquin R, et al. Nuclear accumulation of the AT1 receptor in a rat vascular smooth muscle cell line: effects upon signal transduction and cellular proliferation. J Mol Cell Cardiol 2006;40:696–707 [Epub 2006 Mar 6].

57. Cook JL, Giardina JF, Zhang Z, et al. Intracellular angiotensin II increases the long isoform of PDGF mRNA in rat hepatoma cells. J Mol Cell Cardiol 2002;34: 1525–37.

58. Kumar R, Singh VP, Baker KM. The intracellular renin-angiotensin system: implications in cardiovascular remodeling. Curr Opin Nephrol Hypertens 2008;17: 168–73.

59. Singh VP, Le B, Bhat VB, et al. High-glucose-induced regulation of intracellular ANG II synthesis and nuclear redistribution in cardiac myocytes. Am J Physiol Heart Circ Physiol 2007;293:H939–48 [Epub 2007 May 4].

60. Frustaci A, Kajstura J, Chimenti C, et al. Myocardial cell death in human diabetes. Circ Res 2000;87:1123–32.

61. De Mello WC. Influence of intracellular renin on heart cell communication. Hypertension 1995;25:1172–7.

62. De Mello WC. Cardiac arrhythmias: the possible role of the renin-angiotensin system. J Mol Med 2001;79:103–8.

63. Eto K, Ohya Y, Nakamura Y, et al. Intracellular angiotensin II stimulates voltage-operated Ca channels in arterial myocytes. Hypertension 2002;39:474–8.

64. Haller H, Lidschau C, Quass P, et al. Intracellular actions of angiotensin II in vascular smooth muscle cells. J Am Soc Nephrol 1999;10(Suppl 11):S75–83.

65. De Mello WC, Gerena Y. Eplerenone inhibits the intracrine and extracellular actions of angiotensin II on the inward calcium current in the failing heart. On the presence of an intracrine renin angiotensin aldosterone system. Regul Pept 2008;151:54–60.

66. De Mello WC. Intracellular and extracellular renin have opposite effects on the regulation of heart cell volume. Implications for myocardial ischaemia. J Renin Angiotensin Aldosterone Syst 2008;9:112–8.

The Renin Angiotensin Aldosterone System in Hypertension: Roles of Insulin Resistance and Oxidative Stress

Camila Manrique, MD[a],*, Guido Lastra, MD[a],
Michael Gardner, MD[a], James R. Sowers, MD[a,b,c]

KEYWORDS

- Reactive oxygen species • Insulin resistance • Angiotensin II
- Endothelial dysfunction • Hypertension

Despite major advances in the understanding of the pathogenesis and treatment of hypertension (HTN) and other components of the cardiometabolic syndrome (CMS), these entities continue to contribute to major morbidity and mortality from cardiovascular disease (CVD) and chronic kidney disease (CKD). There is an increasing prevalence of HTN in the United States, and this disease currently affects 29% of the population or approximately 65 million persons.[1] In the adult United States population, the prevalence of overweight and obesity is reported to be 66%, and that of the CMS between 35% and 40%.[2] Approximately 28 million persons in the United States have CKD defined as either proteinuria or estimated glomerular filtration rate of less than 60. HTN, CMS, and diabetes all play important roles in this increase in CKD.

It is estimated that at least 50% of hypertensive patients are insulin resistant, and insulin resistance is one fundamental abnormality in the pathogenesis of the CMS.[3,4] In this context, patients with HTN have higher fasting and postprandial insulin levels, independent of body mass index or body fat distribution.[5] Moreover, both insulin resistance and HTN are implicated in the pathophysiology of CKD and CVD.

[a] Department of Internal Medicine, Diabetes and Cardiovascular Center, University of Missouri, One Hospital Drive Columbia, Columbia, MO 65212, USA
[b] Department of Physiology and Pharmacology, Diabetes and Cardiovascular Center, University of Missouri, One Hospital Drive Columbia, Columbia, MO 65212, USA
[c] Harry S. Truman VA Hospital, D109 HSC Diabetes Center, 800 Hospital Drive, Columbia, MO 65201, USA
* Corresponding author. Harry S. Truman VA Hospital, D109 HSC Diabetes Center, One Hospital Drive, Columbia, MO 65212.
E-mail address: manriquec@health.missouri.edu (C. Manrique).

Med Clin N Am 93 (2009) 569–582
doi:10.1016/j.mcna.2009.02.014
medical.theclinics.com

Studies in humans demonstrate that improving insulin resistance, with insulin sensitizers, has a positive effect on blood pressure control.

Several pathophysiologic factors are involved in the relationship between HTN and the other components of the CMS, including inappropriate activation of the renin angiotensin aldosterone system (RAAS), oxidative stress, and inflammation. Other factors include impaired insulin-mediated vasodilatation, enhanced sympathetic nervous system (SNS) activation, and abnormal sodium handling by the kidney. The purpose of this article is to present the current state of knowledge, focusing on the role of insulin resistance and RAAS-mediated oxidative stress on endothelial dysfunction and the pathogenesis of HTN.

RENAL SODIUM HANDLING

Several abnormalities in renal handling of sodium have been demonstrated in both HTN and the CMS. Initially, it was demonstrated that insulin enhances sodium reabsorption in the diluting segment of the distal nephron, in part, through increased expression of sodium transporters, such as the epithelial sodium channel, with consequent decrease in sodium excretion.[6,7] This effect could potentially contribute to the genesis of hypertension under hyperinsulinemic conditions secondary to selective insulin resistance of nonrenal tissues. In opposition to this hypothesis, using a murine model of selective knockout of the insulin receptor in the renal tubule epithelial cells, it was reported that the absence of insulin action results in impaired natriuresis and increased blood pressure, findings that were correlated with reduced renal nitric oxide (NO) production.[8] This novel evidence can explain how decreased NO production would lead to renal vasoconstriction and increased sodium reabsorption with resultant HTN in conditions of insulin resistance. The significance of these contradictory results is not clear yet, and further studies are needed to clarify the significance of insulin signaling in sodium and water metabolism.

SYMPATHETIC NERVOUS SYSTEM ACTIVATION

Clinical studies have shown that individuals with CMS have increased SNS activity, and this increased activity is correlated with insulin resistance.[9] A number of mechanisms are involved in the activation of the SNS in the CMS. In states of insulin resistance compensatory hyperinsulinemia can cause enhanced sympathetic output in humans through ventromedial hypothalamus mechanisms.[10,11] Additionally leptin, which is elevated in obesity, increases sympathetic nerve activation.[12] The role of leptin in the control of sympathetic tone and blood pressure is supported by the observation that humans with leptin deficiency exhibit sympathetic system dysfunction and postural hypotension.[13] More recently, investigators showed in an animal model of obesity that leptin actions to increase renal sympathetic system activity are mediated by phosphoinositol 3-kinase (PI3K) activation.[14] The PI3K enzyme is involved in many of the metabolic actions of insulin.[15]

RAAS also interacts, in a positive feedback fashion, with the SNS (**Fig. 1**). Injection of angiotensin II (Ang II) in the brain of experimental models causes increased sympathetic output. Additionally, the activation of the RAAS facilitates sympathetic ganglia transmission and inhibits the reuptake of noradrenaline in the nerve terminals.[16] In this context, angiotensin-converting enzyme (ACE) inhibition promotes reuptake of noradrenaline in nerve terminals, perhaps explaining one of the beneficial effects of RAAS blockade.[17] Thus, enhancement of the SNS and the RAAS act in a positive feedback regulatory mechanism in the setting of HTN and the CMS.

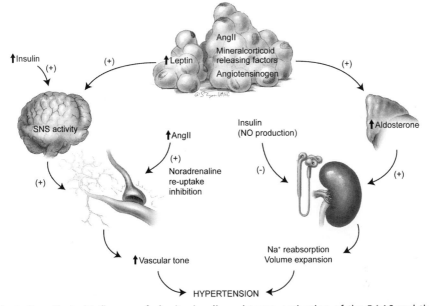

Fig. 1. Coordinated influence of obesity, insulin resistance, activation of the RAAS and the SNS in the pathophysiology of hypertension in the CMS.

RENIN ANGIOTENSIN ALDOSTERONE SYSTEM

The interaction between the RAAS and the SNS is at least partially responsible for the development of HTN in states of insulin resistance, such as the CMS. Often in the CMS there is an increase in visceral adipose tissue and the increased inflammation and oxidative stress in this tissue leads to increased production of components of the adipose renin angiotensin system.[18] In animal models, overexpression of angiotensinogen (AGT), restricted to adipose tissue, increases total body fat mass. Further, mice that overexpress adipose AGT are also hypertensive.[19] These data provide new evidence that AGT and Ang II produced in adipose tissue have local affects to enhance adipocyte tissue growth and expansion, and systemic effects on blood pressure regulation. These findings contribute to the understanding of the role of adipose tissue in development of HTN and other components of the CMS.[20]

Ang II exerts many of its detrimental effects through its interaction with the Ang II type 1 receptor (AT$_1$R). AT$_1$R activation in the zona glomerulosa of the adrenal cortex stimulates the production of mineralocorticoids. Furthermore, the activation of AT$_1$R, in nonadrenal tissues, results in a myriad of intracellular events including production of reactive oxygen species (ROS), which contribute to reduced insulin metabolic signaling, and proliferative and inflammatory responses. These AT$_1$R-mediated signals can cause impaired vascular insulin metabolic signaling and endothelial dysfunction, with secondary increases in blood pressure.[21]

Aldosterone is also increased in conditions of increased adiposity and insulin resistance.[22] Indeed, human and rodent adipose tissue is capable of secreting potent mineralocorticoid-releasing factors.[23] Aldosterone increases blood pressure both by its classic actions, mainly sodium retention and plasma volume expansion, and through nongenomic mineralocorticoid receptor (MR) mediated actions.[15]

OXIDATIVE STRESS

One mechanism by which an activated RAAS increases insulin resistance is through increased generation of reactive oxygen species ROS. These charged products are involved in the regulation of normal cell signaling and cell growth, proliferation, and expansion of the extracellular matrix. ROS can be produced in different vascular cell types, including endothelial cells (ECs) and vascular smooth muscle cells (VSMCs), by activation of xanthine oxidase, nitric oxide synthase, the mitochondrial respiratory chain, and the nicotinamide adenine dinucleotide phosphate (NADPH) oxidase enzymatic complex, resulting in increased production of superoxide (O_2^-) (**Fig. 2**). These ROS can, in turn, directly inflict tissue injury or can contribute to the

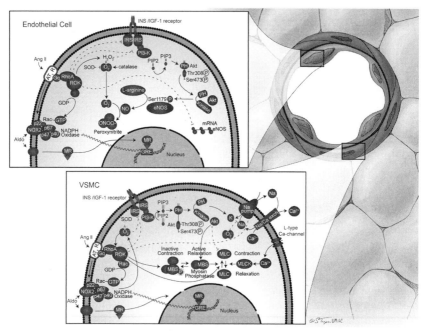

Fig. 2. (*Upper inset*) Vascular effects of insulin (INS) or insulinlike growth factor (IGF)-1 and counterregulatory effects of AT_1R and MR activation in endothelial cells. Insulin actions on the blood vessel are partially mediated by increased production of NO through phosphorylation and secondary activation of endothelial NO synthase (eNOS). AT_1R activation decreases the availability of NO by way of the induction of insulin resistance, diminishing eNOS mRNA stability, and promoting NADPH oxidase-induced ROS production. Mineralocorticoids also activate NAPDH oxidase with secondary O2- production and consequent generation of peroxinitrite (ONOO-). Akt, PI3K/protein kinase B; GRE, glucocorticoid response element; Gq, G_q subunit; IRS, insulin receptor substrate; NOX2, catalytic subunit of NADPH oxidase; p22, p47, p40, and p67, subunits of NADPH oxidase; PH, pleckstrin homology domain; PIP, phosphatidylinositol phosphate; PIP2, phosphatidylinositol bisphosphate; PIP3, phosphatidylinositol (3,4,5)-trisphosphate; ROK, Rho kinase; SOD, superoxide dismutase. (*Lower inset*) Opposing effects of ANG II and aldosterone (Aldo) versus insulin/IGF-1 on VSMCs. Insulin and IGF-1 cause VSMC relaxation, whereas ANG II and mineralocorticoids cause contraction. MBS, myosin-bound serine; MLC, myosin light chain; MLCK, MLC kinase; Na/Ca exch, Na_/Ca2_ exchanger. (*From* Cooper SA, Whaley-Connell A, Habibi J, et al. Renin-angiotensin-aldosterone system and oxidative stress in cardiovascular insulin resistance. Am J Physiol Heart Circ Physiol 2007;293:2009–23; with permission.)

production of additional ROS by converting NO into peroxynitrate, which is also injurious to tissues. This results in less bioavailable NO and consequently impaired endothelial function.[24]

Xanthine oxidase (XO), a hypoxia-inducible enzyme, is also expressed in vascular endothelial and VSMCs, and catalyzes the production of O_2^-. Rodents overexpressing the human renin and AGT genes have increased activity of XO in concert with endothelial dysfunction and HTN. In this model HTN is reversible with antioxidant therapy.[25] In salt-fed spontaneously hypertensive rats (SHR), renal XO activity is increased, and chronic treatment with allopurinol reduces its activity, suggesting a role for this enzyme in HTN-related kidney dysfunction.[26] Additional studies employing this XO inhibitor in hyperuricemic individuals with CKD was associated with reduced uric acid levels, and preserved kidney function.[27]

The nitric oxide synthase enzymes, in particular endothelial nitric oxide synthase enzymes (eNOS), are another important source of ROS. In physiologic conditions, eNOS transfers electrons from a heme group in the oxygenase domain to L-arginine, which results in production of L-citrulline and NO. Under conditions of decreased availability of 5,6,7,8-tetrahydrobiopterin (a cofactor in NO production) or the substrate L-arginine, eNOS switches from this coupled state to an uncoupled state, in which electrons from the heme group reduce oxygen, resulting in production of O_2^-.[28] This uncoupling of eNOS appears to play an important role in endothelial dysfunction and the development of HTN in conditions of insulin resistance, such as the CMS.

ROS are also produced in mitochondria, and during enhanced oxidative phosphorylation this production is increased.[29] Most of electron transport is coupled to production of ATP, but approximately 1% to 2% of electrons can be derived to production of O_2^-, which is scavenged by manganese O_2^- dismutase (SOD), a mechanism that can be overwhelmed in pathologic conditions.[28] Oxidative stress can adversely affect mitochondrial DNA, and studies in both humans and atherosclerosis-prone rodents have correlated the extent of mitochondrial DNA injury to vascular damage and atherosclerosis.[30] Excessive mitochondrial generation of ROS contributes to development of insulin resistance, diabetes, CVD, and CKD.[29]

A major source of ROS is the membrane-bound vascular-derived NADPH oxidase enzymatic system. Key components of this highly regulated system are the membrane-bound subunits p22[phox] and Nox2, the cytosolic subunits p47[phox], p67[phox], p40[phox] and the small guanosine triphosphate-binding protein Rac1/Rac2.[31,32] Activation of the complex involves the interaction between cytosolic subunits p47[phox] and p67[phox], followed by their translocation to the plasma membrane along with prenylated Rac1,[33] where they interact with plasma membrane-bound subunits.[34] In vascular tissue, the NADPH oxidase enzymatic complex can be acutely and chronically activated in response to a variety of stimuli, including Ang II and aldosterone, even at low concentrations.[35]

In normal rats, infusion of noradrenaline or Ang II increased blood pressure to similar extent. However, only Ang II-induced hypertension was associated with increased vascular production of O_2^-.[36] Further, antioxidant treatment with liposomal-encapsulated SOD resulted in significantly reduced blood pressure in Ang II-infused animals, but not in those treated with norepinephrine. Additionally, SOD treatment was associated with enhanced endothelium-dependent vasodilatation and hypotensive responses to acetylcholine. Other models of hypertension, such as the SHR, the stroke-prone SHR, the Dahl salt-sensitive rat, and the transgenic Ren2 rat, also display increased NAPDH oxidase-driven production of ROS. In these models, antioxidant treatment results in improvement of endothelial function and HTN.[37]

From a clinical standpoint, patients with HTN or CVD often exhibit increased oxidative stress. For example, the plasma oxidized-reduced glutathione ratio and malondialdehyde levels are significantly higher, and the activity of SOD, catalase, and glutathione peroxidase significantly lower, in blood and mononuclear peripheral cells of hypertensive patients relative to their normotensive counterparts.[38] Finally, NADPH oxidase-driven production of O_2^- is abnormally enhanced in mononuclear cells, from hypertensive individuals, stimulated with Ang II and ET (endothelin)-1.[39]

Many of the vascular maladaptive effects of the RAAS are mediated through Ang II and aldosterone activation of NADPH oxidase system in vascular tissue (see **Fig. 2**).[5] In addition, Ang II and aldosterone can directly activate NADPH oxidase through stimulation of Rac1 activity and translocation to the membrane in VSMCs or through activation of p47[phox].[28] On the other hand, treatment of hypertensive rats with an hydroxymethylglutaryl-CoA reductase inhibitor results in less activation of vascular NADPH oxidase subunits and reduced generation of ROS, in concert with improved endothelial function and blood pressure.[40] Direct inhibition of NADPH oxidase in a mouse model of Ang II-induced hypertension, by blocking the interaction of p47[phox] and gp91[phox] or the employment of p47[phox] knockout methodology results in blunting of O_2^- production.[41,42] In addition, in rodent models of HTN and increased NADPH activity, use of antioxidants results in improved blood pressure.[43]

Aldosterone can also activate NADPH oxidase and trigger oxidative stress.[44] Other mineralocorticoids such as deoxycorticosterone acetate can also induce increased production of O_2^- in different experimental models of HTN.[45] Furthermore, in the transgenic Ren2 rat, which overexpresses the mouse renin gene in numerous tissues, and exhibits significantly increased plasma aldosterone levels; MR inhibition can reduce cardiac, renal, skeletal muscle, pancreas and vascular NADPH oxidase-ROS generation. This reduction in ROS occurs in concert with improved insulin metabolic signaling and regression of tissue structure abnormalities.[32] MR activation increases skeletal muscle NADPH oxidase activity, in part by way of activation of membrane-bound Nox2 and p22[phox] as well as the cytosolic p47[phox] subunits. The resulting oxidative stress leads to systemic insulin resistance, impaired intracellular insulin signaling, and defective insulin-stimulated glucose transport in skeletal muscle. These changes are reversed by in vivo treatment with a MR inhibitor, at a dose that does not reduce blood pressure.[32]

ROLE OF OXIDATIVE STRESS IN INSULIN RESISTANCE

Binding of insulin to its receptor triggers signaling through the PI3K/protein kinase B (Akt) cascade, which results in glucose transporter-4 (GLUT4) translocation to the plasma membrane and facilitated glucose uptake. In addition, Akt phosphorylates and activates eNOS resulting in NO production and vasodilatation.[46] Therefore, insulin resistance states exhibit impaired insulin-mediated vasodilatation.[46]

On the other hand, data from experimental animal models have shown that insulin can stimulate vasoconstriction through production of ET-1, a process that requires intact mitogen-activated protein kinase (MAPK) signaling.[47] It has been proposed that in insulin-resistant states while the PI3K/Akt pathway signaling is impaired with consequent decreased production of NO, the MAPK pathway is stimulated by hyperinsulinemia resulting in elevated ET-1 production.[48] Nevertheless, a recent study examining obese patients did not confirm a role for hyperinsulinemia in ET-1–mediated vasoconstriction in states of insulin resistance.[49] Thus, the potential role of increased ET-1 in the CMS is still unclear.

The impact of ROS and oxidative stress on insulin metabolic signaling and systemic insulin sensitivity is a field of intense research. The main tissues involved in the pathophysiology of insulin resistance are skeletal muscle and adipose tissue. However, decreased insulin metabolic signaling in vascular tissue can also contribute to endothelial dysfunction, HTN, and atherosclerosis. Increased oxidative stress and resulting impairment in insulin metabolic signaling may play a key role in the pathogenesis of HTN, CMS, and CVD.[50]

In vitro and in vivo studies have demonstrated an association between increased ROS production and insulin resistance. Prolonged exposure of adipose cells to oxidative stress results in decreased insulin-stimulated glucose transport, lipogenesis, and activity of glycogen synthase, consistent with impaired insulin action.[51] In cultured skeletal muscle cells overexpressing GLUT4, pretreatment with the antioxidant α-lipoic acid is protective against oxidative stress-induced impaired insulin-stimulated glucose uptake.[52] Adipocytes obtained from high-fat diet-induced insulin resistance display increased production of ROS and stimulation of the protein kinase C delta, a serine/threonine kinase implicated in impaired cellular insulin metabolic signaling.[53] This, in turn, results in blunted insulin-stimulated glucose uptake and severely decreased expression/activation of GLUT4 and facilitated glucose transport. Other studies conducted in vitro and in animal models have reported a beneficial effect of antioxidants on insulin sensitivity.

Some studies in humans with insulin resistance report similar beneficial effects of vitamin C, E, or glutathione on insulin metabolic signaling.[50] Oxidative stress is strongly associated with increased adiposity and impaired insulin sensitivity in humans, suggesting a role for ROS in the generation of obesity-related insulin resistance.[54] Conversely, it has been demonstrated in humans that insulin resistance is associated with reduced endogenous intracellular antioxidant mechanisms.[55]

The mechanisms implicated in oxidative stress-mediated insulin resistance remain to be fully elucidated, but several experimental studies support a role for activation of redox-sensitive serine (Ser) kinases, including Janus kinase.[56] Activation of these Ser kinases promotes Ser phosphorylation of substrates, including the insulin receptor and the docking proteins insulin receptor substrate (IRS)-1 or 2. This increased Ser phosphorylation of IRS-1 results in decreased engagement of IRS-1 with PI3K and impaired downstream insulin metabolic signaling. In addition, increases in inflammatory molecule NK-kB, a key mediator of inflammation, is triggered by activation of the Ser kinase IKK-β, a process that is reversed by salicylates.[57] In this context, treatment with high doses of aspirin results in increased insulin sensitivity, reduced hepatic glucose output, and improved glucose homeostasis in patients with type 2 diabetes (T2DM).[58]

RENIN ANGIOTENSIN ALDOSTERONE SYSTEMS BLOCKADE IN THE CARDIOMETABOLIC SYNDROME: BEYOND BLOOD PRESSURE NUMBERS

There is increasing evidence for the beneficial effects of RAAS inhibition on metabolic signaling, CVD, and CKD in patients with insulin resistance or overt T2DM. ACE inhibitors and ANG II-receptor blockers (ARBs) have been studied extensively in HTN, congestive heart failure, coronary artery disease, and CKD and are recommended to prevent CVD and nephropathy in patients with T2DM.[59,60] In addition, some of these studies have also suggested reduced incidence of new-onset T2DM, through secondary outcomes and post hoc analysis. In the Heart Outcomes Prevention Evaluation, a double-blind, randomized, placebo-controlled trial assessing the use of ramipril in preventing cardiovascular death in high-risk patients, the incidence of new-onset diabetes was 34% lower in the ramipril-treated group relative to placebo.[61] In the Captopril Prevention Project, a prospective, randomized trial comparing cardiovascular morbidity and mortality in hypertensive patients using an ACE inhibitor or conventional antihypertensive treatment, the prevalence of new-onset T2DM in the captopril-treated arm was significantly lower.[62] In the Candesartan in Heart failure Assessment of Reduction in Mortality and Morbidity study,[63] candesartan reduced the onset of diabetes by 19% compared with placebo when used in patients with chronic heart failure. Other studies that have demonstrated reduction in incidence of new-onset diabetes with the use of ACE inhibitors and ANG II-receptor blockers include the Antihypertensive and Lipid-Lowering Treatment to Prevent Heart Attack Trial,[64] Studies Of Left Ventricular Dysfunction,[65] and Losartan Intervention For Endpoint Reduction in Hypertension Study.[66] Possible mechanisms responsible for the reduced incidence of diabetes in these trials include improvement in insulin-mediated glucose uptake, enhanced endothelial function, increased NO activity, reduced inflammatory response, and increased bradykinin levels.

The only prospective randomized double-blind clinical trial to specifically address the role of ACE inhibition on development of T2DM is the Diabetes Reduction Assessment with Ramipril and Rosiglitazone Medication.[67] This study randomly assigned 5269 participants without CVD but with impaired fasting glycemia or impaired glucose tolerance to receive ramipril or placebo (and rosiglitazone or placebo in another arm of the study) for a median of 3 years. Use of ramipril was not associated with a significant reduction in the incidence of T2DM. However, treatment with ramipril resulted in significantly increased regression to normoglycemia, relative to placebo (hazard ratio, 1.16; 95% CI, 1.07 to 1.27; $P < .05$), and reduced markers of hepatosteatosis suggesting a beneficial effect of RAAS blockade on glucose homeostasis.

MR blockade may improve insulin metabolic signaling,[32] and positively affect CVD outcomes, as demonstrated in the clinical trials: Randomized Aldactone Evaluation Study (RALES) and Eplerenone Post-Acute Myocardial Infarction Heart Failure Efficacy and Survival Study (EPHESUS). The RALES was a double-blind trial that included patients who had severe heart failure and left ventricular ejection fraction below 35%. Participants were randomized to receive 25 mg of spironolactone or placebo plus conventional treatment with an ACE I, a loop diuretic, and in most cases digoxin. In this trial, there was 30% reduction in the relative risk of death in spironolactone group.[68] In the EPHESUS trial, a multicenter, randomized, double-blind, placebo-controlled trial, there was a significant reduction in CVD mortality (relative risk, 0.83; 95% CI, 0.72 to 0.94; $P = .005$) and the rate of death from cardiovascular causes or hospitalization for cardiovascular events (relative risk, 0.87; 95% CI, 0.79 to 0.95; $P = .002$) among patients assigned to eplerenone.[69]

The mechanisms by which MR blockade provides myocardial protection include reduction of coronary vascular inflammation and the risk of subsequent development of interstitial myocardial fibrosis, reduced oxidative stress, improved endothelial dysfunction, attenuated platelet aggregation, decreased activation of matrix metalloproteinases, and improved ventricular remodeling. In addition, MR antagonism results in decreased NADPH oxidase activity and oxidative stress, in concert with improved insulin-stimulated glucose uptake, and attenuated whole-body insulin resistance in the setting of an active RAAS.[32] MR blockade may also improve insulin metabolic signaling.[32]

As the CMS is a strong predictor for development of T2DM, the metabolic effects related to the use of antihypertensive medications should be taken into account.[70] In this regard, antihypertensive therapy with thiazide diuretics and β-blockers have been implicated in the development of new-onset diabetes as well as in the worsening of glycemic control in known diabetic patients.[71] A recent systematic review of 22 clinical trials, with 143,153 participants, reported that the association of different antihypertensives with new-onset diabetes was lower with ARB and ACE I and higher with β-blockers and diuretics.[72] Interestingly, a meta-analysis by Zillich and colleagues[73] that examined studies with thiazide diuretics found an important correlation between the degree of diuretic-induced hypokalemia and increased glycemia; prevention of hypokalemia resulted in a lesser degree of blood glucose elevation. More recently, a small clinical study with 26 centrally obese, hypertensive patients compared the effects of candesartan and hydrochlorothiazide (HCTZ) on insulin resistance or sensitivity, and fat distribution. The authors reported that HCTZ worsens insulin resistance in association with visceral fat redistribution, increased liver fat content, and elevated markers of inflammation when compared with placebo or candesartan. These authors hypothesized that the deleterious effects seen are likely secondary to activation of the RAAS by HCTZ.[74] The adverse metabolic effects of the β-blockers seem to be related to the type of agent used, rather than to a class effect,[75] and new vasodilatory agents as carvedilol and nebivolol are expected to have a better metabolic profile.

The recently published Avoiding Cardiovascular Events through Combination Therapy in Patients Living with Systolic Hypertension trial[76] randomized 11,506 hypertensive patients at high risk for CVD events to receive the combination of benazepril-amlodipine or benazepril-hydrochlorothiazide, and reported a similar reduction in blood pressure between the two groups. However, there was a significant difference concerning the occurrence of cardiovascular events that favor the amlodipine-treated group.[76] The relation between CVD and insulin metabolic effects of these drugs remains to be reported. Nevertheless, it would appear reasonable to suggest an RAAS-blocker agent as first line of therapy for patients with the CMS.

SUMMARY

The relationship between HTN and other components of the CMS is complex. However, there is growing evidence that enhanced activation of the RAAS is a key factor in the development of endothelial dysfunction and HTN. Insulin resistance is induced by activation of the RAAS and resulting increases in ROS. This insulin resistance occurs in cardiovascular tissue and in tissues traditionally considered as targets for the action of insulin, such as muscle and liver. Indeed, there is a mounting body of evidence that the resultant insulin resistance in cardiovascular tissue and kidneys contributes to the development of endothelial dysfunction, HTN, atherosclerosis, CKD, and CVD.[77]

RAAS-associated signaling by way of the AT_1R and MR, triggers tissue activation of the NADPH oxidase enzymatic activation and increased production of ROS. Oxidative stress in cardiovascular tissue is derived from both NADPH oxidase and mitochondrial generation of ROS, and is central to the development of insulin resistance, endothelial dysfunction, HTN, and atherosclerosis.

Pharmacologic blockade of the RAAS not only improves blood pressure, but also has a beneficial impact on inflammation, oxidative stress, insulin sensitivity, and glucose homeostasis. Several strategies are available for RAAS blockade, including ACE inhibitors, ARBs, and MR blockers, which have been proven in the clinical trials to result in improved CVD and CKD outcomes. New research in these areas will allow for a better understanding of the relationship between HTN, insulin resistance, and activation of the RAAS, which could result in newer alternatives for a more comprehensive management of HTN in the setting of the CMS.

REFERENCES

1. Cutler JA, Sorlie PD, Wolz M, et al. Trends in hypertension prevalence, awareness, treatment, and control rates in United States adults between 1988–1994 and 1999–2004. Hypertension 2008;52:818–27.

2. Ford ES. Prevalence of the metabolic syndrome defined by the International Diabetes Federation among adults in the US. Diabetes Care 2005;28:2745–9.
3. Ferrannini E, Buzzigoli G, Bonadonna R, et al. Insulin resistance in essential hypertension. N Engl J Med 1987;317:350–7.
4. Bonora E, Capaldo B, Perin PC, et al. Hyperinsulinemia and insulin resistance are independently associated with plasma lipids, uric acid and blood pressure in non-diabetic subjects. The GISIR database. Nutr Metab Cardiovasc Dis 2008;18:624–31.
5. Manrique C, Lastra G, Whaley-Connell A, et al. Hypertension and the cardiometabolic syndrome. J Clin Hypertens (Greenwich) 2005;7:471–6.
6. Song J, Hu X, Riazi S, et al. Regulation of blood pressure, the epithelial sodium channel (ENaC), and other key renal sodium transporters by chronic insulin infusion in rats. Am J Physiol Renal Physiol 2006;290:F1055–64.
7. DeFronzo RA, Cooke CR, Andres R, et al. The effect of insulin on renal handling of sodium, potassium, calcium, and phosphate in man. J Clin Invest 1975;55:845–55.
8. Tiwari S, Sharma N, Gill PS, et al. Impaired sodium excretion and increased blood pressure in mice with targeted deletion of renal epithelial insulin receptor. Proc Natl Acad Sci U S A 2008;105:6469–74.
9. Grassi G, Dell'Oro R, Quarti-Trevano F, et al. Neuroadrenergic and reflex abnormalities in patients with metabolic syndrome. Diabetologia 2005;48:1359–65.
10. Anderson EA, Hoffman RP, Balon TW, et al. Hyperinsulinemia produces both sympathetic neural activation and vasodilation in normal humans. J Clin Invest 1991;87:2246–52.
11. Landsberg L. Insulin-mediated sympathetic stimulation: role in the pathogenesis of obesity-related hypertension (or, how insulin affects blood pressure, and why). J Hypertens 2001;19:523–8.
12. Haynes WG, Morgan DA, Walsh SA, et al. Receptor-mediated regional sympathetic nerve activation by leptin. J Clin Invest 1997;100:270–8.
13. Ozata M, Ozdemir IC, Licinio J. Human leptin deficiency caused by a missense mutation: multiple endocrine defects, decreased sympathetic tone, and immune system dysfunction indicate new targets for leptin action, greater central than peripheral resistance to the effects of leptin, and spontaneous correction of leptin-mediated defects. J Clin Endocrinol Metab 1999;84:3686–95.
14. Morgan DA, Thedens DR, Weiss R, et al. Mechanisms mediating renal sympathetic activation to leptin in obesity. Am J Physiol Regul Integr Comp Physiol 2008;295:R1730–6.
15. Cooper SA, Whaley-Connell A, Habibi J, et al. Renin-angiotensin-aldosterone system and oxidative stress in cardiovascular insulin resistance. Am J Physiol Heart Circ Physiol 2007;293:H2009–23.
16. Grassi G. Renin-angiotensin-sympathetic crosstalks in hypertension: reappraising the relevance of peripheral interactions. J Hypertens 2001;19:1713–6.
17. Raasch W, Betge S, Dendorfer A, et al. Angiotensin converting enzyme inhibition improves cardiac neuronal uptake of noradrenaline in spontaneously hypertensive rats. J Hypertens 2001;19:1827–33.
18. Engeli S, Negrel R, Sharma AM. Physiology and pathophysiology of the adipose tissue renin-angiotensin system. Hypertension 2000;35:1270–7.
19. Massiera F, Bloch-Faure M, Ceiler D, et al. Adipose angiotensinogen is involved in adipose tissue growth and blood pressure regulation. FASEB J 2001;15:2727–9.
20. Boustany CM, Bharadwaj K, Daugherty A, et al. Activation of the systemic and adipose renin-angiotensin system in rats with diet-induced obesity and hypertension. Am J Physiol Regul Integr Comp Physiol 2004;287:R943–9.

21. Mehta PK, Griendling KK. Angiotensin II cell signaling: physiological and pathological effects in the cardiovascular system. Am J Physiol, Cell Physiol 2007;292: C82–97.

22. Rossi GP, Belfiore A, Bernini G, et al. Body mass index predicts plasma aldosterone concentrations in overweight-obese primary hypertensive patients. J Clin Endocrinol Metab 2008;93:2566–71.

23. Ehrhart-Bornstein M, Lamounier-Zepter V, Schraven A, et al. Human adipocytes secrete mineralocorticoid-releasing factors. Proc Natl Acad Sci U S A 2003; 100:14211–6.

24. Taniyama Y, Griendling KK. Reactive oxygen species in the vasculature: molecular and cellular mechanisms. Hypertension 2003;42:1075–81.

25. Mervaala EMA, Cheng ZJ, Tikkanen I, et al. Endothelial dysfunction and xanthine oxidoreductase activity in rats with human renin and angiotensinogen genes. Hypertension 2001;37:414–8.

26. Laakso J, Mervaala E, Himberg JJ, et al. Increased kidney xanthine oxidoreductase activity in salt-induced experimental hypertension. Hypertension 1998;32:902–6.

27. Siu YP, Leung KT, Tong MK, et al. Use of allopurinol in slowing the progression of renal disease through its ability to lower serum uric acid level. Am J Kidney Dis 2006;47:51–9.

28. Madamanchi NR, Vendrov A, Runge MS. Oxidative stress and vascular disease. Arterioscler Thromb Vasc Biol 2005;25:29–38.

29. Kim J, Wei Y, Sowers JR. Role of mitochondrial dysfunction in insulin resistance. Circ Res 2008;102:401–14.

30. Ballinger SW, Patterson C, Knight-Lozano CA, et al. Mitochondrial integrity and function in atherogenesis. Circulation 2002;106:544–9.

31. Javesghani D, Magder SA, Barreiro E, et al. Molecular characterization of a superoxide-generating NAD(P)H oxidase in the ventilatory muscles. Am J Respir Crit Care Med 2002;165:412–8.

32. Lastra G, Whaley-Connell A, Manrique C, et al. Low-dose spironolactone reduces reactive oxygen species generation and improves insulin-stimulated glucose transport in skeletal muscle in the TG(mRen2)27 rat. Am J Physiol Endocrinol Metab 2008;295:E110–6.

33. Sigal N, Gorzalczany Y, Sarfstein R, et al. The guanine nucleotide exchange factor trio activates the phagocyte NADPH oxidase in the absence of GDP to GTP exchange on Rac. "The emperor's new clothes." J Biol Chem 2003;278: 4854–61.

34. Abo A, Pick E, Hall A, et al. Activation of the NADPH oxidase involves the small GTP-binding protein p21rac1. Nature 1991;353:668–70.

35. Griendling KK, Minieri CA, Ollerenshaw JD, et al. Angiotensin II stimulates NADH and NADPH oxidase activity in cultured vascular smooth muscle cells. Circ Res 1994;74:1141–8.

36. Laursen JB, Rajagopalan S, Galis Z, et al. Role of superoxide in angiotensin II-induced but not catecholamine-induced hypertension. Circulation 1997;95:588–93.

37. Touyz RM. Reactive oxygen species, vascular oxidative stress, and redox signaling in hypertension: what is the clinical significance? Hypertension 2004; 44:248–52.

38. Redon J, Oliva MR, Tormos C, et al. Antioxidant activities and oxidative stress byproducts in human hypertension. Hypertension 2003;41:1096–101.

39. Fortuno A, Olivan S, Beloqui O, et al. Association of increased phagocytic NADPH oxidase-dependent superoxide production with diminished nitric oxide generation in essential hypertension. J Hypertens 2004;22:2169–75.

40. Wassmann S, Laufs U, Baumer AT, et al. HMG-CoA reductase inhibitors improve endothelial dysfunction in normocholesterolemic hypertension via reduced production of reactive oxygen species. Hypertension 2001;37:1450–7.

41. Rey FE, Cifuentes ME, Kiarash A, et al. Novel competitive inhibitor of NAD(P)H oxidase assembly attenuates vascular O2- and systolic blood pressure in mice. Circ Res 2001;89:408–14.

42. Landmesser U, Cai H, Dikalov S, et al. Role of p47phox in vascular oxidative stress and hypertension caused by angiotensin II. Hypertension 2002;40:511–5.

43. Gregg D, Rauscher FM, Goldschmidt-Clermont PJ. Rac regulates cardiovascular superoxide through diverse molecular interactions: more than a binary GTP switch. Am J Physiol, Cell Physiol 2003;285:C723–34.

44. Johar S, Cave AC, Narayanapanicker A, et al. Aldosterone mediates angiotensin II-induced interstitial cardiac fibrosis via a Nox2-containing NADPH oxidase. FASEB J 2006;20:1546–8.

45. Beswick RA, Zhang H, Marable D, et al. Long-term antioxidant administration attenuates mineralocorticoid hypertension and renal inflammatory response. Hypertension 2001;37:781–6.

46. Muniyappa R, Quon MJ. Insulin action and insulin resistance in vascular endothelium. Curr Opin Clin Nutr Metab Care 2007;10:523–30.

47. Potenza MA, Marasciulo FL, Chieppa DM, et al. Insulin resistance in spontaneously hypertensive rats is associated with endothelial dysfunction characterized by imbalance between NO and ET-1 production. Am J Physiol Heart Circ Physiol 2005;289:H813–22.

48. Sarafidis PA, Bakris GL. Insulin and endothelin: an interplay contributing to hypertension development? J Clin Endocrinol Metab 2007;92:379–85.

49. Lteif AA, Fulford AD, Considine RV, et al. Hyperinsulinemia fails to augment ET-1 action in the skeletal muscle vascular bed in vivo in humans. Am J Physiol Endocrinol Metab 2008;295:E1510–7.

50. Ceriello A, Motz E. Is oxidative stress the pathogenic mechanism underlying insulin resistance, diabetes, and cardiovascular disease? The common soil hypothesis revisited. Arterioscler Thromb Vasc Biol 2004;24:816–23.

51. Rudich A, Kozlovsky N, Potashnik R, et al. Oxidant stress reduces insulin responsiveness in 3T3-L1 adipocytes. Am J Phys 1997;272:E935–40.

52. Maddux BA, See W, Lawrence JC Jr, et al. Protection against oxidative stress–induced insulin resistance in rat L6 muscle cells by micromolar concentrations of α-lipoic acid. Diabetes 2001;50:404–10.

53. Talior I, Yarkoni M, Bashan N, et al. Increased glucose uptake promotes oxidative stress and PKC-δ activation in adipocytes of obese, insulin-resistant mice. Am J Physiol Endocrinol Metab 2003;285:E295–302.

54. Urakawa H, Katsuki A, Sumida Y, et al. Oxidative stress is associated with adiposity and insulin resistance in men. J Clin Endocrinol Metab 2003;88: 4673–6.

55. Bruce CR, Carey AL, Hawley JA, et al. Intramuscular heat shock protein 72 and heme oxygenase-1 mRNA are reduced in patients with type 2 diabetes: evidence that insulin resistance is associated with a disturbed antioxidant defense mechanism. Diabetes 2003;52:2338–45.

56. Kyriakis JM, Avruch J. Sounding the alarm: protein kinase cascades activated by stress and inflammation. J Biol Chem 1996;271:24313–6.

57. Yuan M, Konstantopoulos N, Lee J, et al. Reversal of obesity- and diet-induced insulin resistance with salicylates or targeted disruption of IKK beta. Science 2001;293:1673–7.

58. Hundal RS, Petersen KF, Mayerson AB, et al. Mechanism by which high-dose aspirin improves glucose metabolism in type 2 diabetes. J Clin Invest 2002; 109:1321–6.
59. Gillespie EL, White CM, Kardas M, et al. The impact of ACE inhibitors or angiotensin II type 1 receptor blockers on the development of new-onset type 2 diabetes. Diabetes Care 2005;28:2261–6.
60. Scheen AJ. Renin-angiotensin system inhibition prevents type 2 diabetes mellitus. Part 1. A meta-analysis of randomised clinical trials. Diabete Metab 2004; 30:487–96.
61. Yusuf S, Gerstein H, Hoogwerf B, et al. Ramipril and the development of diabetes. JAMA 2001;286:1882–5.
62. Hansson L, Lindholm LH, Niskanen L, et al. Effect of angiotensin-converting-enzyme inhibition compared with conventional therapy on cardiovascular morbidity and mortality in hypertension: the Captopril Prevention Project (CAPP) randomised trial. Lancet 1999;353:611–6.
63. Pfeffer MA, Swedberg K, Granger CB, et al. Effects of candesartan on mortality and morbidity in patients with chronic heart failure: the CHARM-Overall programme. Lancet 2003;362:759–66.
64. The ALLHAT Officers and Coordinators for the ALLHAT Collaborative Research Group. Major cardiovascular events in hypertensive patients randomized to doxazosin vs chlorthalidone: The Antihypertensive and Lipid-Lowering Treatment to Prevent Heart Attack Trial (ALLHAT). JAMA 2000;283:1967–75.
65. Effect of enalapril on mortality and the development of heart failure in asymptomatic patients with reduced left ventricular ejection fractions. The SOLVD investigators. N Engl J Med 1992;327:685–91.
66. Dahlof B, Devereux RB, Kjeldsen SE, et al. Cardiovascular morbidity and mortality in the Losartan Intervention For Endpoint reduction in hypertension study (LIFE): a randomised trial against atenolol. Lancet 2002;359:995–1003.
67. The Dream Trial Investigators. Effect of ramipril on the incidence of diabetes. N Engl J Med 2006;355:1551–62.
68. Pitt B, Zannad F, Remme WJ, et al. The effect of spironolactone on morbidity and mortality in patients with severe heart failure. N Engl J Med 1999;341:709–17.
69. Pitt B, Remme W, Zannad F, et al. Eplerenone, a selective aldosterone blocker, in patients with left ventricular dysfunction after myocardial infarction. N Engl J Med 2003;348:1309–21.
70. Pollare T, Lithell H, Berne C. A comparison of the effects of hydrochlorothiazide and captopril on glucose and lipid metabolism in patients with hypertension. N Engl J Med 1989;321:868–73.
71. Bakris GL, Sowers JR. ASH position paper: treatment of hypertension in patients with diabetes—an update. J Clin Hypertens (Greenwich) 2008;10:707–13.
72. Elliott WJ, Meyer PM. Incident diabetes in clinical trials of antihypertensive drugs: a network meta-analysis. Lancet 2007;369:201–7.
73. Zillich AJ, Garg J, Basu S, et al. Thiazide diuretics, potassium, and the development of diabetes: a quantitative review. Hypertension 2006;48:219–24.
74. Eriksson JW, Jansson PA, Carlberg B, et al. Hydrochlorothiazide, but not candesartan, aggravates insulin resistance and causes visceral and hepatic fat accumulation: the Mechanisms for the Diabetes Preventing Effect of Candesartan (MEDICA) Study. Hypertension 2008;52:1030–7.
75. Bakris GL, Fonseca V, Katholi RE, et al. Metabolic effects of carvedilol vs metoprolol in patients with type 2 diabetes mellitus and hypertension: a randomized controlled trial. JAMA 2004;292:2227–36.

76. Jamerson K, Weber MA, Bakris GL, et al. Benazepril plus amlodipine or hydrochlorothiazide for hypertension in high-risk patients. N Engl J Med 2008;359: 2417–28.
77. Zhang S-L, Chen X, Hsieh TJ, et al. Hyperglycemia induces insulin resistance on angiotensinogen gene expression in diabetic rat kidney proximal tubular cells. J Endocrinol 2002;172:333–44.

Arterial Aging and Subclinical Arterial Disease are Fundamentally Intertwined at Macroscopic and Molecular Levels

Edward G. Lakatta, MD*, Mingyi Wang, MD, PhD, Samer S. Najjar, MD

KEYWORDS

- Arterial aging • Angiotensin II • Intimal-medial thickening
- Arteriosclerosis • Hypertension

The structure and function of arteries change throughout the lifetime of humans and animals. Epidemiologic studies have found unequivocally that age is the dominant risk factor for hypertension, coronary heart disease, congestive heart failure, and stroke. Specifically, the greatest risk is posed by the most advanced age-associated changes in the arteries, which reflect unsuccessful aging.[1] It is reasonable to hypothesize that specific mechanisms that underlie the arterial substrates that have been altered during aging are intimately linked to the aforementioned cardiovascular diseases. The age-associated arterial changes include lumenal dilation, diffuse intimal and medial thickening, increased stiffness, reduced compliance of central arteries, endothelial dysfunction, impaired nitric oxide (NO) availability, increased reactive oxygen species (ROS), inflammation, and angiogenesis. These age-associated alterations impair arterial regulatory mechanisms and the ability of arteries to adapt, repair, and remodel through the integration of multiple signaling mechanisms.

A megacept emerges with the realization that evolution of these age-associated profiles within the arterial wall is strikingly similar to that which develops in arteries

This research was supported by the Intramural Research Program of the National Institute on Aging, National Institutes of Health.

Laboratory of Cardiovascular Science, Intramural Research Program, National Institute on Aging, National Institutes of Health, 5600 Nathan Shock Drive, Baltimore, MD 21224, USA

* Corresponding author.

E-mail address: lakattae@grc.nia.nih.gov (E.G. Lakatta).

Med Clin N Am 93 (2009) 583–604

doi:10.1016/j.mcna.2009.02.008

0025-7125/09/$ – see front matter. Published by Elsevier Inc.

medical.theclinics.com

of younger animals in response to experimental induction of early atherosclerosis or hypertension. Thus, "aging"-associated arterial changes and those associated with the aforementioned "diseases" are fundamentally intertwined at the cellular and molecular levels. In humans, other well-known risk factors (eg, altered lipid metabolism, smoking, and lack of exercise) interact with this arterial substrate that has been altered during aging and that renders the aging artery a fertile soil facilitating the initiation and progression of arterial diseases. The cellular/molecular proinflammatory alterations that underlie arterial aging thus become novel putative candidates to be targeted by interventions aimed at attenuating arterial aging as a major risk factor for cardiovascular diseases. This approach is similar to those aimed at lifestyle and pharmacologic interventions that already have proved effective in preventing or ameliorating arterial diseases associated with aging.

This review provides a landscape of central arterial aging and age-disease interactions by attempting to integrate perspectives that range from humans to molecules, with the goal that future therapies for cardiovascular diseases, such as hypertension, also will target the prevention or amelioration of unsuccessful arterial aging.

AGE-ASSOCIATED CHANGES IN CENTRAL ARTERIAL STRUCTURE AND FUNCTION
Aortic Macroscopic Structure

The structure and function of the central arteries change throughout the lifetime of humans.[2–8] Cross-sectional studies show that central elastic arteries dilate with age, leading to an increase in lumen size (**Fig. 1**A). The thickness of the arterial wall also increases with advancing age (**Fig. 1**B). Postmortem studies indicate that in humans, this increase mainly is the result of intimal thickening.[6] Studies of experimental animal models have increased understanding of age-associated alterations in arterial structure in humans. Age-associated restructuring of the central arteries of rats, rabbits, and nonhuman primates includes diffuse intimal thickening in the absence of clinical arterial diseases and is similar to that observed in grossly normal arterial segments in humans (**Table 1**).[1,3–8]

Aortic Microscopic Structure

Viewed microscopically, age predominantly alters the intima, which is located between the lumen-endothelial interface and the internal elastic lamina of the artery. A series of studies show that age dramatically alters the volume and contents of this zone in rats, nonhuman primates, and humans.[9–16] Small disoriented vascular smooth muscle cells (VSMC) and collagen types I and III all increase markedly within the thickened intima of old FXBN rats. Because nonhuman primate cardiovascular structure and function is similar to those of humans, primates are an ideal model in which to study arterial aging.[9] Old monkeys (approximately 20 years) have a thickened intima containing cells and matrix beneath an intact endothelium, and nearly all of these cells stain positively for α-smooth muscle actin (α-SMA), a marker of VSMC (**Fig. 2**A).[10,11] Aging also increases intimal cells in humans (**Fig. 2**B), which stain positively with an antibodies to α-SMA (see **Fig. 2**B) and to SMemb, a marker for the fetal-type VSMC.[12] SMemb is a non–muscle-type myosin heavy chain that is expressed predominantly in undifferentiated VSMC in the fetal stage and is remarkably reduced in adults[17] but reemerges in response to arterial injury.[17]

In nonhuman primates and rats, inflammatory cells have not been detected in the thickened intima.[9–11,13–16] In grossly normal specimens from humans over age 65, aortic intimal cell infiltration and matrix deposition are increased dramatically compared with specimens from younger individuals (approximately 20 years) (see

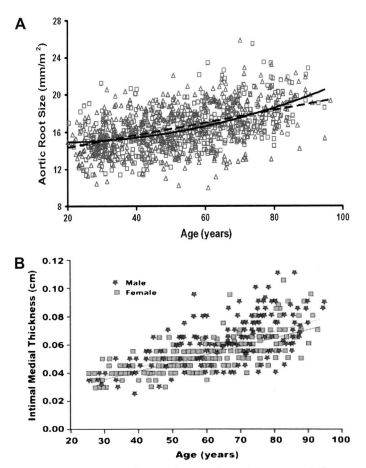

Fig. 1. Age-associated macroscopic changes in central arterial structure in humans. Central arterial lumen (*A*) and intimal-medial wall thickness (*B*) increase with advancing age in men (red) and women (blue). Best-fitting age regression curves are shown for men (*solid lines*) and women (*dashed lines*).

Fig. 2B).[12] The vast majority of cells within the intima stain positively for α-SMA.[12] Unlike aged rats and monkeys, sporadic clusters of macrophages (CD-68 stained cells) are more numerous (see **Fig. 2**B) and mast cells also are detected occasionally in the older intima of the human aortic walls (**Fig. 2**C), even in the absence of lipid deposition.[12] These mast cells within the older human aorta exhibit signs of activation and release a large number of enzymatic granules, including chymase.[11,18] These findings suggest that intimal thickening and VSMC cellularity are characteristic of arterial aging in various species.

The age-associated increase of intimal VSMC cellularity is assumed to be the result of the migration/invasion of VSMC from the tunica media to the intima where they proliferate.[1,3–6] This resembles experimental mechanical arterial injury.[17,19] Early passage (discussed later) medial VSMC of old rats do exhibit an exaggerated chemotactic response to platelet-derived growth factor-BB (PDGF-BB), whereas medial VSMC from young aorta require several additional passages in culture to generate

Table 1
Arterial remodeling: impact of dietary sodium, aging, hypertension, and artherosclerosis and angiotensin II signaling

	Aging				Hypertension	Artherosclerosis	Angiotensin II signaling
	Humans (>65 y)	Monkeys (15–20 y)	Rats (24–30 mo)	Rabbits (3–6 y)			
	+	+	+	+	?	?	?
↑ Stiffness	+	+	+	+	+	+	+
Endothelial dysfunction	+	+	+	+	+	+	+
Diffuse intimal thickening	+	+	+	+	+	+	+
Lipid involvement	—	—	—	—	±	+	+
↑ VSMC number	+	+	+	+	+	+	+
Macrophages	+	—	—	+	+	+	+
↑ Matrix	+	+	+	+	+	+	+
↑ Local ACE-ANGII-AT1	+	+	+	+	+	+	+
MMP/calpain dysregulation	+	+	+	?	+	+	+
↑ MCP-1/CCR2	+	+	+	+	+	+	+
↑ ICAM-1	?	?	+	?	+	+	+
↑ TGF-β	+	+	+	?	+	+	+
↑ NAD(P)H oxidase	?	?	+	?	+	+	+
↓ NO bioavailability	?	?	+	+	+	+	+
HYPERTENSION	±	±	±	?	+	±	+
ARTHEROSCLEROSIS	±	—	—	—	±	+	+

?, information unknown.

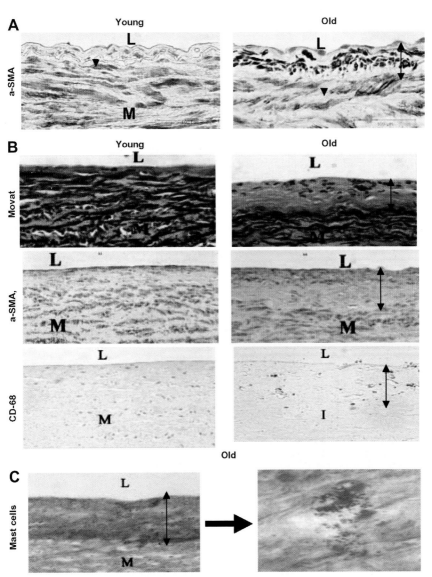

Fig. 2. Age-associated aortic structural remodeling. (*A*) Arterial immunostaining for α-SMA (brown) from monkeys. Arrowhead indicates internal elastin lamina. (*B*) Movat staining (*upper panels*) and immunohistochemical staining (brown color) for α-SMA (*middle panels*) and for CD68 (brown color) (*lower panels*) in aorta from humans. (*C*) Toludine blue staining for mast cells in old human aorta (*left panel*) and observed under an oil lens (*right panel*). I, intima; L, lumen; M, media. Up-down arrows indicate thickened intima. (*From* Wang M, Takagi G, Asai K, et al. Aging increases aortic MMP-2 activity and angiotensin II in nonhuman primates. Hypertension 2003;41(6):1308–16 and Wang M, Zhang J, Jiang LQ, et al. Proinflammatory profile within the grossly normal aged human aortic wall. Hypertension 2007;50(1):219–7; with permission.)

an equivalent response (**Fig. 3**A).[19] Furthermore, as early as 3 days in culture, VSMC from old rats display a faster growth rate than VSMC from young rats (**Fig. 3**B).[20] Old VSMC have a greater percentage of their population in the S phase of the cell cycle and a reduced number in G2/M or G0G1 compared with young VSMC.[21] Thus, early passage cultured VSMC of old aorta do not exhibit the in vitro cell senescence pattern of some other cell types in which proliferative capacity wanes.

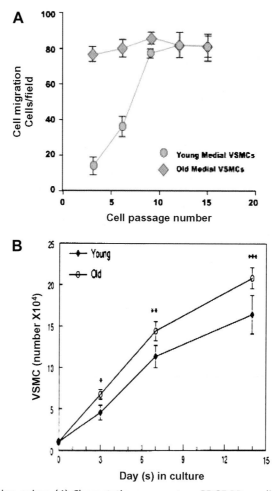

Fig. 3. VSMC during aging. (*A*) Chemotatic response to a PDGF-BB gradient is increased in early passage VSMC from the aortic media of old rats compared with those from younger rats. VSMC within the older aorta are primed to respond to the growth factor. (*From* Pauly RR, Passaniti A, Crow M, et al. Experimental models that mimic the differentiation and dedifferentiation of vascular cells. Circulation 1992;86(Suppl):III68–73; with permission.) (*B*) Growth curves of VSMC cultured from young and old rat aortae. The number of VSMC obtained from old rats was significantly higher at days 3, 7, and 14. (*From* Li Z, Cheng H, Lederer WJ, et al. Enhanced proliferation and migration and altered cytoskeletal proteins in early passage smooth muscle cells from young and old rat aortic explants. Exp Mol Pathol 1997;64(1):1–11; with permission.)

Human Endothelial Function In Vivo

Endothelial cells (EC) play a pivotal role in regulating several arterial properties, including vascular tone, permeability, and the response to inflammation. Several features of these endothelial properties undergo age-associated alterations in function via endothelial-derived substances (eg, NO) and ROS. In brachial or coronary arteries, endothelial function, as assessed by agonist- or flow-mediated vasoreactivity, has been shown to decline with advancing age[22] in the absence of clinical disease (**Fig. 4A**).

Molecular and Cellular Studies of Endothelial Function

Studies of endothelia in experimental animal models have increased understanding of age-associated arterial endothelial dysfunction in humans. Many molecular and cellular alterations in arterial EC structure and function that occur with aging likely are implicated in age-associated endothelial dysfunction.[23] Morphologically, aortic EC from older donors are flattened and enlarged, and the number of EC with polyploid nuclei increases with advancing age.[10,24] Age alters the amount, arrangement, and structural integrity of the EC cytoskeleton, which affects the mobility, migration, proliferation, and secretory proteomic profile of EC.[10,23–25] In addition, simple end-to-end inter-EC connections increase, but stronger more complex overlapping or interdigitating connections decrease with advancing age, suggesting an age-associated deficiency in intercellular communication and in endothelial barrier function.[26] Advancing age also is associated with decreased EC capacity for replication and repair, which has been linked to increased apoptosis,[10] telomere shortening,[27,28] proinflammatory state,[23] reduced NO bioavailability,[29] and decreased number[30] and the function[31] of endothelial progenitor cells.

As in humans, mechanical vasodilation and agonist-induced NO-dependent endothelial vasodilation are attenuated in older versus younger rats and monkeys.[10,32] The impairment of endothelial-mediated vasodilatation with aging in humans can, in part, be reversed by L-arginine administration, suggesting that NO production becomes reduced with aging.[33] Plasma levels of asymmetric dimethylarginine, which reduces NO synthase (NOS) activity, also increase with age in humans. In rats, arterial arginase activity increases with age and may deplete local substrates for NOS.[32]

Some animal studies show that the marked age-associated reduction in arterial NO bioavailability occurs in the context of an increase in endothelial NOS expression, whereas other studies have noted that the expression of endothelial NOS isoform is markedly reduced with aging.[29–34] ROS are important modulators of NO bioavailability. Nicotinamide adenine dinucleotide phosphate (NAD[P]H) oxidase is a major source of ROS in vascular cells and within the rat arterial wall, where NADH-driven O_2^- generation increases with aging.[29,34] NAD(P)H oxidase is composed of six subunits: Rho guanosine triphosphatase (GTPase), usually Rac1 or Rac2, and five phagocyte oxidase (phox) units of p90, p22, p40, p47, and p67. Among NAD(P)H subunits, p22 phox is higher in the aortic endothelium of old compared with young rats.[35] In addition, arterial wall activities of the ROS scavengers, Cu/Zn superoxide dismutase (SOD), Mg SOD, and extracellular matrix SOD, do not change or decrease with increasing age in rats.[29] Thus, an imbalance between oxidase and dismutase results in increased in situ levels of superoxide and hydrogen peroxide and a decrease in NO bioavailability in the coronary and aortic walls of rats with aging.

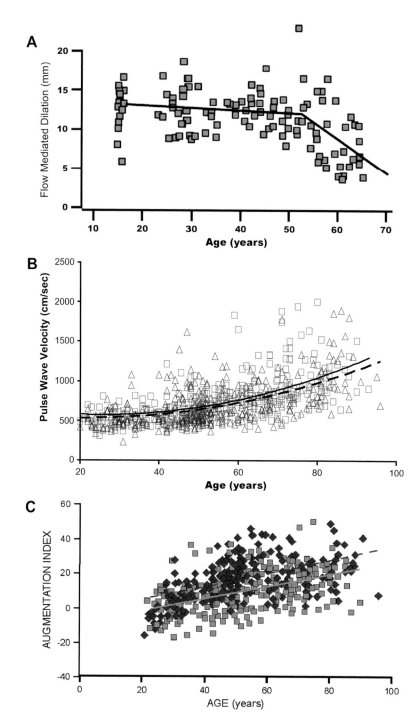

Fig. 4. Age-associated changes in arterial function in humans. (*A*) Flow-mediated induced dilation in the brachial artery of apparently healthy women. (*Adapted from* Celermajer DS, Sorensen KE, Spiegelhalter DJ, et al. Aging is associated with endothelial dysfunction in healthy men years before the age-related decline in women. J Am Coll Cardiol 1994;24(2):471–6; with permission.) Age-associated increase in carotid-femoral PWV (*B*), an index of central arterial stiffness, and in augmentation index (*C*) in healthy men (red) and women (blue). Best-fitting age regression curves are shown for men (*solid lines*) and women (*dashed lines*).

Noninvasive Evaluation of Arterial Mechanical Properties in Humans

Arterial stiffness and compliance

The increase in arterial wall thickening and reduction in endothelial function with advancing age are accompanied by an increase in arterial stiffening (**Fig. 4**B).[36] Arterial stiffness depends on intrinsic stress/strain relationships that are determined by structural properties of the blood vessel wall and by smooth muscle tone. Among the various indexes of arterial stiffness, carotid-femoral pulse wave velocity (PWV) has emerged as the gold standard for noninvasive assessment of central arterial stiffness.[37] PWV is assessed as the distance between the carotid and femoral sampling sites divided by the time delay for the onset of the pressure wave between these two sites.

In contrast to central arteries, the stiffness of muscular arteries does not increase with advancing age.[38] Thus, the manifestations of arterial aging may vary among the different vascular beds, reflecting differences in the structural compositions of the arteries and, perhaps, differences in the age-associated signaling cascades that modulate the arterial properties (discussed later) or differences in the response to these signals across the arterial tree. Organs with high flow and low resistance, however, such as the heart, kidney, and brain, are particularly vulnerable to the increased pulsatility that is associated with central arterial stiffening, because this pulsatility can be transmitted to the microvasculature where it my cause damage.[39] For example, a longitudinal study showed that age-associated accelerated progression of arterial stiffness is an independent predictor of longitudinal decline in some aspects of cognitive function, such as verbal learning, nonverbal memory, and a measure of cognitive screening in nondemented individuals.[40]

Reflected pulse waves

PWV assesses the velocity of the forward pulse wave that is generated with each cardiac cycle. When this wave reaches an area of impedance mismatch, a reflected wave is generated, which travels back up the arterial tree toward the central aorta. This reflected wave alters the central arterial pressure waveform. The velocity of the reflected flow wave is proportional to the stiffness of the arterial wall. Thus, in young individuals whose vascular wall is compliant, the reflected wave does not reach the large elastic arteries until late systole. With advancing age and increasing arterial stiffening, the velocity of the reflected wave increases, and the wave reaches the central circulation earlier in the cardiac cycle during the early phase of systole (ascending limb of pressure waveform). This reflected wave can be assessed noninvasively from recordings of the carotid or radial arterial pulse waveforms by arterial applanation tonometry and high-fidelity micromanometer probes.[41] Inspection of the recorded arterial pulse wave contour often shows an inflection point, which heralds the arrival of the reflected wave (**Fig. 4**C). The height from the inflection point to the peak of the arterial waveform is the pressure pulse augmentation that is due to the early arrival of the reflected wave. Dividing this augmentation by the height from the peak to the trough of the arterial waveform (corresponding to the pulse pressure) yields the augmentation index. Unlike PWV, which increases quadratically with age in older individuals, the augmentation index increases with age (see **Fig. 4**C) but seems to plateau at older ages.[42]

The pressure pulse augmentation provided by the early return of the reflected wave is an added load against which the ventricle must contract. Furthermore, the loss of diastolic augmentation that is observed with the early return of the reflected wave leads is associated with a drop in diastolic blood pressure, which has the potential to compromise coronary blood flow, because the latter occurs almost exclusively during diastole.

Although the augmentation index traditionally has been considered an index of arterial stiffness, it is increasingly recognized that because reflected waves originate, in part, in small arteries, the age-associated changes in the augmentation index also probably are determined, in part, by age-associated changes in the structure and function of these small arteries. Evaluation of the diastolic decay of pulse wave contour may provide insights into the characteristics and the pathology of more distal vessels in which reflected waves originate.[43]

Arterial Stiffness Under the Microscope

Arterial mechanical properties are influenced by alterations in the arterial extracellular matrix.[6] The arrangement and interrelation of the macromolecular matrix and cellular components of the aorta determine the viscoelastic characteristics that account for many of the static and dynamic mechanical features of the aorta. At physiologic blood pressures, aortic medial elastin and collagen fibers and smooth muscle cells form well-defined layers: thick elastin bands form concentric plates or lamellae, between which elastin microfibers form networks; collagen fibers align circumferentially and are dispersed in the interstices of the elastic network; and VSMC extend circumferentially between adjacent elastin lamellae among the finer elastin and collagen fibers.

Elastin, which constitutes approximately 30% of the dry weight of the arteries, decreases with aging. An imbalance between the synthesis and degradation of the precursor tropoelastin leads to a reduction in the formation of mature elastin within the aged arterial wall.[44,45] The steady-state level of aortic tropoelastin mRNA decreases dramatically with increasing age.[45] Furthermore, because of the age-associated reduction in lysyl oxidase, tropoelastin in older animals is insufficiently cross-linked, thus has a diminished capacity to form a meshwork of mature elastin fibers.[46] In addition, with maturation and aging, the glycoprotein component of elastin fibrils decreases and eventually disappears; elastin (in rats) becomes fragile and its Ca^{2+} content increases.[47]

In addition to mature collagen fiber deposition (an increase in the distribution of immature collagen occurs with age), it has been proposed that age-associated changes involve a decrease in the coiling and twisting of molecular chains and a reduction in effective chain length.[48,49] With increasing age, free amino groups on collagen proteins become more vulnerable to nonenzymatic glycation, oxidation, and nitration to form advanced glycated end products via the Maillard reaction.[50] These can lead to covalent cross-linking of adjacent collagen molecules, which further increases their tensile strength.[50]

Thus, the alterations in mechanical properties of aged vessels are consistent with a relative loss or damage of elastin and an increase in collagen deposition and cross-linking.[51]

Angiotensin II Signaling Molecules within the Aortic Wall

In addition to the structural alterations (described previously), arterial function is governed by age-associated changes in several signaling cascades, most prominently the renin-angiotensin system (RAS). The classic RAS is composed of angiotensinogen, renin, angiotensin (Ang) I and II, angiotensin-converting enzyme (ACE), chymase, angiotensin, and Ang II receptor (AT1). All of these components have been found to increase within the aged arterial wall in various species.[9,11,12,16] The local Ang II concentration is more than 1000-fold that of circulating Ang II, is independently regulated, and plays an important role in vascular pathophysiology with aging.[9,16,52,53] Ang II protein abundance increases in the aged aortic wall in rats (**Fig. 5**A).[16] Studies of nonhuman primates also show that Ang II (**Fig. 5**B), ACE (**Fig. 5**C), and chymase

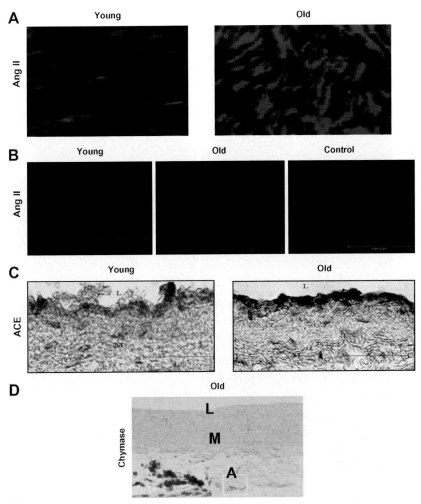

Fig. 5. Ang II and its converting enzymes increase in the aged aortic wall from rats and nonhuman primates. (*A*) Immunolabeled Ang II (red) in the en face medial aortic sections from young (*left panel*) and old rats (*right panels*). (*From* Jiang L, Wang M, Zhang J, et al. Increased aortic calpain-1 activity mediates age-associated angiotensin II signaling of vascular smooth muscle cells. PLoS ONE 2008;3:e2231.) (*B*) The immunofluorescent staining for Ang II (red color) on frozen sections of aortae from monkeys. (*C*) The immunostaining for ACE (red color) on frozen sections of aortae from monkeys. (*D*) The immunostaining for chymase in an old monkey aorta. Inset, rectangular region under high power. A, adventitia; L, lumen; M, media. (*From* Wang M, Takagi G, Asai K, et al. Aging increases aortic MMP-2 activity and angiotensin II in nonhuman primates. Hypertension 2003;41(6): 1308–16; with permission.)

(**Fig. 5**D) staining are increased in the thickened intima of older monkey aorta.[11] Studies also show that in humans, Ang II (**Fig. 6**A), AT1 (**Fig. 6**B), ACE (**Fig. 6**C), and chymase immunofluorescence increase within the grossly normal aortic wall of samples from older donors.[12] Further, double immunolabeling demonstrates that intimal Ang II is co-localized with ACE or chymase staining in older aorta.[12] These

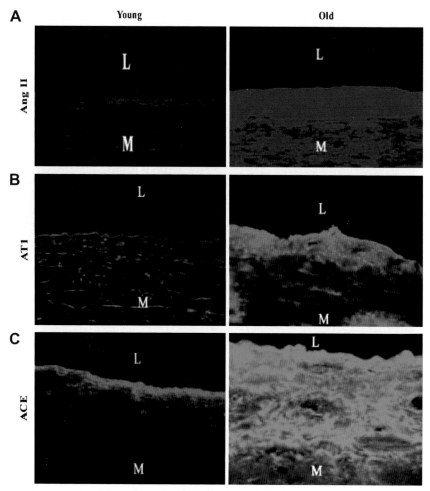

Fig. 6. Components of the RAS in the human aortic wall. Immunofluorescence staining for (*A*) Ang II (red color); (*B*) AT1 (green color) (*upper panels*); and (*C*) ACE (*green color*) (upper panel). L, lumen; M, media. (*From* Wang M, Zhang J, Jiang LQ, et al. Proinflammatory profile within the grossly normal aged human aortic wall. Hypertension 2007;50(1):219–7; with permission.)

findings demonstrate that elements of the classic RAS are all up-regulated in the aged arterial wall.

The molecules linked to the Ang II signaling cascade, including calpain-1, matrix metalloproteinase types 2 and 9 (MMP-2 and MMP-9), monocyte chemotactic protein-1 (MCP-1), and transforming growth factor-beta 1 (TGF-β1) are up-regulated within the aged arterial wall (**Fig. 7**) (see **Table 1**).[9,11–16]

Calpain-1

Calpain-1 is a ubiquitous cytosolic Ca^{2+} activated neutral protease. Arterial calpain-1 transcript levels and protein abundance are enhanced with aging, and increased calpain-1 protein within the old rat aorta is co-localized with VSMC.[16] Calpain -1 activity also increases within the aged aorta in rats.[16]

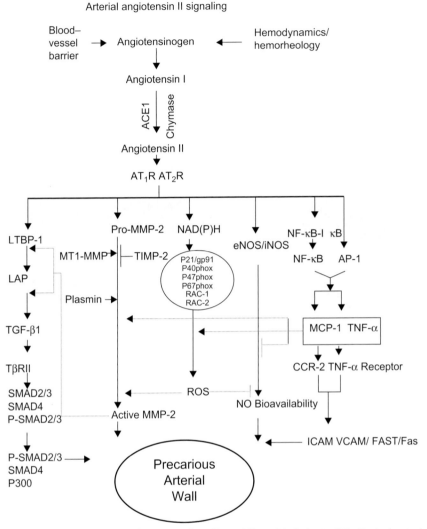

Fig. 7. Simplified Ang II signaling cascades. (*From* Wang M, Lakatta EG. Central arterial aging: humans to molecules. In: Safar M, editor. Handbook of hypertension: arterial stiffness in hypertension. Amsterdam: Elsevier; 2006. p. 137–60; with permission.)

Matrix metalloproteinase types 2 and 9

MMP-2 and MMP-9 are members of the zinc-containing endopeptidase family. They degrade native and denatured collagen and elastin, promote matrix protein degradation in vascular disease remodeling, and facilitate VSMC migration. Aortic MMP-2 activation in situ is progressively enhanced with aging, mainly localized to the intima, and co-localized with EC and VSMC in rats[9,14] and monkeys (**Fig. 8A**).[11] A recent study shows that in humans, MMP-2 and MMP-9 activity also is enhanced in situ in the grossly normal aortic segments with aging (**Fig. 8B**).[12]

Transforming growth factor-beta 1

TGF-β1 is a pluripotent growth factor implicated in various aspects of vascular development and structural remodeling in health and disease. TGF-β1 is a key regulator of

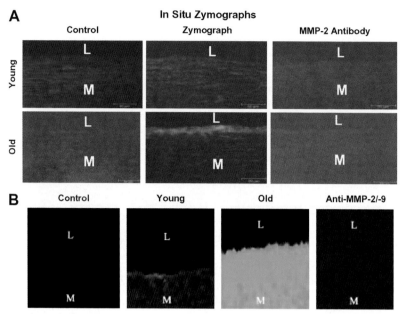

Fig. 8. In situ gelatin zymograms. (*A*) In situ gelatin zymographs of monkey aorta. Protease activity (green color) is localized mainly in the older aortic intima (*middle panel*). (*From* Wang M, Takagi G, Asai K, et al. Aging increases aortic MMP-2 activity and angiotensin II in nonhuman primates. Hypertension 2003;41(6):1308–16.) (*B*) In situ gelatin zymographs (green color) of humans. I, intimae; L, lumen; M, media. *P<.05, young versus old. (*From* Wang M, Zhang J, Jiang LQ, et al. Proinflammatory profile within the grossly normal aged human aortic wall. Hypertension 2007;50(1):219–7; with permission.)

collagen and fibronectin expression.[14] TGF-β1, transcription, translation, and activity are increased within the aorta of old rats, particularly within the thickened intima.[14]

Activated TGF-β1 exerts its biologic effects by binding to its receptor TGF-β type II receptor (TβRII) via SMAD signaling. Aortic TβRII transcription and translation also are increased with aging. TβRII is increased within the wall of the aged aorta. Furthermore, the SMAD proteins, the receptor-regulated phosphorylated p-SMAD2/3, and the common-mediator SMAD4, are increased within the aged aortic wall, whereas the antagonistic or inhibitory SMAD7 protein decreases by 20% with age within the arterial media.[14]

Monocyte chemotactic protein-1

MCP-1/CCL2 (chemokine [C-C motif] ligand 2), a well-known chemokine, plays multiple roles in proinflammatory responses through the activation of its receptor, CCR2. Aortic MCP-1 and CCR2 transcriptome and protein abundance increase in rats with aging, mainly within the intima.[15] As in rats, the increased MCP-1 within human old aorta resides predominantly within the intima, resulting in a markedly increased, age-associated intimal-medial gradient of the MCP-1, which potentially can induce migration of medial VSMC to intima.[12]

Up-Regulation of Angiotensin II Signaling Mimics Arterial Aging

In young FXBN rats, in vivo chronic infusion of Ang II at concentrations sufficient to elicit an increase in arterial pressure similar to that observed with age increases

MMP-2, calpain-1, and TGF-β1 activity and imparts to their central arteries structural and molecular characteristics of arteries of old, untreated rats.[9,16] Even a subpressor infusion of Ang II increases MMP-2 expression and activity and increases collagen production within the arterial wall.[9] Administration of phenylephrine, an adrenergic receptor agonist, to young rats increases arterial Ang II levels and reproduces Ang II effects on arteries.[9] These results demonstrate that Ang II signaling can cause structural, biochemical, and functional alterations of the arterial wall of young rats that resemble those that occur with aging and that the effects of phenylephrine signaling are mediated, in part at least, by Ang II.

In vitro Ang II treatment of VSMC from young rats induces MMP-2 and calpain-1 activity, reaching the levels of untreated VSMC from old rats.[9,11,16] These Ang II- and age-associated effects are reduced by losartan, an AT1 receptor blocker.[9,11,16] The increased MMP-2 activity driven by Ang II or aging also is abolished by Ci 1, a calpain inhibitor.[9,11,16]

Other in vitro studies show that the age-associated increase in VSMC invasion/migration could be modulated by concurrent alterations in Ang II signaling molecules.[9,11,15,16] Relative to young VSMC, those isolated from old aorta exhibit increased invasion of a synthetic basement membrane in response to a gradient of PDGF-BB or MCP-1, and this age difference is abolished or substantially reduced by losartan, an AT1 receptor blocker; vCCI, an inhibitor of CCR2 signaling; GM 6001, an inhibitor of MMP; and Ci 1.[9,11,15,16] Furthermore, exposure of young aortic medial VSMC to Ang II, MCP-1, or calpain-1, induces an increase in invasion ability in a dose-dependent manner, up to the level of untreated, old medial VSMC.[9,11,15,16] These effects are inhibited by losartan, vCCI, GM6001, and Ci 1.[9,11,15,16]

Thus, these results support the concept that Ang II signaling is a central pathway that mediates the cellular and molecular mechanisms that underlie arterial aging.

Arterial Blood Pressure

Arterial pressure is determined by the interplay of central arterial compliance, peripheral resistance, stroke volume, and the pattern of left ventricular (LV) ejection. A decline in central arterial compliance accompanies the age-associated increase in arterial wall stiffness, but neither peripheral resistance nor stroke volume changes appreciably with advancing age in normotensive individuals,[54] although this normotensive status is maintained in only approximately 30% of older persons. In the face of the age-associated increase in arterial wall stiffness and the early return of reflected waves, a higher systolic blood pressure is required to distend the hardened capacitance vessels and maintain stroke volume. Furthermore, diastolic blood pressure is decreased as a result of the reduced storage capacity of the stiffened central aorta. Thus, with advancing age, systolic blood pressure rises, whereas diastolic blood pressure increases until the fifth decade, after which it plateaus and subsequently decreases. As a result, pulse pressure increases with advancing age throughout life, whereas mean arterial pressure increases with age but seems to plateau at older ages.

Most of the literature on blood pressure has focused on brachial blood pressure, which is readily measurable noninvasively. Central arterial pressure (ie, the pressure that is sensed by the heart) may differ from peripheral blood pressure because of central to peripheral arterial blood pressure amplification. This amplification is attributed to central to peripheral alterations in the properties of the arterial tree.[55] This amplification is attenuated by the early return of reflected waves. Thus central to peripheral systolic pressure (and pulse pressure) amplification is inversely related to age. Emerging evidence suggests that central pressures may carry more robust prognostic information than peripheral pressures[56] and that monitoring of central pressure may provide more accurate reflection of the efficacy of antihypertensive medications and may help explain, in part, the differential impact on outcomes that has been observed with some medications in spite of apparently equivalent changes in peripheral blood pressure.[57]

EXAGGERATED ARTERIAL AGING AND DISEASE

The age-associated alterations in arterial structure, function, molecules, and local signaling cascades, such as endothelial dysfunction, arterial stiffening, and intimal-medial thickening, and Ang II signaling increasingly are recognized as potent risk factors for arterial diseases, even after accounting for traditional cardiovascular risk factors, such as arterial pressure, plasma lipids, and smoking. For example, increased intimal-medial thickness is associated with silent ischemia among asymptomatic older individuals[58] and is an independent predictor of stroke and future myocardial infarction.[59] Several clinical studies recently have shown the adverse cardiovascular effects of accelerated arterial stiffening.[37] In hypertensive patients, PWV is a marker of cardiovascular risk and coronary events and is an independent predictor of mortality. In addition, PWV is an independent predictor of mortality in population-based studies and in subjects over 70 years of age. The augmentation index also has been shown to be a predictor of adverse events in end-stage renal disease patients.[60] A discussion of the interventions to retard or reverse accelerated arterial aging is beyond the scope of this article. Suffice it to mention that these include lifestyle modifications (diet and exercise) and some traditional (eg, angiotensin antagonists) and promising (eg, the advanced glycation end-product cross-link breaker, Alagebrium) pharmacologic agents.[3]

Arterial Aging and Hypertension

Patients who have hypertension exhibit increased central arterial wall thickness, greater carotid wall thickness,[61] and central pressure augmentation[62] than do normotensive subjects, even after adjusting for age. They are believed to have larger central arterial diameters although this is debated.[53–65]

Systolic hypertension is the dominant form of hypertension in older individuals. As discussed previously, central arterial stiffness is one of the main determinants underlying the increase in systolic and pulse pressure. Longitudinal studies in humans have shown that arterial stiffness is an independent predictor of the rise in systolic blood pressure and of incident hypertension.[66] The intimate link and the continuum between measures of arterial aging and hypertension increasingly are being recognized. A recent position article by the American Society of Hypertension Writing Group (HWG)[67] proposed that the classification of hypertension be expanded by integrating additional preclinical and clinical cardiovascular manifestations that stress the structural and functional status of the vasculature and target organ damage. Thus, the HWG implicitly recognizes the role of accelerated arterial aging in the continuum of cardiovascular risk leading to hypertension. It is hoped that, in the future, a composite measure of arterial aging can be developed that would modulate, or at best even replace, chronologic age as a risk factor within this continuum.

Endothelial Dysfunction in Hypertension

Endothelial dysfunction occurs early in several cardiovascular disorders, including atherosclerosis, diabetes, and hypertension. Impaired endothelial vasoreactivity, in the coronary and peripheral arterial beds, is an independent predictor of future cardiovascular events.[68] Hypertensive individuals exhibit endothelial dysfunction,[69] and the mechanisms underlying their endothelial dysfunction are similar to the ones that occur with normotensive aging, although they appear at an earlier age.[70] The normotensive offsprings of hypertensive subjects also exhibit endothelial dysfunction,[71] suggesting that endothelial dysfunction may precede the development of clinical hypertension. Among hypertensive subjects, greater endothelial dysfunction is an independent predictor of adverse cardiovascular outcomes.[68]

Arterial Stiffening in Hypertension

As discussed previously, clinical and epidemiologic studies in several different populations with varying prevalence of cardiovascular diseases have confirmed the prognostic importance of arterial stiffness and of pulse pressure. Furthermore, in several studies, pulse pressure was a stronger predictor of outcomes than systolic or diastolic blood pressures. The implication of this is that the status of the arterial wall, which is a major determinant of pulse pressure, may be an important therapeutic target. In a study of patients who had end-stage renal disease who required dialysis,[72] treatment of hypertension had differing effects on PWV, despite having similar blood pressure–lowering effects in patients. Mortality was higher in the group in whom PWV increased in spite of therapy, and progression of vascular stiffening was an independent predictor of mortality. These observations suggest that treating increases in blood pressure is necessary but not sufficient therapy for the syndrome of hypertension. Whether or not arterial stiffness is a risk factor or a risk marker for cardiovascular diseases awaits intervention studies aimed at reducing arterial stiffness, to determine whether or not this improves outcomes independent of the effects on blood pressure.

Arterial-Ventricular Coupling

The interaction of the LV with the arterial system, termed arterial-ventricular coupling,[73] can be indexed by the ratio of effective arterial elastance (Ea), a measure of the net arterial load exerted on the LV, to LV end-systolic elastance (E_{LV}), a load-independent measure of LV chamber performance. Previous studies of healthy individuals have shown that, at rest, Ea/E_{LV} is tightly controlled within a narrow range across a broad age spectrum and even across species. This tight coupling allows the CV system to optimize energetic efficiency.

Arterial-ventricular coupling and age

During exercise, Ea/E_{LV} decreases because of disproportionate increases in E_{LV} versus Ea to ensure that cardiac performance is augmented sufficiently to meet the increased demands for blood flow. The reduction in Ea/E_{LV} (inversely related to EF) during exercise has been shown to differ by age and gender.[74] In both genders, Ea/E_{LV} decreases during exercise (because E_{LV} increases more than Ea), but the ratio declines to a lesser extent in older subjects. There are gender differences in the components of Ea/E_{LV} during exercise: Ea is greater in older versus young women but is unaffected by age in men. E_{LV} increases to a greater extent in young versus older subjects. Thus, suboptimal ventricular-vascular coupling helps to explain the age-associated blunting of maximal exercise EF, and its underlying mechanisms seem to differ between men and women.

Arterial-ventricular coupling and hypertension

Hypertension is a major risk factor for heart failure, including heart failure with preserved ejection fraction, particularly burdensome in older individuals. The specific mechanisms that underlie the transition of a hypertensive LV to a failing LV have not been elucidated completely. Hypertension is associated with structural and functional alterations in the central arteries and in the LV that are gender specific and believed to be, at least in their early stages, adaptive in nature. It is well established that LV performance is influenced by the arterial load and that the arterial properties are, in turn, influenced by LV performance. Thus, studying the interaction between the LV and the arterial system may provide a useful framework to gain insights into cardiovascular performance.

Compared with normotensive subjects, women who have systolic hypertension have a lower resting Ea/E_{LV}; a higher energetic requirement at rest, at peak exercise, and during recovery; and a markedly attenuated Ea/E_{LV} reserve.[75] No differences were noted between normotensive and hypertensive men. The diminished Ea/E_{LV} reserve in women who have systolic hypertension deserves further study as a possible cause of future functional limitations that could putatively explain the increased incidence of heart failure with preserved ejection fraction in older women who have systolic hypertension.

In summary, the metabolic, enzymatic, cellular, and molecular alterations and lifestyle factors (eg, high dietary sodium) that have been implicated in age-associated structural remodeling (see **Table 1**) are linked to Ang II signaling (see **Fig. 7**) and increasingly are recognized as playing a critical role in the genesis or promotion of inflammatory arterial diseases, including hypertension. In other words, many of the same factors that underlie the age-associated structural and functional alterations of the arterial wall also are implicated in the pathogenesis of hypertension. These and other previously well-defined factors are the culprits that accumulate and underlie the "risky" component of arterial aging and are linked to the increased incidence of the quintessential cardiovascular diseases, such as hypertension, in the elderly.

ACKNOWLEDGMENTS

The authors thank Robert E. Monticone for his assistance in preparing this document.

REFERENCES

1. Najjar SS, Scuteri A, Lakatta EG. Arterial aging: is it an immutable cardiovascular risk factor? Hypertension 2005;46(3):454–62.
2. Lakatta EG, Levy D. Arterial and cardiac aging: major shareholders in cardiovascular disease enterprises: part I: aging arteries: a "set-up" for vascular disease. Circulation 2003;107(1):139–46.
3. Najjar SS, Lakatta EG. Vascular aging: from molecular to clinical cardiology. In: Patterson WC, Runge M, editors. Principles of molecular cardiology. Totowa (NJ): Humana Press; 2005. p. 517–47.
4. Wang M, Lakatta EG. Central arterial aging: humans to molecules. In: Safar M, editor. Handbook of hypertension: arterial stiffness in hypertension. Amsterdam: Elsevier; 2006. p. 137–60.
5. Lakatta EG. Central arterial aging and the epidemic of systolic hypertension and atherosclerosis. J Am Soc Hypertens 2007;1(5):302–40.
6. Virmani R, Avolio AP, Mergner WJ, et al. Effect of aging on aortic morphology in populations with high and low prevalence of hypertension and atherosclerosis. Comparison between occidental and Chinese communities. Am J Pathol 1991; 139(5):1119–29.
7. Lakatta EG. Arterial and cardiac aging: major shareholders in cardiovascular disease enterprises: part III: cellular and molecular clues to heart and arterial aging. Circulation 2003;107(3):490–7.

8. Wang M, Lakatta EG. The salted artery and angiotensin ii signaling: a deadly duo in arterial disease. J Hypertens 2009;27(1):19–21.

9. Wang M, Zhang J, Spinetti G, et al. Angiotensin II activates matrix metalloproteinase type II and mimics age-associated carotid arterial remodeling in young rats. Am J Pathol 2005;167(5):1429–42.

10. Asai K, Kudej RK, Shen YT, et al. Peripheral vascular endothelial dysfunction and apoptosis in old monkeys. Arterioscler Thromb Vasc Biol 2000;20(6):1493–9.

11. Wang M, Takagi G, Asai K, et al. Aging increases aortic MMP-2 activity and angiotensin II in nonhuman primates. Hypertension 2003;41(6):1308–16.

12. Wang M, Zhang J, Jiang LQ, et al. Proinflammatory profile within the grossly normal aged human aortic wall. Hypertension 2007;50(1):219–27.

13. Wang M, Lakatta EG. Altered regulation of matrix metalloproteinase-2 in aortic remodeling during aging. Hypertension 2002;39(4):865–73.

14. Wang M, Zhao D, Spinetti G, et al. Matrix metalloproteinase 2 activation of transforming growth factor-beta1 (TGF-beta1) and TGF-beta1-type II receptor signaling within the aged arterial wall. Arterioscler Thromb Vasc Biol 2006;26(7):1503–9.

15. Spinetti G, Wang M, Monticone R, et al. Rat aortic MCP-1 and its receptor CCR2 increase with age and alter vascular smooth muscle cell function. Arterioscler Thromb Vasc Biol 2004;24(8):1397–402.

16. Jiang L, Wang M, Zhang J, et al. Increased aortic calpain-1 activity mediates age-associated angiotensin II signaling of vascular smooth muscle cells. PLoS ONE 2008;3:1–12.

17. Sekiguchi K, Kurabayashi M, Oyama Y, et al. Homeobox protein Hex induces SMemb/nonmuscle myosin heavy chain-B gene expression through the cAMP-responsive element. Circ Res 2001;88(1):52–8.

18. Miyazaki M, Takai S, Jin D, et al. Pathological roles of angiotensin II produced by mast cell chymase and the effects of chymase inhibition in animal models. Pharmacol Ther 2006;112(3):668–76.

19. Pauly RR, Passaniti A, Crow M, et al. Experimental models that mimic the differentiation and dedifferentiation of vascular cells. Circulation 1992;86(Suppl):III68–73.

20. Li Z, Cheng H, Lederer WJ, et al. Enhanced proliferation and migration and altered cytoskeletal proteins in early passage smooth muscle cells from young and old rat aortic explants. Exp Mol Pathol 1997;64(1):1–11.

21. Hariri RJ, Hajjar DP, Coletti D, et al. Aging and arteriosclerosis. Cell cycle kinetics of young and old arterial smooth muscle cells. Am J Pathol 1988;131(1):132–6.

22. Celermajer DS, Sorensen KE, Spiegelhalter DJ, et al. Aging is associated with endothelial dysfunction in healthy men years before the age-related decline in women. J Am Coll Cardiol 1994;24(2):471–6.

23. Csiszar A, Wang M, Lakatta EG, et al. Inflammation and endothelial dysfunction during aging: role of NF-{kappa} B. J Appl Phys 2008;105(4):1333–41.

24. Shi Q, Aida K, Vandeberg JL, et al. Passage-dependent changes in baboon endothelial cells–relevance to in vitro aging. DNA Cell Biol 2004;23(8):502–9.

25. Wagner M, Hampel B, Bernhard D, et al. Replicative senescence of human endothelial cells in vitro involves G1 arrest, polyploidization and senescence-associated apoptosis. Exp Gerontol 2001;36(8):1327–47.

26. Yeh HI, Chang HM, Lu WW, et al. Age-related alteration of gap junction distribution and connexin expression in rat aortic endothelium. J Histochem Cytochem 2000;48(0):1377–89.

27. Chang E, Harley CB. Telomere length and replicative aging in human vascular tissues. Proc Natl Acad Sci U S A 1995;92(24):11190–4.

28. Iwama H, Ohyashiki K, Ohyashiki JH, et al. Telomeric length and telomerase activity vary with age in peripheral blood cells obtained from normal individuals. Hum Genet 1998;102(4):397–402.

29. Van der Loo B, Labugger R, Skepper JN, et al. Enhanced peroxynitrite formation is associated with vascular aging. J Exp Med 2000;192(12):1731–44.

30. Rauscher FM, Goldschmidt-Clermont PJ, Davis BH, et al. Aging, progenitor cell exhaustion, and atherosclerosis. Circulation 2003;108(4):457–63.

31. Conboy IM, Conboy MJ, Wagers AJ, et al. Rejuvenation of aged progenitor cells by exposure to a young systemic environment. Nature 2005;433(7027):760–4.

32. Berkowitz DE, White R, Li D, et al. Arginase reciprocally regulates nitric oxide synthase activity and contributes to endothelial dysfunction in aging blood vessels. Circulation 2003;108(16):2000–6.

33. Bode-Boger SM, Muke J, Surdacki A, et al. Oral L-arginine improves endothelial function in healthy individuals older than 70 years. Vasc Med 2003;8(2):77–81.

34. Cernadas MR, Sanchez de Miguel L, Garcia-Duran M, et al. Expression of constitutive and inducible nitric oxide synthases in the vascular wall of young and aging rats. Circ Res 1998;83(3):279–86.

35. Hamilton CA, Brosnan MJ, McIntyre M, et al. Superoxide excess in hypertension and aging: a common cause of endothelial dysfunction. Hypertension 2001;37(2 Part 2):529–34.

36. Vaitkevicius PV, Fleg JL, Engel JH, et al. Effects of age and aerobic capacity on arterial stiffness in healthy adults. Circulation 1993;88(4 Part 1):1456–62.

37. Laurent S, Cockcroft J, Van Bortel L, et al. Expert consensus document on arterial stiffness: methodological issues and clinical applications. Eur Heart J 2006; 27(21):2588–605.

38. Laurent S, Lacolley P, Girerd X, et al. Arterial stiffening: opposing effects of age- and hypertension-associated structural changes. Can J Physiol Pharmacol 1996; 74(7):842–9.

39. Mitchell GF. Effects of central arterial aging on the structure and function of the peripheral vasculature: implications for end-organ damage. J Appl Phys 2008; 105(5):1652–60.

40. Waldstein SR, Rice SC, Thayer JF, et al. Pulse pressure and pulse wave velocity are related to cognitive decline in the Baltimore Longitudinal Study of Aging. Hypertension 2008;51(1):99–104.

41. Kelly R, Hayward C, Avolio A, et al. Noninvasive determination of age-related changes in the human arterial pulse. Circulation 1989;80(6):1652–9.

42. Mitchell GF, Parise H, Benjamin EJ, et al. Changes in arterial stiffness and wave reflection with advancing age in healthy men and women: the Framingham Heart Study. Hypertension 2004;43(6):1239–45.

43. McVeigh GE, Allen PB, Morgan DR, et al. Nitric oxide modulation of blood vessel tone identified by arterial waveform analysis. Clin Sci (Lond) 2001;100(4):387–93.

44. Foster JA, Rich CB, Miller M, et al. Effect of age and IGF-I administration on elastin gene expression in rat aorta. J Gerontol 1990;45(4):B113–8.

45. Quaglino D, Fornieri C, Nanney LB, et al. Extracellular matrix modifications in rat tissues of different ages. Correlations between elastin and collagen type I mRNA expression and lysyl-oxidase activity. Matrix 1993;13(6):481–90.

46. Behmoaras J, Slove S, Seve S, et al. Differential expression of lysyl oxidases LOXL1 and LOX during growth and aging suggests specific roles in elastin and collagen fiber remodeling in rat aorta. Rejuvenation Res 2008;11(5):883–9.

47. Kaplan D, Meyer K. Mucopolysaccharides of aorta at various ages. Proc Soc Exp Biol Med 1960;105:78–81.

48. Harding SE, Jones SM, O'Gara P, et al. Isolated ventricular myocytes from failing and nonfailing human heart: the relation of age and clinical status of patients to isoproterenol response. J Mol Cell Cardiol 1992;24(5):549–64.
49. King AL. Pressure-volume relation for cylindrical tubes with elastomeric walls: the human aorta. J Appl Phys 1946;17:501–5.
50. Brownlee M. Advanced protein glycosylation in diabetes and aging. Annu Rev Med 1995;46:223–34.
51. Roach MR, Burton AC. The effect of age on the elasticity of human iliac arteries. Can J Biochem Physiol 1959;37(4):557–70.
52. Navar LG, Harrison-Bernard LM, Wang CT, et al. Concentrations and actions of intraluminal angiotensin II. J Am Soc Nephrol 1999;10(Suppl 11):S189–95.
53. Diz D, Lewis K. Dahl memorial lecture: the renin-angiotensin system and aging. Hypertension 2008;52(1):37–43.
54. Lakatta EG, Levy D. Arterial and cardiac aging: major shareholders in cardiovascular disease enterprises: part II: the aging heart in health: links to heart disease. Circulation 2003;107(2):346–54.
55. Nichols WW, O'Rourke MF. McDonald's blood flow in arteries: theoretical, experimental and clinical principles. 4th edition. London: Edward Arnold; 1998.
56. Wang KL, Cheng HM, Chuang SY, et al. Central or peripheral systolic or pulse pressure: which best predicts target-organ damage and mortality? J Hypertens, in press.
57. Williams B, Lacy PS, Thom SM, et al. Differential impact of blood pressure-lowering drugs on central aortic pressure and clinical outcomes: principal results of the Conduit Artery Function Evaluation (CAFE) study. Circulation 2006;113(9): 1213–25.
58. Nagai Y, Metter EJ, Earley CJ, et al. Increased carotid artery intimal-medial thickness in asymptomatic older subjects with exercise-induced myocardial ischemia. Circulation 1998;98(15):1504–9.
59. O'Leary DH, Polak JF, Kronmal RA, et al. Carotid-artery intima and media thickness as a risk factor for myocardial infarction and stroke in older adults. Cardiovascular Health Study Collaborative Research Group. N Engl J Med 1999;340(1): 14–22.
60. London GM, Blacher J, Pannier B, et al. Arterial wave reflections and survival in end-stage renal failure. Hypertension 2001;38(3):434–8.
61. Arnett DK, Tyroler HA, Burke G, et al. Hypertension and subclinical carotid artery atherosclerosis in blacks and whites: the Atherosclerosis Risk in Communities Study. ARIC Investigators. Arch Intern Med 1996;156(17):1983–9.
62. Nichols WW, Nicolini FA, Pepine CJ. Determinants of isolated systolic hypertension in the elderly. J Hypertens Suppl 1992;10(6):S73–7.
63. O'Rourke MF, Nichols WW. Aortic diameter, aortic stiffness, and wave reflection increase with age and isolated systolic hypertension. Hypertension 2005;45(4): 652–8.
64. Mitchell GF, Lacourciere Y, Ouellet JP, et al. Determinants of elevated pulse pressure in middle-aged and older subjects with uncomplicated systolic hypertension: the role of proximal aortic diameter and the aortic pressure-flow relationship. Circulation 2003;108(13):1592–8.
65. Farasat SM, Morrell CH, Scuteri A, et al. Pulse pressure is inversely related to aortic root diameter implications for the pathogenesis of systolic hypertension. Hypertension 2008;51(2):196–202.
66. Najjar SS, Scuteri A, Shetty V, et al. Pulse wave velocity is an independent predictor of the longitudinal increase in systolic blood pressure and of incident

hypertension in the Baltimore Longitudinal Study of Aging. J Am Coll Cardiol 2008;51(14):1377–83.

67. Giles TD, Berk BC, Black HR, et al. Expanding the definition and classification of hypertension (Greenwich). J Clin Hypertens 2005;7(9):505–12.

68. Perticone F, Ceravolo R, Pujia A, et al. Prognostic significance of endolethial dysfunction in hypertensive patients. Circulation 2001;104(2):191–6.

69. Laurent S, Boutouyrie P, Asmar R, et al. Aortic stiffness is an independent predictor of all-cause and cardiovascular mortality in hypertensive patients. Hypertension 2001;37(5):1236–41.

70. Taddei S, Virdis A, Mattei P, et al. Hypertension causes premature aging of endothelial function in humans. Hypertension 1997;29(3):736–43.

71. Taddei S, Virdis A, Mattei P, et al. Defective Larginine-nitric oxide pathway in offspring of essential hypertensive patients. Circulation 1996;94(6):1298–303.

72. Guerin AP, Blacher J, Pannier B, et al. Impact of aortic stiffness attenuation on survival of patients in end-stage renal failure. Circulation 2001;103(7):987–92.

73. Chantler PD, Lakatta EG, Najjar SS. Arterial-ventricular coupling: mechanistic insights into cardiovascular performance at rest and during exercise. J Appl Phys 2008;105(4):1342–51.

74. Najjar SS, Schulman SP, Gerstenblith G, et al. Age and gender affect ventricular-vascular coupling during aerobic exercise. J Am Coll Cardiol 2004;44(3):611–7.

75. Chantler PD, Melenovsky V, Schulman SP, et al. The sex-specific impact of systolic hypertension and systolic blood pressure on arterial-ventricular coupling at rest and during exercise. Am J Physiol Heart Circ Physiol 2008;295(1):H145–53.

Hypertension, Systolic Blood Pressure, and Large Arteries

Michel E. Safar, MD

KEYWORDS

- Hypertension • Pulse pressure • Larges arteries
- Arterial stiffness • Wave reflections

The authors of epidemiologic studies have long emphasized the close relationship between high systolic blood pressure (SBP) or diastolic blood pressure (DBP) and the incidence of cardiovascular (CV) disease.[1-3] In the past, clinical hypertension was principally diagnosed based on the DBP level.[1-3] The hemodynamic characteristics of the disease were attributed to a reduction of the caliber and/or number of small arteries, causing elevated peripheral vascular resistance and secondary adaptive changes of the structure and function of arterioles and the heart. Later, prospective studies on Framingham Heart Study populations[4] redirected attention to SBP as a better guide than DBP to evaluate CV and all-cause mortality. In 1988 and later,[5,6] we investigated a large population of patients treated for hypertension and where DBP was consistently and adequately controlled ($\leq$90 mm Hg). Approximately one third of the subjects exhibited a high SBP ($\geq$140 mm Hg) and pulse pressure (PP = SBP − DBP) for the same mean arterial pressure (MAP) as the remaining two thirds of the total population. The former group was characterized by significantly higher aortic pulse wave velocity (PWV) and degree of cardiac hypertrophy than the latter. Finally, it was shown that, in large populations, antihypertensive therapy frequently achieved adequate DBP control but that SBP was much more difficult to control.[7,8] Those findings focused attention on the factors that modulate SBP and PP levels in hypertensive individuals, and therefore on the potential role of increased arterial stiffness and/or wave reflections in SBP and PP control, and hence CV morbidity and mortality.

A major function of the large arteries is to change the pulsatile pressure and flow coming from the heart into a steady pressure and flow at the periphery, to obtain optimal oxygenation of tissues.[1,2,9,10] This major modification is a consequence of

This work was performed with the help of INSERM (Institut de la Santé et de la Recherche Médicale) and GPH-CV (Groupe de Pharmacologie et d'Hémodynamique Cardiovasculaire), Paris. We thank Dr. Anne Safar for helpful and stimulating discussions.
Université Paris Descartes, Assistance Publique-Hôpitaux de Paris, Hôtel-Dieu, Centre de Diagnostic et de Thérapeutique, 1 place du Parvis Notre-Dame, 5181 Paris Cedex 04, Paris, France
E-mail address: michel.safar@htd.aphp.fr

Med Clin N Am 93 (2009) 605–619
doi:10.1016/j.mcna.2009.02.011
0025-7125/09/$ – see front matter © 2009 Elsevier Inc. All rights reserved.

the so-called "Windkessel" effect. During systole, part of the stroke volume directly flows toward the periphery, causing systolic perfusion. The other part of the stroke volume is stored within the elastic thoracic aorta wall and restored during diastole, causing the resultant diastolic perfusion. The association of systolic and diastolic flows is responsible for continuous and steady peripheral perfusion, which contrasts with the alternative cyclic movement initiated by the heart. This "Windkessel" effect has major impact on SBP regulation, through the mechanisms of wave reflections and the development of systolic hypertension. This article is composed of the following four parts:

(1) Factors modulating central and peripheral SBP and PP in hypertensive subjects;
(2) Mechanisms enhancing PP variations in this population;
(3) Analysis of pulsatile arterial hemodynamics as predictors of CV risk; and
(4) Pulsatile hemodynamics and strategies lowering CV risk in the treatment of hypertension.

FUNCTIONAL AND STRUCTURAL FACTORS INFLUENCING CENTRAL SYSTOLIC BLOOD PRESSURE AND PULSE PRESSURE

This section summarizes briefly the principal factors modulating SBP and PP and acting on large arteries in hypertensive subjects. Increased SBP and PP are the main clinical characteristics of hypertension in the elderly.

The Systolic Blood Pressure and Pulse Pressure Arterial and Arteriolar Circuit

As we mentioned earlier, at the end of ventricular ejection, the pressure in the aorta falls much more slowly than in the left ventricle because the large central arteries, particularly the aorta, are elastic, and thus act as a reservoir during systole, storing part of the ejected blood, which is then forced out into the peripheral vessels during diastole.[1,2,9,10] More specifically, the pulsatile load is borne primarily by elastin-containing arteries, which fulfill the bulk of the cushioning function by expanding during systole to store some, but not all, of each stroke volume, and then contracting during diastole to facilitate peripheral run-off of the stored blood, thereby supporting diastolic blood flow to peripheral tissues.

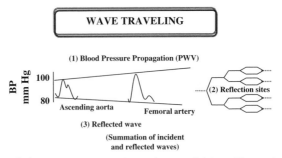

Fig. 1. Progression of the pressure wave along the arterial tree. Three steps are involved: propagation, reflection, and summation of the incident and the reflected waves. (*From* Safar ME, Lacolley P. Disturbance of macro- and microcirculation: relation with pulse pressure and cardiac organ damage. Am J Physiol Heart Circ Physiol 2007;293:H1–7; with permission.)

Then, the pressure pulse generated by ventricular contraction travels along the aorta as a wave (**Fig. 1**). It is possible to calculate the velocity of this wave (ie, pulse wave velocity, PWV) from the interval between two BP curves located at two different sites in the arterial tree, particularly the aorta. Because a fundamental principle is that pulse waves travel faster in stiffer arteries, PWV measurement is considered the best surrogate to evaluate arterial stiffness. It estimates 3 to 5 m/s in young persons at rest, but increases considerably with age. Given that peripheral arteries are markedly stiffer than central arteries, an important limitation of PWV determinations is the large heterogeneity of the arterial wall components at its different sites.

When several BP measurements are made simultaneously at different points all along the aorta, the pressure wave changes shape as it travels down the aorta. Whereas SBP actually rises with distance from the heart, the DBP and MAP fall slightly (about 4 mm Hg) during the same course along the aorta trajectory (see **Fig. 1**). Thus, pressure-oscillation amplitude between systole and diastole, which is PP, nearly doubles. This SBP and PP amplification along the vascular tree is a physiologic finding, approximating 14 mm Hg between the thoracic aorta root and the brachial artery, and continuing in aortic ramifications out to about the third-generation level of branches. Thereafter, both PP and MAP drop sharply to the levels found in the microcirculation, a territory in which steady flow is nearly achieved.

If an individual's body length is about 2 m at most, and aortic PWV is approximately 5 m/s, something must happen to the BP-curve shape within each beat if heart rate is 60/min. What happens is the generation of wave reflections and their summation with the incident wave, as summarized in **Fig. 1**. The incident wave is driven away from the heart through the highly conductive arteries. However, it encounters an impedance mismatch at the junction of the high conductive artery and high resistance arterioles, blocking its entry into the arterioles and it is reflected, traveling backward toward the heart. Thus, the shape of every pulse wave results from the summation of the incident (forward-traveling) and reflected (backward-traveling) pressure waves.

Age, Wave Reflections, and Systolic Hypertension

Reflected waves may be initiated from any discontinuity of the arterial or arteriolar wall, but are mainly issued from high-resistance vessels.[1,9,10] Pulse-wave propagation and

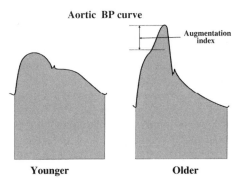

Fig. 2. Characteristics of the pressure wave in young and old subjects for the same cross-sectional area of the blood pressure curve (ie, the same mean arterial pressure). Aix: Augmentation index is the supplement of SBP owing to the reflected wave and located between the two arrows indicated within the figure. (*From* Nichols WW, O'Rourke MF, McDonald DA. McDonald's blood flow in arteries. Theoretical, experimental and clinical principles. 4th edition. Sydney: Hodder Arnold; 1998. p. 54–401. Copyright © 1998. Reproduced by permission of Edward Arnold (Publishers) Ltd.)

reflection vary considerably according to age. In young adults at their maximum height and maximum elasticity of their central arteries (low PWV), the summation of the incident arterial pressure wave and the reflected wave results in progressive PP amplification, so that SBP is higher in the brachial artery than the ascending aorta (**Figs. 1 and 2**). This hemodynamic profile contrasts with MAP and DBP, which decline minimally in vessels at increasing distance from the heart at all ages (see **Figs. 1 and 2**). Note that, in the thoracic aorta, because PWV is relatively low, the reflected wave comes back during diastole, thereby maintaining DBP and boosting coronary perfusion. Hence, an optimal arterial function is maintained, along with adequate coronary perfusion.

The pattern of wave reflections and the pulse wave shape are directly dependent on aging and arterial stiffness. The development of increasing arterial stiffness (high PWV) and altered wave reflections with aging and hypertension completely abolishes the differences between central and peripheral PP by age 50 to 60 years (see **Fig. 2**), with major consequences on ventricular load and coronary perfusion. The increased velocity of the aortic pulse wave means that the reflected waves return to the aortic root earlier, during late systole. In that situation, the reflected waves summate with the forward-traveling wave to create an increase or "augmentation" of the central SBP and ventricular load (see **Fig. 2**). In elderly persons with isolated systolic hypertension, aortic SBP can be elevated by as much as 30 to 40 mm Hg as a result of the early return of the wave reflection.[1,2] Furthermore, because the backward pressure returns in systole, and not in diastole, as a consequence of enhanced PWV, DBP and coronary blood flow tend to be reduced, a situation favoring coronary ischemia.

Arterial Remodeling, Wave Reflections, and Their Cardiovascular Consequences

An arterial wall is a complex tissue composed of different cell populations capable of structural and functional changes, in response to direct injury and atherogenic factors, or to modifications of long-term hemodynamic conditions. The principal geometric modifications induced by hemodynamic alterations are changes of the arterial radius (r) lumen and/or arterial wall thickness (h) owing to activation, proliferation, and migration of vascular smooth muscle (VSM) cells, and rearrangements of cellular elements and extracellular matrix (ECM).[11–18] Whereas acute changes of tensile or shear stress (= v/r, with v = blood velocity) induce transient vasomotor-tone and arterial diameter adjustments, chronic alterations of mechanical forces lead to modifications of the geometry and composition of the vessel walls, as observed in hypertension, particularly in the elderly.[13,14] To maintain tensile stress (T) within physiologic limits, arteries respond by thickening their walls (Laplace's law: $T = P \times r/h$, where P = pressure). Experimental and clinical data indicate that acute and chronic augmentations of arterial blood flow induce proportional increases of the vessel lumen, whereas diminished flow leads to reduction of the inner arterial diameter.[14,15] The presence of the endothelium is a major prerequisite for normal vascular adaptation to chronic changes of blood flow and pressure. Finally, although the alterations of tensile and shear stresses are interrelated, tensile stress changes primarily induce (as in hypertension) hypertrophy and sclerosis of the arterial media, whereas shear stress changes principally modify the dimensions and structure of the intima (atherosclerosis).

Hypertensive remodeling is characterized by the increased wall/lumen (h/r) ratio of arterioles, which represent the site of vascular resistance and also the origin of wave reflections (see **Figs. 1 and 2**).[14–18] Regression of arteriolar hypertrophy is associated with diminution of vascular resistance and reflection coefficients, and thereby lower SBP, PP, and augmentation index (Aix), a classical marker of wave reflections (see **Fig. 2**).[16–18] This process occurs approximately after 1 year of treatment with angiotensin or calcium blockade, but not under most of the beta-blocking agents.[18] Endothelial dysfunction may sometimes participate to this process, mainly through nitrite oxide (NO) deficiency and development of oxidative stress.[11,14–18]

MECHANISMS OF PULSE PRESSURE DIFFUSION AND VARIATION

It has recently been shown that PP interacts with the arterial wall through transduction mechanisms independent of MAP. Indeed, at any given MAP value, the arterial wall becomes much stiffer in the presence than in the absence of pulsatile stimulus.[2,9,11] Furthermore, calcifications and attachment molecules are able to enhance arterial stiffness independently of both systemic MAP and changes in elastin and/or collagen within the vessel wall.[2] All these factors contribute to PP widening.

Cyclic Mechanical Factors and the Arterial Wall

Since the pioneering studies of Glagov,[19] many investigations[17,20,21] have examined the effect of cyclic forces on the arterial wall, particularly on endothelial cells exposed to pulsatile shear stress in vitro.[17,20–23] The role of cyclic shear stress (as opposed to steady stress), and the importance of stimulus duration and graded responses to mechanical forces have been demonstrated especially concerning NO and super oxide anions.[20] Cyclic mechanical strain has also been analyzed, mostly using cultured VSM cells. Long-term cyclic distention enhances the mechanical properties of collagen-based medial components and even heightens collagen and fibronectin (Fn) accumulations in animal or human VSM models.[17,21] The vessel-wall materials become stronger and stiffer than those obtained under static conditions.

A distinct feature of VSM cells is their phenotypic plasticity, particularly during the transition from the contractile to the synthetic phenotype of VSM-cell cultures in the absence of mechanical forces.[21] Exposing cultured VSM cells to cyclic stretch can restore the expression of high-molecular-weight caldesmon and other markers of differentiated VSM cells. A certain degree of stretch is required to preserve the VSM contractile state.[21] Hence, the failure to maintain a threshold level stretch is likely to contribute to VSM-cell transformation.

Stretch initiates complex signal-transduction cascades leading to gene transcription and functional responses, via interaction of integrins with extra cellular matrix (ECM) proteins, or by stimulating G-protein receptors, tyrosine kinase receptors, or ion channels (reviewed in Lehoux and colleagues[23]). The intracellular pathways reported to be activated in VSM cells by cyclic stretch include, mainly, the mitogen-activated protein kinase cascades and nuclear factor-kappa B,[2,21] which has been studied at both VSM and endothelial levels. More recently, steady and cyclic modes of stretch were shown to transduce differently in the aorta: the former implicating focal adhesion kinase and the latter free radicals derived from oxidative stress and the presence of inflammatory factors[23,24] (**Fig. 3**).

Finally, the transcriptional profile of mechanically induced genes in VSM cells subjected to a uniform biaxial cyclic strain was studied.[25] Cyclic stretch was found to stimulate the expression of a number of genes, including vascular endothelial growth factor and plasminogen activator inhibitor-1, but to negatively regulate others, such as ECM metalloproteinase-1 and thrombomodulin.

Wall Material, Stiffness, Calcifications, and the Role of Attachment Molecules

In recent years, studies on rodents showed that, particularly in old age, diabetes mellitus and/or in subjects on a high-sodium diet, arterial calcifications (not addressed in this article) and attachment molecules (between VSM cells, or VSM cells and ECM

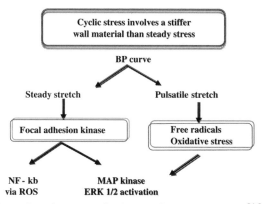

Fig. 3. Simplified view of mechanotransduction mechanisms. See text.[21,23,24]

proteins, or between collagen fibers), contribute per se to stiffening the vascular wall.[2,26]

Cross-links may stabilize collagen fibrils, preventing slippage of adjacent molecules under applied tensile stress[2] and contributing to increased arterial stiffness through the formation of end-glycation products.[27] In elderly subjects with systolic hypertension, drugs involving collagen cross-link breakers acutely reduce arterial stiffness and PP, without any change of MAP.[27] Glycosaminoglycans exhibit viscoelastic properties, which make them good candidates for flow-sensing molecules, binding sodium and calcium ions in their helicoidal chains.[28] In the carotid arteries of spontaneously hypertensive rats (SHR), chronic high-sodium diet results in the reduction of arterial hyaluron and enhanced aortic stiffness.[29]

Because integrins transmit inside-out and outside-in signals capable of modulating vascular responses, it has been suggested that adhesion molecules, such as Fn and its integrin receptor(s), might contribute per se to changing arterial wall stiffness. For instance, Fn-ECM polymerization increases tensile strength of model tissue.[30–32] In young and old SHR, aortic Fn measurements indicate that more attachment sites between VSM cells and ECM proteins might contribute to enhanced arterial rigidity.[2,26] On a normal-sodium diet, angiotensin-converting enzyme inhibition (ACEI) led to lower MAP and PP, together with reduction of aortic Fn and $\alpha_5\beta_1$ integrin, and increase of isobaric arterial distensibility.[31] On ACEI plus high-sodium diet, MAP was significantly reduced, but PP, arterial stiffness, and aortic Fn remained elevated. Similar results were obtained when chronic aldosterone administration was combined with high-sodium diet for Sprague - Dawley rats.[32] In the latter experiment, the enhancements of Fn and stiffness were reversed by administration of the selective aldosterone-antagonist eplerenone.[32]

Local changes of the attachments between VSM cells and ECM proteins along with arterial calcifications might independently modulate the stiffness of each artery taken individually. All these pathophysiological mechanisms might also contribute to the development of new wave-reflection sites, particularly in aged people. Finally, the extent of abnormal arterial stiffness and wave reflections in each individual is largely influenced by the vascular territories involved and the subject's age. In some cases, as in obese persons and/or those with insulin resistance, arterial stiffness is enhanced with minor changes in wave reflections.[1,2] In most cases, both parameters are increased in parallel. For all patients, bidirectional interactions develop between higher PP and enhanced wall stiffness, thereby creating a vicious circle and raising the risk of

CV complications.[1,2] Finally, increased stiffness and pulsatility may lead to target-organ damage every time PP is transmitted to the corresponding organ. This process requires the loss of organ autoregulatory mechanisms, whose study is beyond the scope of this article.

PULSATILE ARTERIAL HEMODYNAMICS AS INDEPENDENT PREDICTORS OF CARDIOVASCULAR RISK

This paragraph shows that brachial PP, aortic PWV, and even at a higher extent, central PP and wave reflections are independent predictors of CV risk in the elderly.

Brachial Pulse Pressure

In a 1989 French study including normotensive and untreated hypertensive adults,[33] a pulsatile-component index, defined as a strong correlate of brachial PP, was derived by principal-components analysis of SBP and DBP measurements. An association was found between the pulsatile-component index and electrocardiographic evidence of left ventricular hypertrophy. During 10 years of follow-up, the pulsatile-component index was independently associated with an increased risk of death from coronary artery disease (CAD), but not from stroke. The relationship was found to be particularly consistent for women older than 55. In another prospective study evaluating hypertensive subjects,[34,35] those in the highest brachial PP tertile before starting therapy ($\geq$ 63 mm Hg) had an enhanced risk of myocardial infarction and, to a lesser extent, stroke. This result was obtained during an average follow-up of 5 years. In a later study, multivariate analysis revealed that brachial PP as a categorical (but not continuous) variable was an independent predictor of myocardial infarction. Finally, that association was observed, regardless of whether PP was measured by sphygmomanometry or ambulatory BP measurements over 24 hours.[36]

Franklin and colleagues[37] for the Framingham Heart Study, Millar and colleagues[38] for the Medical Research Council trial, and Blacher and colleagues[39] for the European Working Party on High Blood Pressure in the Elderly, Syst-China, and Syst-Eur trials, showed, almost simultaneously, that, after 50 to 60 years of age, brachial PP was a stronger CV risk factor than SBP alone for myocardial infarction in populations of hypertensive individuals. The best predictor function of all possible linear combinations of SBP and DBP was shown to be similar to that of PP, indicating that their association was not a statistical artifact caused by the correlation between SBP and PP.[37–39] Furthermore, one report[39] clearly indicated that CV risk was not only attributable to a SBP increase but also specifically to a DBP decline. As shown in **Fig. 4**, CV risk rises sharply with SBP. However, at any given SBP value, CV risk is higher when DBP is lower.[39] This important finding was confirmed by the result of a longitudinal study,[40] which indicated that, during 20 years of follow-up, subjects with higher CV mortality were those whose SBP rose and DBP declined, and their CV-mortality rate was significantly higher than that for those individuals whose SBP and DBP increased.[41] Finally, it was demonstrated that, in the elderly, neither SBP nor DBP was superior to PP for predicting coronary risk[37] and PP was found to be an independent predictor of CV mortality, even for individuals with recurrent myocardial infarction, congestive heart failure, or myocardial dysfunction.[41–45] Finally, brachial PP was shown also to be an independent predictor of CV risk in subjects with end-stage renal disease, diabetes mellitus,[46,47] or even systemic vasculitis.[48]

In a population of 19,083 normo- or hypertensive men followed for 20 years, Benetos and colleagues[49,50] not only confirmed that elevated brachial PP was a strong predictor of myocardial infarction but also that this predictive value was even observed in

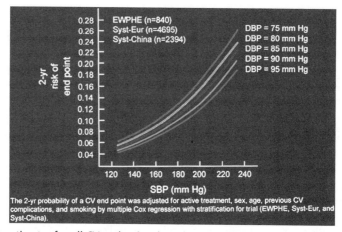

The 2-yr probability of a CV end point was adjusted for active treatment, sex, age, previous CV complications, and smoking by multiple Cox regression with stratification for trial (EWPHE, Syst-Eur, and Syst-China).

Fig. 4. Risk estimates for all CV end points based on 3 trials. Risk associated with increasing SBP at fixed levels of DBP. Curves plotting the 2-year risk of CV events in the elderly as function of increasing SBP. Note that, at each given SBP value, the CV risk was higher when baseline DBP was lower. (*From* Blacher J, Staessen JA, Girerd X, et al. Pulse pressure not mean pressure determines cardiovascular risk in older hypertensive patients. Arch Intern Med 2000;160:1085–9; with permission.)

a normotensive population, especially in men older than 55. Those findings were also applied to treated hypertensive individuals.[51] Pertinently, even when normotensive BP values (SBP ≤ 140 mm Hg; DBP ≤ 90 mm Hg) were obtained with successful drug therapy, elevated PP predicted a higher CV-mortality rate, especially for diabetic patients.[51] Furthermore, according to many therapeutic trials conducted on elderly hypertensive subjects, CV mortality was indeed substantially lowered but, at the end of the trials, the population was characterized by low DBP as opposed to SBP, which remained high (> 140 mm Hg). These findings suggest to what extent the presence of drug treatment might be partly responsible, together with age, for the hemodynamic profile associating low DBP and high SBP, ie, increased PP.[52,53]

Aortic Pulse Wave Velocity

In older populations, PP is poorly influenced by ventricular ejection, which tends to decline with age, whereas, in contrast, arterial stiffness tends to increase.[1,2] However, until recently, it was not known whether aortic PWV, a classic index of arterial stiffness and wave reflections, was an independent predictor of CV mortality in hypertensive individuals.

Based on the characteristics of 201 patients[54] with end-stage renal disease (ESRD), logistic-regression and Cox analyses identified three predictors of CV mortality: aortic (and not limb) PWV, and age and duration of hemodialysis before entry. Lipid abnormalities, anemia, and low DBP influenced risk to much smaller degrees. After adjusting for age, duration of hemodialysis, preexisting CV disease, left ventricular hypertrophy, BP, serum albumin, and hemoglobin levels, the odds ratios for PWV (> 12 m/s) were 5.6 (95% confidence interval [CI] 2.4–11.9) for all-cause mortality, and 5.9 (95% CI 2.3–15.5) for CV mortality. These results provided the first evidence that, in ESRD patients on hemodialysis, enhanced aortic stiffness (but also PP) was a major independent predictor of CV mortality. Similar findings were observed in this population using, in the place of aortic PWV, carotid wall–material stiffness as an index of vascular wall–material stiffness. That analysis indicated that, while the wall/lumen ratio of the common carotid artery did not predict CV risk, carotid stiffness itself (and not wall thickness) was a highly significant predictor of CV mortality.[55] Finally, the predictive value of carotid stiffness was subsequently extended to carotid wave reflections.[56] Similar observations were obtained for ESRD patients with diabetes mellitus[57] and in kidney-transplant recipients.[58]

Identifying predictive factors contributing to essential hypertension is complex because long-term longitudinal studies with aortic PWV measurements are difficult to conduct, mainly because of patient mobility but also to the paucity of mechanisms involved. However, the calculating CV risk with Framingham equations can partly resolve this difficulty.[59] In a study on 530 hypertensive subjects,[60] the odds ratio of carrying a high CV risk based on various known factors was evaluated. The CV risk assessed using Framingham equations was linearly associated with the PWV increase. Furthermore, aortic PWV was shown to be the best predictor of CV mortality. The odds ratio of being at high risk of CV mortality (> 5% for 10 years) for patients with PWV greater than 13.5 m/s was 7.1 (95% CI 4.5–11.3). That study[60] provided the first evidence that a single aortic PWV measurement could be a strong independent predictor of CV risk for hypertensive patients. The results of longitudinal studies[61,62] confirmed that aortic PWV is a significant and independent predictor of CV risk, more potent than PP itself.

To assess the prognostic significance of aortic PWV above and beyond the other traditional CV risk factors, a sex- and age-stratified random sample of 1678 Danish subjects, 40 to 70 years old, was investigated.[63] Cox regression was used to evaluate the prognostic value of PWV, office PP, and 24-hour ambulatory PP, with adjustment for MAP and other covariates. Over a median follow-up of 9.4 years, fatal and nonfatal CV end points, CV mortality, and fatal and nonfatal CAD concerned 154, 62, and 101 patients respectively. Adjustments were made for sex, age, body mass index, MAP measured in the office (conventional PP and PWV), or by ambulatory monitoring (24-hour PP), smoking, and alcohol consumption. After these adjustments, PWV maintained its prognostic significance for each end point ($P < .05$), whereas office and 24-hour PP lost their predictive value ($P > .19$), except for office PP in a context of CAD ($P = .02$) (**Fig. 5**). For each increment of one PWV standard deviation (3.4 m/s), the risk of an event increased 16% to 20%. According to sensitivity analyses, PWV still predicted all CV events after standardizing to a heart rate of 60 beats per minute, after adjustment for 24-hour MAP instead of office MAP, and/or after additional adjustment for the total-to-HDL serum cholesterol ratio and diabetes mellitus at baseline. Thus, in a general Danish population, PWV predicted a composite of CV outcomes above and beyond traditional CV risk factors, including 24-hour MAP. Similar findings were obtained for other populations of diabetic and nondiabetic subjects.[64–66]

Central Pulse Pressure, Aortic Stiffness, and Coronary Artery Disease

Numerous studies have shown in the past significant associations between CAD and enhanced aortic or carotid stiffness.[1,2,67,68] Because, in most cases of CAD, brachial, and not aortic, BP was measured[1,2,67,68] and because brachial PP is physiologically higher than aortic PP for the same MAP,[1,2] most of those earlier studies did not clearly demonstrate that aortic PP was the main hemodynamic parameter significantly predicting CAD.

As we stated previously, studies on pulsatile arterial hemodynamics showed that, whereas MAP remains nearly constant along the arterial tree, PP rises markedly from central (thoracic aorta and carotid artery) to peripheral (brachial) arteries. That

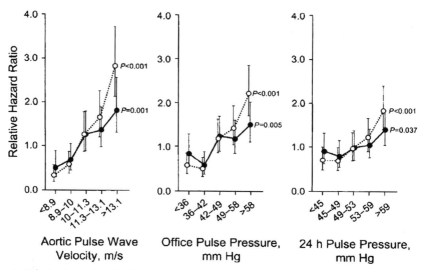

Fig. 5. Relative hazard ratios for the composite CV end point by quintiles of the distribution of PWW, office, or 24-hour PP unadjusted (*open symbols*) or adjusted for sex and age (*closed symbols*). The hazard ratios express the risk for each quintile versus the average risk for the whole population. Vertical lines denote 95% confidence intervals. *P* values are for trend. (*From* Willum-Hansen T, Staessen JA, Torp-Pedersen C, et al. Prognostic value of aortic pulse wave velocity as index of arterial stiffness in the general population. Circulation 2006;113:664–70; with permission.)

physiologic amplification can be explained by the pressure-wave propagation along arterial vessels associated with the progressive artery-diameter decline and arterial stiffness increase, resulting in modifications of wave-reflections timing and/or amplitude. Therefore, aortic PP is expected to be more relevant to the investigation of CV risk than brachial PP, because it is closer to the heart, coronary arteries, and carotid arteries, which are the most important sites of CV events.[1,2] Aortic, but not brachial, pulsatility has been shown to be independently associated with CAD in patients undergoing coronary angiography after angioplasty.[69–72] In 409 subjects followed for 4 to 5 years by Jankowski and colleagues,[73] a 10-mm Hg aortic PP increase was associated with a corresponding 13% increase of CV events. In atherosclerotic subjects, central wave reflections were shown to be independent predictors of CAD.[74] In ESRD patients, aortic PWV and carotid wave reflections (and/or central PP) were shown to predict independently CV mortality.[1,2,74] Finally, in the same patients and in elderly subjects with essential hypertension, central PP was demonstrated to be an independent predictor of mortality.[75] Taken together, all these findings suggested that central PP was superior to brachial PP to predict coronary risk and indicated that, during long-term antihypertensive drug therapy, serial central BP determinations are required to predict CV complications.[2]

PULSATILE ARTERIAL HEMODYNAMICS AND RISK-REDUCTION STRATEGIES IN HYPERTENSION

The main therapeutic trial demonstrating the predictive role of aortic stiffness in hypertensive subjects was conducted on ESRD patients on hemodialysis.[76] The objective of that trial was to lower CV morbidity and mortality through a therapeutic regimen involving, successively, salt and water depletion by dialysis; then, after randomization,

ACE inhibition or calcium-channel blockade; and, finally, the combination of the two agents and/or their association with a beta-blocker. Using that protocol, it was possible to evaluate, over long-term follow-up (51 months), whether or not the drug-induced MAP reduction was associated with a parallel diminution of arterial stiffness impacting on CV risk. During follow-up, it was clearly shown that survivors' MAP, PP and aortic PWV were lowered in parallel. In contrast, for patients who died from CV events, MAP had been reduced to the same extent as in survivors, but neither PWV nor PP had been significantly modified by drug treatment. Thus, survival of ESRD patients was significantly better when aortic PWV declined in response to BP lowering. The adjusted relative risks for all-cause and CV mortality rates in those with unchanged PWV in response to BP changes were, respectively, 2.59 (95% CI, 1.51–4.43) and 2.35 (95% CI, 1.23–4.51) ($P < .01$). The prognostic value of PWV sensitivity to BP reduction on survival was independent of age, BP changes, and blood-chemistry abnormalities. The results indicated that arterial stiffness was not only a risk factor contributing to the development of CV disease but that it was also a marker of established, more advanced, and less reversible arterial lesions. This interpretation was supported by the loss of aortic PWV sensitivity to BP lowering for non-survivors, compared with survivors whose arterial stiffness remained responsive to BP reduction. Finally, in that trial, prolonged survival seemed to be more closely associated with the use of an ACEI than other drugs or the number of drugs per se. The use of beta-blockers and/or dihydropyridine calcium-channel blocker had no direct impact on the outcomes.[76]

The Reason study[16,77] was the first to investigate the long-term interactions among PP, arterial stiffness, and wave reflections in relationship to drug treatment and end-organ damage (cardiac mass) in hypertensive subjects. ACEI perindopril (Per), associated with low-dose indapamide (Ind) was compared for 1 year of treatment with the beta-blocking agent atenolol. For the same DBP and MAP decreases, Per/Ind lowered SBP and PP more than atenolol. The reduction was more pronounced centrally (carotid artery) than peripherally (brachial artery). Although the two drug regimens lowered PWV equally, only Per/Ind reduced the Aix.[77] In addition, Per/Ind decreased cardiac hypertrophy more than atenolol, and that diminution was attributed to Aix, indicating that the reduction of cardiac end-organ damage mainly reflected the effect on central wave reflections.[77]

The Conduit Artery Function Evaluation (CAFE) study, a subanalysis of the Anglo-Scandinavian Cardiac Outcomes Trial,[78] conducted on 2073 subjects, showed that aortic PP, recorded noninvasively by radial tonometry and the application of generalized transfer functions, is a determinant of clinical outcome, independently of age, other traditional CV risk factors, and even peripheral PP.[78] In agreement with the REASON study,[17,18] the CAFE study results showed that treating subjects with a regimen based on the beta blocker atenolol and a diuretic versus one based on the calcium-channel blocker amlodipine and an ACEI had similar effects on brachial SBP and PP but different impacts on central aortic pressures.[78] Even though brachial pressure reductions were similar for the two arms of the study, central SBP and PP decreases were greater for the perindopril (ACEI) arm. That study's results not only demonstrated that brachial PP does not always reflect the impact of different pressure-lowering treatments on central aortic pressures, but also suggested that central changes in pressure might better predict clinical outcomes other than brachial pressures.[78] Therefore, antihypertensive drug therapy should selectively lower SBP and PP through complex interactions between small and large artery effects, thereby opening the way to the development of new long-term CV-treatment strategies involving both small and large arteries.

REFERENCES

1. Nichols WW, O'Rourke M. McDonald's blood flow in arteries. Theoretical, experimental and clinical principles. 4th edition. Sydney: Arnold E; 1998. p. 54–401.
2. Safar ME, O'Rourke ME. Arterial stiffness in hypertension. In: Birkenhäger WH, Reid JL, editors. Handbook of hypertension. vol. 23. Edinburgh (UK): Elsevier; 2006. p. 3–62, 75–136, 459–501.
3. Kannel WB, Stokes JLL. Hypertension as a cardiovascular risk factor. In: Bulpitt CJ, editor. Handbook of hypertension. Epidemiology of hypertension. Amsterdam: Elsevier Science; 1985. p. 15–34.
4. Kannel WB, Gordon T, Schwartz MJ. Systolic versus diastolic blood pressure and risk of coronary disease. The Framingham study. Am J Cardiol 1971;27:335–46.
5. Safar ME. Therapeutic trials and large arteries in hypertension. Am Heart J 1988; 115:702–10.
6. Asmar R, Benetos A, London G, et al. Aortic distensibility in normotensive untreated and treated hypertensive patients. Blood Press 1995;4:48–54.
7. Black HR. The paradigm has shifted to systolic blood pressure. Hypertension 1999;34:386–7.
8. Mancia G, Seravalle G, Grassi G. Systolic blood pressure: an underestimated cardiovascular risk factor. J Hypertens 2002;20:S21–7.
9. Safar ME, Levy BI, Struijker Boudier H. Current perspectives on arterial stiffness and pulse pressure in hypertension and cardiovascular diseases. Circulation 2003;107:2864–9.
10. Caro CG, Pedley TJ, Schroter RC, et al. The mechanics of the circulation. New York: Oxford University Press; 1978. p. 243–349.
11. Safar ME, Lacolley P. Disturbance of macro- and microcirculation: relation with pulse pressure and cardiac organ damage. Am J Physiol Heart Circ Physiol 2007;293:H1–7.
12. Levy BI, Ambrosio G, Pries AR, et al. Microcirculation in hypertension. A new target for treatment? Circulation 2001;104:735–40.
13. Langille BL. Remodeling of developing and mature arteries: endothelium, smooth muscles, and matrix. J Cardiovasc Pharmacol 1993;21(suppl I):S11–7.
14. Kamiya A, Togowa T. Adaptative regulation of wall shear stress to flow change in the carotid artery. Am J Physiol 1980;239:H14–21.
15. Gibbons GH, Dzau VJ. The emerging concept of vascular remodeling. N Engl J Med 1994;330:1431–8.
16. London GM, Asmar RG, O'Rourke MF, et al. on behalf of the REASON Project Investigators. Mechanism(s) of selective systolic blood pressure reduction after a low-dose combination of perindopril/indapamide in hypertensive subjects: comparison with atenolol. J Am Coll Cardiol 2004;43:92–9.
17. Williams B. Mechanical influences on vascular smooth muscle cell function. J Hypertens 1998;16:1921–9.
18. Safar ME, Rizzoni D, Blacher J, et al. Macro and microvasculature in hypertension: therapeutic aspects. J Hum Hypertens 2008;22:590–5.
19. Glagov S. Hemodynamic risk factors: mechanical stress, mural architecture, medial nutrition and vulnerability of arteries to atherosclerosis. In: Wissler RW, Geer JC, editors. The pathogenesis of atherosclerosis. Baltimore (MD): Williams and Wilkins; 1972. p. 164–99.
20. Hishikawa K, Oemar BS, Yang Z, et al. Pulsatile stretch stimulates superoxide production and activates nuclear factor-kappa B in human coronary smooth muscle. Circ Res 1997;81:797–803.

21. Lehoux S, Tedgui A. Cellular mechanics and gene expression in blood vessels. J Biomech 2003;36:631–43.
22. Chien S, Li S, Shyy YJ. Effects of mechanical forces on signal transduction and gene expression in endothelial cells. Hypertension 1998;31:162–9.
23. Lehoux S, Esposito B, Merval R, et al. Pulsatile stretch-induced extracellular signal-regulated kinase 1/2 activation in organ culture of rabbit aorta involves reactive oxygen species. Arterioscler Thromb Vasc Biol 2000;20:2366–72.
24. Lehoux S, Esposito B, Merval R, et al. Differential regulation of vascular focal adhesion kinase by steady stretch and pulsatility. Circulation 2005;111:643–9.
25. Lee RT. Functional genomics and cardiovascular drug discovery. Circulation 2001;104:1441–6.
26. Bezie Y, Lamaziere JM, Laurent S, et al. Fibronectin expression and aortic wall elastic modulus in spontaneously hypertensive rats. Arterioscler Thromb Vasc Biol 1998;18:1027–34.
27. Susic D, Varagic J, Ahn J, et al. Crosslink breakers: a new approach to cardiovascular therapy. Curr Opin Cardiol 2004;19:336–40.
28. Bevan JA. Flow regulation of vascular tone. Its sensitivity to changes in sodium and calcium. Hypertension 1993;22:273–81.
29. Et-Taouil K, Schiavi P, Levy BI, et al. Sodium intake, large artery stiffness and proteoglycans in the SHR. Hypertension 2001;38:1172–6.
30. Gildner CD, Lerner AL, Hocking DC. Fibronectin matrix polymerization increases tensile strength of model tissue. Am J Physiol Heart Circ Physiol 2004;287:H46–53.
31. Labat C, Lacolley P, Lajemi M, et al. Effects of valsartan on mechanical properties of the carotid artery in spontaneously hypertensive rats under high-salt diet. Hypertension 2001;38:439–43.
32. Lacolley P, Labat C, Pujol A, et al. Increased carotid wall elastic modulus and fibronectin in aldosterone-salt-treated rats: effects of eplerenone. Circulation 2002;106:2848–53.
33. Darné B, Girerd X, Safar M, et al. Pulsatile versus steady component of blood pressure: a cross-sectional analysis and a prospective analysis on cardiovascular mortality. Hypertension 1989;13:392–400.
34. Madhavan S, Ooi WL, Cohen H, et al. Relation of pulse pressure and blood pressure reduction to the incidence of myocardial infarction. Hypertension 1994;23:395–401.
35. Fang J, Madhavan S, Cohen H, et al. Measures of blood pressure and myocardial infarction in treated hypertensive patients. J Hypertens 1995;13:413–9.
36. Verdecchia P, Schillaci G, Borgioni C, et al. Ambulatory pulse pressure. A potent predictor of total cardiovascular risk in hypertension. Hypertension 1998;32:983–8.
37. Franklin SS, Khan SA, Wong ND, et al. Is pulse pressure useful in predicting risk for coronary heart disease? The Framingham heart study. Circulation 1999;100:354–60.
38. Millar JA, Lever AF, Burke V. Pulse pressure as a risk factor for cardiovascular events in the MRC mild hypertension trial. J Hypertens 1999;17:1065–72.
39. Blacher J, Staessen JA, Girerd X, et al. Pulse pressure not mean pressure determines cardiovascular risk in older hypertensive patients. Arch Intern Med 2000;160:1085–9.
40. Domanski MJ, Davis BR, Pfeffer MA, et al. Isolated systolic hypertension, prognostic information provided by pulse pressure. Hypertension 1999;34:375–80.

41. Benetos A, Zureik M, Morcet J, et al. A decrease in diastolic blood pressure combined with an increase in systolic blood pressure is associated with high cardiovascular mortality. J Am Coll Cardiol 2000;35:673–80.
42. Mitchell GF, Moye LA, Braunwald E, et al. Sphygmomanometrically determined pulse pressure is a powerful independent predictor of recurrent events after myocardial infarction in patients with impaired left ventricular function. Circulation 1997;96:4254–60.
43. Chae CU, Pfeffer MA, Glynn RJ, et al. Increased pulse pressure and risk of heart failure in the elderly. JAMA 1999;281:634–9.
44. Domanski MJ, Mitchell GF, Norman JE, et al. Independent prognostic information provided by sphygmomanometrically determined pulse pressure and mean arterial pressure in patients with left ventricular dysfunction. J Am Coll Cardiol 1999; 33:951–8.
45. Haider AW, Larson MG, Franklin SS, et al. Systolic blood pressure, diastolic blood pressure, and pulse pressure as predictors of risk for congestive heart failure in the Framingham Heart Study. Ann Intern Med 2003;138:10–6.
46. Klassen PS, Lowrie EG, Reddan DN, et al. Association between pulse pressure and mortality in patients undergoing hemodialysis. JAMA 2002;287:1548–55.
47. Schram MT, Kostense PJ, van Dijk RA, et al. Diabetes, pulse pressure and cardiovascular mortality: the Hoorn Study. J Hypertens 2002;20:1743–51.
48. Booth AD, Wallace S, McEniery CM, et al. Inflammation and arterial stiffness in systemic vasculitis: a model of vascular inflammation. Arthritis Rheum 2004;50: 3398–9.
49. Benetos A, Safar M, Rudnichi A, et al. Pulse pressure: a predictor of long-term cardiovascular mortality in a French male population. Hypertension 1997;30:1410–5.
50. Benetos A, Rudnichi A, Safar M, et al. Pulse pressure and cardiovascular mortality in normotensive and hypertensive subjects. Hypertension 1998;32:560–4.
51. Alderman MH, Cohen H, Madhavan S. Distribution and determinants of cardiovascular events during 20 years of successful antihypertensive treatment. J Hypertens 1998;16:761–9.
52. Somes GW, Pahor M, Shorr RI, et al. The role of diastolic blood pressure when treating isolated systolic hypertension. Arch Intern Med 1999;159:2004–9.
53. Greenberg J. Antihypertensive treatment alters the predictive strength of pulse pressure and other blood pressure measures. Am J Hypertens 2005;18:1033–9.
54. Blacher J, Guérin A, Pannier B, et al. Impact of aortic stiffness on survival in end-stage renal failure. Circulation 1999;99:2434–9.
55. Blacher J, Pannier B, Guérin A, et al. Carotid arterial stiffness as a predictor of cardiovascular and all-cause mortality in end-stage renal disease. Hypertension 1998;32:570–4.
56. London G, Blacher J, Pannier B, et al. Arterial wave reflections and survival in end-stage renal failure. Hypertension 2001;38:434–8.
57. Shoji T, Emoto M, Shinohara K, et al. Diabetes mellitus, aortic stiffness, and cardiovascular mortality in end-stage renal disease. J Am Soc Nephrol 2001; 12:2117–24.
58. Barenbrock M, Kosch M, Jöster E, et al. Reduced arterial distensibility is a predictor of cardiovascular disease in patients after renal transplantation. J Hypertens 2002;20:79–84.
59. Anderson KM, Odell PM, Wilson PWF, et al. Cardiovascular disease risk profiles. Am Heart J 1991;121:293–8.
60. Blacher J, Asmar R, Djane S, et al. Aortic pulse wave velocity as a marker of cardiovascular risk in hypertensive patients. Hypertension 1999;33:1111–7.

61. Laurent S, Boutouyrie P, Asmar R, et al. Aortic stiffness is an independent predictor of all-cause and cardiovascular mortality in hypertensive patients. Hypertension 2001;37:1236–41.
62. Meaume S, Benetos A, Henry OF, et al. Aortic pulse wave velocity predicts cardiovascular mortality in subjects > 70 years of age. Arterioscler Thromb Vasc Biol 2001;21:2046–50.
63. Willum-Hansen T, Staessen JA, Torp-Pedersen C, et al. Prognostic value of aortic pulse wave velocity as index of arterial stiffness in the general population. Circulation 2006;113:664–70.
64. Mattace-Raso FUS, van der Cammen TJM, Hofman A, et al. Arterial stiffness and risk of coronary heart disease and stroke: the Rotterdam Study. Circulation 2006; 113:657–63.
65. Tedesco MA, Natale F, Di Salvo G, et al. Effects of coexisting hypertension and type II diabetes mellitus on arterial stiffness. J Hum Hypertens 2004;18:469–73.
66. Cruickshank K, Riste L, Anderson SG, et al. Aortic pulse-wave velocity and its relationship to mortality in diabetes and glucose intolerance: an integrated index of vascular function? Circulation 2002;106:2085–90.
67. Hirai T, Sasayama S, Kawasaki T, et al. Stiffness of systemic arteries in patients with myocardial infarction. A noninvasive method to predict severity of coronary atherosclerosis. Circulation 1989;80:78–86.
68. Gatzka CD, Cameron JD, Kingwell BA, et al. Relation between coronary artery disease, aortic stiffness, and left ventricular structure in a population sample. Hypertension 1998;32:575–8.
69. Stefanadis C, Wooley CF, Bush CA, et al. Aortic distensibility abnormalities in coronary artery disease. Am J Cardiol 1987;59:1300–4.
70. Nishijima T, Nakayama Y, Tsumura K, et al. Pulsatility of ascending aortic blood pressure waveform is associated with an increased risk of coronary heart disease. Am J Hypertens 2001;14:469–73.
71. Nakayama Y, Tsumura K, Yamashita N, et al. Pulsatility of ascending aortic pressure waveform is a powerful predictor of restenosis after percutaneous transluminal coronary angioplasty. Circulation 2000;101:470–2.
72. Philippe F, Chemaly E, Blacher J, et al. Aortic pulse pressure and extent of coronary artery disease in percutaneous transluminal coronary angioplasty candidates. Am J Hypertens 2002;15:672–7.
73. Jankowski P, Kawecka-Jaszcz K, Czarnecka D, et al. Pulsatile but not steady component of blood pressure predicts cardiovascular events in coronary patients. Hypertension 2008;51:848–55.
74. Weber T, Auer J, O'Rourke MF, et al. Arterial stiffness, wave reflections, and the risk of coronary artery disease. Circulation 2004;109:184–9.
75. Safar ME, Blacher J, Pannier B, et al. Central pulse pressure and mortality in end-stage renal disease. Hypertension 2002;39:735–8.
76. Guérin A, Blacher J, Pannier B, et al. Impact of aortic stiffness attenuation on survival of patients in end-stage renal disease. Circulation 2001;103:987–92.
77. de Luca N, Asmar RG, London GM, et al. REASON Project Investigators. Selective reduction of cardiac mass and central blood pressure on low-dose combination perindopril/indapamide in hypertensive subjects. J Hypertens 2004;22:1623–30.
78. Williams B, Lacy PS, Thom SM, et al. CAFE Investigators, Anglo-Scandinavian Cardiac Outcomes Trial Investigators, CAFE Steering Committee and Writing Committee. Differential impact of blood pressure-lowering drugs on central aortic pressure and clinical outcomes: principal results of the Conduit Artery Function Evaluation (CAFE) study. Circulation 2006;113:1213–25.

Oxidative Stress and Hypertension

David G. Harrison, MD*, Maria Carolina Gongora, MD

KEYWORDS

- Blood pressure • Superoxide • Sympathetic
- Angiotensin II • NADPH oxidase • Sodium
- Inflammation

Reactive oxygen species (ROS) are metabolites of oxygen that can either strip electrons away from other molecules (oxidize), donate electrons to molecules (reduce), or react with and become part of molecules (ie, oxidative modification). Many ROS possess an unpaired electron in their outer orbital and are, therefore, radicals. A particularly important radical for cardiovascular biology is superoxide ($O_2^{\cdot-}$), which is formed by the one-electron reduction of oxygen (**Fig. 1**). $O_2^{\cdot-}$ is important because it can serve as both an oxidant and as a reductant in biologic systems and is a progenitor for other ROS. Other radicals include the hydroxyl radical ($HO^{\cdot}$), lipid peroxy- ($LOO^{\cdot}$) radical, and alkoxy- radicals ($LO^{\cdot}$). Other molecules, including peroxynitrite ($ONOO^-$), hypochlorous acid ($HOCl^-$), and hydrogen peroxide (H_2O_2) are not radicals but have strong oxidant properties and are, therefore, included as ROS. Another relevant group of molecules are the reactive nitrogen species (RNS) including nitric oxide (NO), the nitrogen dioxide radical (NO_2), and the nitrosonium cation (NO^+). Peroxynitrite is considered both an ROS and RNS and is formed by the near diffusion-limited reaction between $O_2^{\cdot-}$ and NO. RNS are important, because they often react with and modify proteins and other cellular structures and alter function of these targets. The topic of ROS and protective mechanisms has been discussed in depth elsewhere.[1]

Although originally considered toxic by-products of cellular metabolism, both ROS and RNS are now recognized to have signaling roles that are important for normal cell function, including growth, migration, apoptosis, and remodeling. An interesting recent example is that H_2O_2 has been implicated as an endothelium-derived hyperpolarizing factor important for maintenance of vascular tone.[2] Various ROS, including H_2O_2, stimulate cellular proliferation and migration.[3] These events are important in development in utero, growth of new vessels in the adult animal, and wound repair.

Supported by NIH grants R01 HL390006, P01 HL58000, and P01 HL075209 and a Department of Veterans Affairs Merit Review Grant.

Division of Cardiology, Department of Medicine, Emory University School of Medicine and the Atlanta Veterans Administration Hospital, Room 319 WMRB, Atlanta, GA 30322, USA

* Corresponding author.

E-mail address: dharr02@emory.edu (D.G. Harrison).

Med Clin N Am 93 (2009) 621–635
doi:10.1016/j.mcna.2009.02.015
0025-7125/09/$ – see front matter. Published by Elsevier Inc.

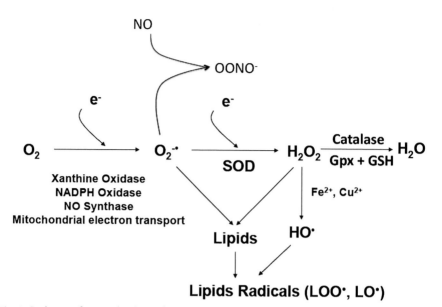

Fig. 1. Pathways for production of ROS in mammalian cells. Shown are enzymes thought important in hypertension, which can donate electrons to oxygen to form $O_2^{·-}$. A 2-electron of oxygen can form H_2O_2. H_2O_2 can also be formed by the action of (SOD) on $O_2^{·-}$ and is further reduced to water by either catalase or glutathione peroxidases (Gpx). $O_2^{·-}$ and H_2O_2 can undergo reactions with transition metals to form OH. ROS can react with lipids to form biologically active lipid radicals. Gpx, glutathione peroxidases; H_2O_2, hydrogen peroxide; OH, hydroxyl radical; SOD, superoxide dismutase.

The normal inflammatory response that permits rejection of foreign organisms is greatly dependent on ROS. Thus, ROS represent a component of the innate immune system, and they are not only involved in the respiratory burst of neutrophils but also signal inflammatory cell chemotaxis into sites of inflammation.[4] These responses, which are important for health, become exaggerated in disease states and contribute to pathologic processes.

In cardiovascular organs, the most relevant enzyme systems that produce ROS are the nicotinamide adenine dinucleotide phosphate (NADPH) oxidases, the mitochondria, xanthine oxidase, and, under certain conditions, the nitric oxide synthases (see **Fig. 1**).[5] There are numerous examples of these enzymes being activated in a variety of disease states, including atherosclerosis, hypertension, diabetes, and renal disease. Angiotensin II is well known to activate the NADPH oxidase via its action on the AT_1 receptor, and many of the pathophysiological effects of angiotensin II have at least in part been attributed to promotion of oxidative stress via this mechanism.[6]

Importantly, there is a great deal of interaction between these various enzyme systems, such that the ROS produced by one enzyme can activate others. As an example, peroxynitrite can oxidize the critical co-factor for nitric oxide synthase, tetrahydrobiopterin, which leads to a condition known as nitric oxide synthase (NOS) uncoupling, in which the nitric oxide synthases produce $O_2^{·-}$ rather than nitric oxide.[7,8]

In addition to ROS-forming enzymes, mammalian cells produce myriad molecules and enzymes that remove ROS. Some of these are small molecules, such as the thiol-containing tripeptide glutathione. Others are enzymes that catalyze removal of

ROS, such as the superoxide dismutases (SODs), which catalyze dismutation of $O_2^{\cdot-}$ to H_2O_2 and water; catalase, which converts H_2O_2 to oxygen and water; the glutathione peroxidases, which use H_2O_2 and glutathione as co-substrates to form water and glutathione disulfide; thioredoxin; and others. These have been extensively reviewed elsewhere.[9]

GENERAL CONSIDERATIONS REGARDING REACTIVE OXYGEN SPECIES IN DISEASE

Although there is an enormous amount of basic information supporting a role of ROS in various animal models of disease, it has been difficult to prove a role of these molecules in human disease. In particular, antioxidant trials, using large amounts of vitamin E, vitamin C, or combinations of antioxidants, have failed to show a beneficial effect in a variety of diseases. Surprisingly, high-dose vitamin E has worsened cardiovascular outcomes in some studies.[10,11] In hypertensive humans, although a few small studies have shown benefit,[12,13] larger trials have failed to confirm an effect of antioxidant vitamins on either the development or control of blood pressure.[14,15]

The results of these clinical trials have raised questions and doubt about the oxidation theory of disease. One clear message is that, as mentioned here, the role of ROS is far more complex than simply one of causing pathology. As can be gleaned from the following discussion, these molecules have essential functions, without which survival is impossible. Thus, the notion that removal of these is always beneficial is clearly incorrect. Therefore, the reader is urged to consider this article in terms of understanding how ROS and oxidative events affect both normal and pathophysiological functions in various organs associated with hypertension rather than viewing this as describing only deleterious effects of these molecules.

ROLE OF REACTIVE OXYGEN SPECIES IN HYPERTENSION

A large body of literature has shown that excessive production of ROS contributes to hypertension and that scavenging of ROS decreases blood pressure. In an initial study, Nakazono and colleagues[16] showed that bolus administration of a modified form of SOD acutely lowered blood pressure in hypertensive rats. Membrane-targeted forms of SOD and SOD mimetics such as tempol lower blood pressure and decrease renovascular resistance in hypertensive animal models.[17–21] There is ample evidence suggesting that ROS not only contribute to hypertension but that the NADPH oxidase is their major source. Components of this enzyme system are up-regulated by hypertensive stimuli, and NADPH oxidase enzyme activity is increased by these same stimuli. Moreover, both angiotensin II-induced hypertension and deoxycorticosterone acetate (DOCA)-salt hypertension are blunted in mice lacking this enzyme.[22,23]

Despite the substantial evidence that oxidative stress contributes to hypertension, there is not a clear understanding of exactly how this happens. Hypertension is associated with increased ROS formation in multiple organs, including the brain, the vasculature, and the kidney, all of which could contribute to hypertension. A major problem is that we currently lack a complete understanding of which of these organs or cell types predominate in the genesis of hypertension or if there is important interplay between them that causes this disease. In this review, we discuss the evidence that hypertension is associated with oxidative stress that occurs in the central nervous system (CNS), the kidney, and the vasculature and attempt to provide evidence for how this contributes to hypertension. Finally, we show recent data suggesting that the adaptive immune system can contribute to hypertension by interacting with these organs.

REACTIVE OXYGEN SPECIES, THE KIDNEY, AND HYPERTENSION

There is ample evidence that hypertension increases oxidative stress in the kidney and that this in turn augments blood pressure elevations. Virtually all cells in the kidney, including vessels, glomeruli, podocytes, interstitial fibroblasts, the medullary thick ascending limb (mTAL), the macula densa, the distal tubule, and the collecting duct express components of the NADPH oxidase,[24] and various stimuli have been shown to activate these. Some of the documented effects of ROS in the kidney are summarized in **Fig. 2**. For purposes of discussion, we first focus on oxidative events in the renal cortex and then in the medulla.

Several studies have examined the effect of various hypertensive stimuli on the renal cortex and how these are modulated by ROS. The structures that are targets of oxidant stress include the afferent arteriole, the glomerulus, the proximal tubule, and the cortical collecting duct. As with other vessels, an increase in $O_2{}^{\cdot-}$ in the afferent arteriole can oxidatively degrade NO, which could enhance afferent arteriolar vasoconstriction and reduce glomerular filtration rate (GFR). Indeed, studies in rabbits have shown that angiotensin II-induced hypertension increases expression of the

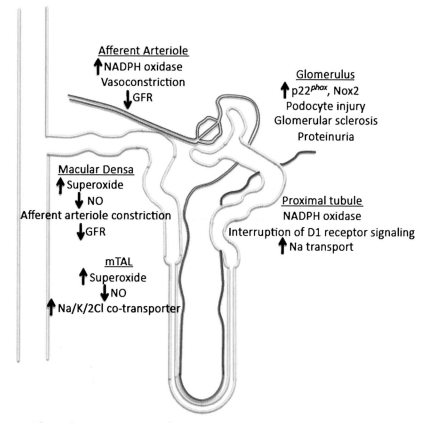

Fig. 2. Schematic representation of a juxtamedullary glomerulus showing sites of ROS production and potential roles in sodium transport, reabsorption, and blood pressure regulation. D1, Dopamine type 1 receptor; GFR, glomerular filtration rate; mTAL, medullary thick ascending limb; Na, sodium; NO, nitric oxide.

NADPH oxidase subunit p22^{phox}, activates the NADPH oxidase, and causes endothelial dysfunction in afferent arterioles.[25] Studies of isolated afferent arterioles have also shown that $O_2^{\cdot-}$ generated by the NADPH oxidase potentiates intracellular calcium.[26] The beneficial effects of $O_2^{\cdot-}$ scavenging in hypertensive animals have, at least in part, been attributed to alleviation of renal vasoconstriction and improved renal perfusion.[27]

Podocyte injury, a precursor to proteinuria, is evident early after salt loading in Dahl salt-sensitive rats and is reversed by aldosterone blockade but not by an equi-hypotensive dose of hydralazine. There is up-regulation of glomerular p22^{phox} and Nox2 in the glomeruli of these animals.[28] The antioxidant tempol reduces glomerular sclerosis and proteinuria in Dahl salt-sensitive rats, further supporting a role for ROS in glomerular injury.[29]

Cells of the proximal tubule also contain components of the NADPH oxidase, particularly in lipid rafts, where they are maintained in an inactive state. Dopamine-1 (D1) receptor agonists inhibit, whereas disruption of lipid rafts and angiotensin II stimulates the proximal tubule NADPH oxidase.[30,31] An important role of ROS and the NADPH oxidase in the proximal tubule is modulation of sodium transport via altering Na/K ATPase and Na/H exchange function on the basal and apical membranes of the proximal tubular cells, respectively.[30,32,33] Sodium transport is stimulated by angiotensin II and inhibited by Dopamine, and oxidant stress enhances the effect of angiotensin II and disrupts dopamine signaling, thus increasing proximal tubular sodium transport.[32,33] The question of how proximal tubular cells are affected by ROS, nitric oxide, and comorbid conditions in hypertension is a subject of substantial recent investigation.[34]

One of the important mechanisms in which ROS in the cortex could modulate sodium handling and ultimately blood pressure is by affecting tubuloglomerular feedback. This is a phenomenon mediated by the interaction of the macula densa of the thick ascending limb as it makes contact with its own glomerulus in the cortex. The macula densa senses sodium concentration in the proximal tubule via its apical Na/K/2Cl co-transporter, which in turn stimulates signaling molecules, one of which is NO produced by the neuronal nitric oxide synthase. This dilates afferent arterioles and increases glomerular filtration.[35,36] An increase in $O_2^{\cdot-}$ within or in the vicinity of the macula densa could inactivate NO, leading to afferent arteriolar vasoconstriction and a reduction of GFR.[37] In this regard, an elegant study of isolated, single nephrons by Nouri and colleagues showed that in vivo silencing RNA deletion of the NADPH oxidase subunit p22^{phox} enhanced single tubular glomerular filtration in angiotensin II-treated rats but not in control rats. By either including or excluding the distal tubule, these authors showed that this effect was likely mediated by ROS produced in the macula densa.[38]

There is ample evidence linking oxidative stress in the renal medulla with sodium reabsorption and modulation of blood pressure. As in the blood vessel, there is a balance between $O_2^{\cdot-}$ and NO produced by cells within the medulla, including the epithelial cells of the mTAL and the pericytes of the vasa recta. Comparison studies indicate that there is markedly more NO synthase activity in the renal medulla compared with that in the cortex.[39] This likely contributes to independent regulation of medullary and cortical perfusion. Elegant studies by Cowley's group have shown that cells of the mTAL release NO that diffuses to nearby pericytes of the adjacent vasa recta to promote dilation of these vessels.[40,41] This increases medullary flow, and by increasing interstitial Starling forces, promotes sodium movement to the tubule and thus natriuresis and diuresis. Inhibition of NO synthase in the medulla with L-Nitro-arginine methyl ester markedly reduces medullary perfusion and promotes sodium reabsorption without changing cortical flow.[42] As discussed earlier, all of the components of the NADPH oxidase are present in the renal medulla and can be activated by either systemic or locally produced angiotensin II.[43] The consequent increase in medullary $O_2{}^{\cdot-}$ leads to vasoconstriction of the vasa recta and reduces Starling forces such that sodium movement into the vasa recta is favored, reducing natriuresis and increasing blood pressure. Another important mechanism whereby medullary $O_2{}^{\cdot-}$ could affect renal sodium relates to changes in medullary sodium transport.[44] Direct exposure of mTAL preparations to $O_2{}^{\cdot-}$ enhance Na/K/2Cl cotransporter activity via a protein kinase C activation.[45] Infusion of angiotensin II in vivo mimics this effect and is prevented by administration of the $O_2{}^{\cdot-}$ scavenger tempol.[46]

These considerations regarding the role of ROS in the control of renal function emphasize an important function of these molecules in that they seem to play a critical role in normal renal physiology and are not simply mediators of pathophysiological events. The ability of the kidney to retain sodium and water during times of salt restriction is an extremely important function in land-dwelling mammals, without which survival would be impossible. It is likely that $O_2{}^{\cdot-}$ and other ROS are generated as needed to modulate sodium balance.

REACTIVE OXYGEN SPECIES, THE CENTRAL NERVOUS SYSTEM, AND HYPERTENSION

It is well established that the CNS is necessary for the production and maintenance of most forms of experimental hypertension, principally by sympathetic efferent nerves, and that even the action of hormones, such as angiotensin II and aldosterone, which have myriad systemic effects, causes hypertension via action on central sites.[47] The most compelling evidence supporting this is that destruction of a region of the forebrain surrounding the anteroventral third cerebral ventricle (AV3-V) prevents development of many forms of experimentally induced hypertension in rodents.[48,49] This region of the forebrain includes the median preoptic eminence, the organum vasculosum of the lateral terminalis, and the preoptic periventricular nucleus (**Fig. 3**).[50] Following disruption of this region of the brain, virtually all of the central actions of

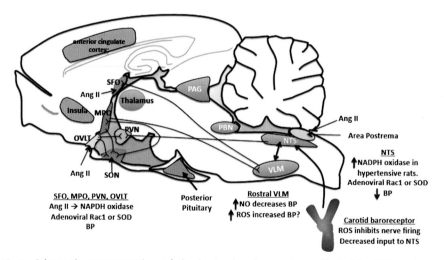

Fig. 3. Schematic representation of the brain showing centers affected by ROS that are thought to participate in hypertension. NTS, nucleus tractis solitarius; OVLT, organum vasculosum lateral terminalis; PAG, periaquaductal gray; PBN, parabrachial nucleus; PVN, paraventricular nucleus; SFO, subfornical organ; VLM, ventral lateral medulla; MPO, median preoptic eminence.

angiotensin II, including drinking behavior, vasopressin secretion, and increased sympathetic outflow, are abrogated.[51] These portions of the brain are also reciprocally connected to other regions involved in central cardiovascular regulation. Important among these is the subfornical organ (SFO), a circumventricular organ (CVO) lacking a blood-brain barrier, allowing peripheral hormonal signals sent to the AV3-V to be translated into increased sympathetic outflow and hypertension.[49] This region also communicates with other important cardiovascular control centers in the mid- and hindbrain, including the parabrachial nucleus, the nucleus tractus solitarii (NTS) and the rostral ventral lateral medulla (VLM) (see **Fig. 3**).

In the past several years, a convincing body of evidence has emerged suggesting that signaling in these brain centers is modulated by local production of ROS and can contribute to hypertension.[52] As an example, intracerebroventricular (ICV) injection of an adenovirus encoding SOD markedly attenuates the hypertension caused by either local injection or systemic infusion of angiotensin II.[53,54] Zimmerman and colleagues[55] have shown that angiotensin II increases $O_2^{·-}$ production and intracellular calcium in cultured neurons. An important regulator of the NADPH oxidase is the small G protein Rac-1, and these investigators showed that the increase in neuronal intracellular calcium caused by angiotensin II was blocked by a dominant negative form of Rac-1 and also by SOD.[55] Moreover, these investigators have also shown that dominant negative Rac1 gene transfer in the CNS prevents hypertension caused by angiotensin II.[56]

As mentioned here, projections from the CVO interact with centers in the hypothalamus. There is evidence that ROS derived from the NADPH oxidase enhances nerve traffic in this region. Erdos and colleagues[57] have shown that ICV injection of angiotensin II increases NADPH oxidase-mediated $O_2^{·-}$ production not only in the SFO but also in anterior hypothalamic nuclei such as the median preoptic eminence and in the paraventricular nucleus of the hypothalamus. These effects were blocked by the NADPH oxidase inhibitor apocynin as were the hemodynamic effects of centrally administered angiotensin II. Thus, angiotensin II and its effects on the NADPH oxidase seem to coordinate activation of several forebrain centers to promote a hypertensive response.

There is also important signaling between the forebrain and pontomedullary cardiovascular control centers in the hindbrain. An important nucleus in the hindbrain that regulates blood pressure is the NTS, which receives input from the CVO and relays inhibitory stimuli from baroreceptors. Angiotensin II inhibits the negative feedback from the baroreceptors to the NTS.[58] In studies of neurons from the NTS, angiotensin II has been shown to augment L-type calcium channel activity via ROS generated by the NADPH oxidase.[59] Nozoe and colleagues showed that the activities of NADPH oxidase and Rac1 are increased in the NTS of stroke-prone, spontaneously hypertensive rats. These investigators further showed that injection of an adenovirus that inhibits Rac-1 or an adenovirus to increase SOD into the NTS reduced blood pressure, heart rate, urinary norepinephrine, and a marker of oxidative stress in these animals.[60] This elegant study provides strong evidence for oxidative stress in the NTS in this model of hypertension.

An important consequence of increased $O_2^{·-}$ production is a loss of NO, which has a critical role in the central regulation of blood pressure. A site that has been studied in this regard is the ventral lateral medulla (VLM). The VLM lies below the NTS and both receives and sends signals to the NTS and, as a result, importantly regulates cardiovascular sympathetic tone.[61] Experimental interventions that increase NO in the rostral VLM lower blood pressure, whereas increases in oxidative stress in this region raises blood pressure.[62,63]

There is also evidence that ROS modulate baroreflex function, which is routinely abnormal in the setting of chronic hypertension. Normally, an increase in blood pressure activates the carotid baroreflex, resulting in bradycardia and sympathetic withdrawal. This response is blunted in chronic hypertension, a phenomenon referred to as baroreflex resetting. Elegant studies by Li and colleagues[64] have shown that ROS generated in the carotid bulb of atherosclerotic rabbits reduce carotid sinus nerve responses to elevations of pressure and that this could be mimicked by exogenous administration of ROS and prevented by ROS scavenging.

REACTIVE OXYGEN SPECIES, THE VASCULATURE, AND HYPERTENSION

Perhaps the most studied target of oxidative injury in hypertension is the vasculature. The major source of $O_2{}^{·-}$ in vessels is the NADPH oxidase,[65,66] and the seminal demonstration that angiotensin II could stimulate the NADPH oxidase was first made in cultured vascular smooth muscle cells[67] and confirmed in vessels of angiotensin II-infused rats.[68] Hypertension of many etiologies increases vascular production of ROS in all layers of the vessel wall. The NADPH oxidase and uncoupled nitric oxide synthase are major sources of ROS in vessels of hypertensive animals.[22,69]

Increased vascular $O_2{}^{·-}$ production is in large part responsible for reducing endothelium-dependent vasodilatation. Scavenging of $O_2{}^{·-}$ with membrane-targeted forms of SOD or SOD mimetics markedly improves endothelium-dependent vasodilatation in vessels from hypertensive animals, whereas having minimal effects in normal vessels.[68,70] In keeping with this, genetic deletions of SOD isoforms impair endothelium-dependent vasodilatation in nonhypertensive animals.[71,72] In human studies, intra-arterial administration of large amounts of vitamin C improves the vasodilatation caused by acetylcholine.[73]

At first glance, it is compelling to speculate that the increase in vascular $O_2{}^{·-}$ is the key to causing hypertension. The concomitant loss of bioavailable NO could reduce vasodilatation, increase vasoconstriction, and cause an increase in systemic vascular resistance. Assuming that cardiac output is unchanged (the usual situation in hypertension), this increase in systemic vascular resistance would lead to hypertension. Despite the attractiveness of this scenario, a major argument against this is that experimental models of diabetes and hypercholesterolemia severely alter endothelium-dependent vasodilatation; however, they do not generally cause hypertension in the absence of other stimuli. It is quite likely that the increase in vascular $O_2{}^{·-}$ enhances vascular lesion formation and might, therefore, help explain the common occurrence of atherosclerosis and hypertension.

An important consequence of vascular ROS formation is vascular smooth muscle hypertrophy (**Fig. 4**). In particular, H_2O_2 has been implicated in the hypertrophic effect of angiotensin II in cultured cells,[74] and vascular smooth muscle hypertrophy is strikingly increased in mice overexpressing NADPH oxidase in the vascular smooth muscle.[75] The hypertrophic response of vascular smooth muscle is a critical component of vascular remodeling in hypertension. More than half a century ago, Folkow suggested that structural changes such as these in resistance vessels could add to the increased systemic vascular resistance that occurs in established hypertension and, therefore, worsen the disease.[76]

A common cause of hypertension, particularly in the elderly, is an increase in vascular stiffness, which alters pulse wave contour and augments systolic pressure. The secretion of collagen by vascular smooth muscle is increased by ROS,[77,78] and inhibition of the NADPH oxidase reduces aldosterone-induced vascular collagen deposition in experimental animals.[79] This effect of ROS has not been extensively studied.

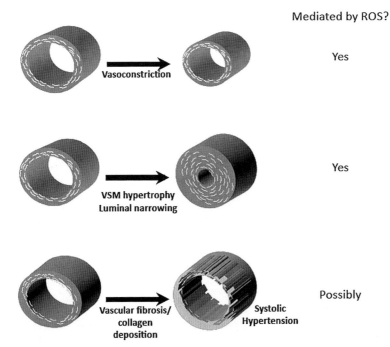

Fig. 4. Vascular effects of ROS contributing to hypertension.

REACTIVE OXYGEN SPECIES, INFLAMMATION, AND HYPERTENSION

Diverse stimuli common to the hypertensive milieu, including angiotensin II, aldosterone, catecholamines, increased vascular stretch, and endothelin, promote ROS production, which then increases expression of proinflammatory molecules that cause rolling, adhesion, and transcytosis of inflammatory cells.[80–82] As a result, there is a striking accumulation of inflammatory cells in the vessel and kidney.[83–85] In keeping with this, there is an increase in plasma markers of inflammation in hypertensive humans.[86,87]

Although macrophages are commonly considered important in the genesis of cardiovascular disease, increasing evidence has accumulated suggesting that the adaptive immune response and, in particular, T lymphocytes are important in atherosclerosis and hypertension. Recent studies from our own laboratory have emphasized a role of T cells in the genesis of hypertension.[88] We found that RAG-1$^{-/-}$ mice, that lack both T and B cells, have markedly blunted hypertensive responses to angiotensin II and DOCA-salt challenges, and that these are normalized by restoring T cells, but not B cells, to these animals. Moreover, the increase in vascular $O_2{}^{\cdot-}$ and altered endothelium-dependent vasodilatation seems dependent on T cells. These studies show that angiotensin II stimulates accumulation of effector-like T cells in the perivascular fat, and we hypothesize that these cells release cytokines that cause vascular and renal dysfunction, promoting hypertension.

The observation that a circulating cell, such as the T cell, is important in the genesis of hypertension might help provide a unifying link between oxidative events in the CNS, the vasculature, and the kidney. These interactions, illustrated in **Fig. 5**, are dependent on activation of the NADPH oxidase in all of these sites. Centrally, in the

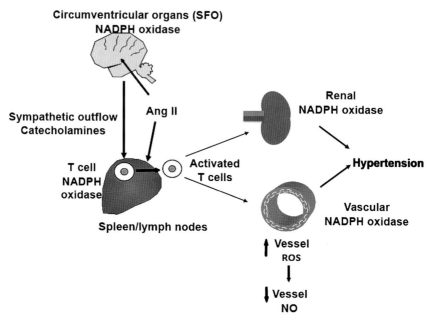

Fig. 5. Proposed role of T cells in the genesis of hypertension and the role of the NADPH oxidase in multiple cells/organs in modulating this effect. In this scenario, angiotensin II stimulates an NADPH oxidase in the CVOs of the brain, increasing sympathetic outflow. Sympathetic nerve terminals in lymph nodes activate T cells, and angiotensin II also directly activates T cells. These stimuli also activate expression of homing signals in the vessel and likely the kidney, which attract T cells to these organs. T cells release cytokines that stimulate the vessel and kidney NADPH oxidases, promoting vasoconstriction and sodium retention. SFO, subfornical organ.

SFO, and other CVOs, the NADPH oxidase is activated. This increases sympathetic nerve stimulation of peripheral lymphoid tissues, leading to T cell activation.[89] The NADPH oxidase is essential for T cell activation in hypertension, as T cells lacking this enzyme mediate this response in an incomplete fashion.[90] The NADPH oxidase in the kidney and vessels initiates signals that cause T cell homing and infiltration.[83] Finally, cytokines released by T cells diffuse to renal and vascular cells, promoting further NADPH oxidase activation, sodium retention, and vasoconstriction, leading to overt hypertension.

SUMMARY

This review has summarized some of the data supporting a role of ROS and oxidant stress in the genesis of hypertension. There is evidence that hypertensive stimuli, such as high salt and angiotensin II, promote the production of ROS in the brain, the kidney, and the vasculature and that each of these sites contributes either to hypertension or to the untoward sequelae of this disease. Although the NADPH oxidase in these various organs is a predominant source, other enzymes likely contribute to ROS production and signaling in these tissues. A major clinical challenge is that the routinely used antioxidants are ineffective in preventing or treating cardiovascular disease and hypertension. This is likely because these drugs are either ineffective or act in a non-targeted fashion, such that they remove not only injurious ROS but also those involved in normal cell signaling. A potentially important and relatively new direction is the concept that inflammatory cells such as T cells contribute to hypertension. Future studies are needed to understand the interaction of T cells with the CNS, the kidney, and the vasculature and how this might be interrupted to provide therapeutic benefit.

REFERENCES

1. Harrison DG, Dikalov S. Oxidative events in cell and vascular biology. In: Re RN, DiPette DJ, Schriffrin EL, et al, editors. Molecular mechanisms in hypertension. 1st edition. Abingdon (UK): Taylor & Francis Medical Books; 2006. p. 297–320.
2. Miura H, Bosnjak JJ, Ning G, et al. Role for hydrogen peroxide in flow-induced dilation of human coronary arterioles. Circ Res 2003;92(2):e31–40.
3. Lyle AN, Griendling KK. Modulation of vascular smooth muscle signaling by reactive oxygen species. Physiology (Bethesda) 2006;21:269–80.
4. Bogdan C, Rollinghoff M, Diefenbach A. Reactive oxygen and reactive nitrogen intermediates in innate and specific immunity. Curr Opin Immunol 2000;12(1): 64–76.
5. Mueller CF, Laude K, McNally JS, et al. ATVB in focus: redox mechanisms in blood vessels. Arterioscler Thromb Vasc Biol 2005;25(2):274–8.
6. Mehta PK, Griendling KK. Angiotensin II cell signaling: physiological and pathological effects in the cardiovascular system. Am J Physiol Cell Physiol 2007; 292(1):C82–97.
7. Laursen JB, Somers M, Kurz S, et al. Endothelial regulation of vasomotion in apoE-deficient mice: implications for interactions between peroxynitrite and tetrahydrobiopterin. Circulation 2001;103(9):1282–8.
8. Munzel T, Daiber A, Ullrich V, et al. Vascular consequences of endothelial nitric oxide synthase uncoupling for the activity and expression of the soluble guanylyl cyclase and the cGMP-dependent protein kinase. Arterioscler Thromb Vasc Biol 2005;25(8):1551–7.
9. Wassmann S, Wassmann K, Nickenig G. Regulation of antioxidant and oxidant enzymes in vascular cells and implications for vascular disease. Curr Hypertens Rep 2006;8(1):69–78.
10. Lonn E, Bosch J, Yusuf S, et al. Effects of long-term vitamin E supplementation on cardiovascular events and cancer: a randomized controlled trial. JAMA 2005; 293(11):1338–47.
11. Miller ER 3rd, Pastor-Barriuso R, Dalal D, et al. Meta-analysis: high-dosage vitamin E supplementation may increase all-cause mortality. Ann Intern Med 2005;142(1):37–46.
12. Duffy SJ, Gokce N, Holbrook M, et al. Treatment of hypertension with ascorbic acid. Lancet 1999;354(9195):2048–9.
13. Mullan BA, Young IS, Fee H, et al. Ascorbic acid reduces blood pressure and arterial stiffness in type 2 diabetes. Hypertension 2002;40(6):804–9.
14. Czernichow S, Bertrais S, Blacher J, et al. Effect of supplementation with antioxidants upon long-term risk of hypertension in the SU.VI.MAX study: association with plasma antioxidant levels. J Hypertens 2005;23(11):2013–8.
15. Kim MK, Sasaki S, Sasazuki S, et al. Lack of long-term effect of vitamin C supplementation on blood pressure. Hypertension 2002;40(6):797–803.
16. Nakazono K, Watanabe N, Matsuno K, et al. Does superoxide underlie the pathogenesis of hypertension? Proc Natl Acad Sci U S A 1991;88(22):10045–8.

17. Fukui T, Ishizaka N, Rajagopalan S, et al. p22phox mRNA expression and NADPH oxidase activity are increased in aortas from hypertensive rats. Circ Res 1997; 80(1):45–51.

18. Laursen JB, Rajagopalan S, Galis Z, et al. Role of superoxide in angiotensin II-induced but not catecholamine-induced hypertension. Circulation 1997;95(3): 588–93.

19. Schnackenberg CG, Welch WJ, Wilcox CS. Normalization of blood pressure and renal vascular resistance in SHR with a membrane-permeable superoxide dismutase mimetic: role of nitric oxide. Hypertension 1998;32(1):59–64.

20. Schnackenberg CG, Wilcox CS. Two-week administration of tempol attenuates both hypertension and renal excretion of 8-Iso prostaglandin f2 alpha. Hypertension 1999;33(1 Pt 2):424–8.

21. Adeagbo AS, Zhang X, Patel D, et al. Cyclo-oxygenase-2, endothelium and aortic reactivity during deoxycorticosterone acetate salt-induced hypertension. J Hypertens 2005;23(5):1025–36.

22. Landmesser U, Cai H, Dikalov S, et al. Role of p47(phox) in vascular oxidative stress and hypertension caused by angiotensin II. Hypertension 2002;40(4): 511–5.

23. Matsuno K, Yamada H, Iwata K, et al. Nox1 is involved in angiotensin II-mediated hypertension: a study in Nox1-deficient mice. Circulation 2005;112(17):2677–85.

24. Chabrashvili T, Tojo A, Onozato ML, et al. Expression and cellular localization of classic NADPH oxidase subunits in the spontaneously hypertensive rat kidney. Hypertension 2002;39(2):269–74.

25. Wang D, Chen Y, Chabrashvili T, et al. Role of oxidative stress in endothelial dysfunction and enhanced responses to angiotensin II of afferent arterioles from rabbits infused with angiotensin II. J Am Soc Nephrol 2003;14(11):2783–9.

26. Fellner SK, Arendshorst WJ. Angiotensin II, reactive oxygen species, and Ca2+ signaling in afferent arterioles. Am J Physiol Renal Physiol 2005;289(5):F1012–9.

27. Kopkan L, Castillo A, Navar LG, et al. Enhanced superoxide generation modulates renal function in ANG II-induced hypertensive rats. Am J Physiol Renal Physiol 2006;290(1):F80–6.

28. Nagase M, Shibata S, Yoshida S, et al. Podocyte injury underlies the glomerulopathy of Dahl salt-hypertensive rats and is reversed by aldosterone blocker. Hypertension 2006;47(6):1084–93.

29. Meng S, Cason GW, Gannon AW, et al. Oxidative stress in Dahl salt-sensitive hypertension. Hypertension 2003;41(6):1346–52.

30. Banday AA, Lokhandwala MF. Loss of biphasic effect on Na/K-ATPase activity by angiotensin II involves defective angiotensin type 1 receptor-nitric oxide signaling. Hypertension 2008;52(6):1099–105.

31. Han W, Li H, Villar VA, et al. Lipid rafts keep NADPH oxidase in the inactive state in human renal proximal tubule cells. Hypertension 2008;51(2):481–7.

32. Banday AA, Fazili FR, Lokhandwala MF. Oxidative stress causes renal dopamine D1 receptor dysfunction and hypertension via mechanisms that involve nuclear factor-kappaB and protein kinase C. J Am Soc Nephrol 2007;18(5):1446–57.

33. Banday AA, Lau YS, Lokhandwala MF. Oxidative stress causes renal dopamine D1 receptor dysfunction and salt-sensitive hypertension in Sprague-Dawley rats. Hypertension 2008;51(2):367–75.

34. Beltowski J, Borkowska E, Wojcicka G, et al. Regulation of renal ouabain-resistant Na+-ATPase by leptin, nitric oxide, reactive oxygen species, and cyclic nucleotides: implications for obesity-associated hypertension. Clin Exp Hypertens 2007; 29(3):189–207.

35. Deng A, Baylis C. Locally produced EDRF controls preglomerular resistance and ultrafiltration coefficient. Am J Physiol 1993;264(2 Pt 2):F212–5.

36. Vallon V, Traynor T, Barajas L, et al. Feedback control of glomerular vascular tone in neuronal nitric oxide synthase knockout mice. J Am Soc Nephrol 2001;12(8): 1599–606.

37. Liu R, Ren Y, Garvin JL, et al. Superoxide enhances tubuloglomerular feedback by constricting the afferent arteriole. Kidney Int 2004;66(1):268–74.

38. Nouri P, Gill P, Li M, et al. p22phox in the macula densa regulates single nephron GFR during angiotensin II infusion in rats. Am J Physiol Heart Circ Physiol 2007; 292(4):H1685–9.

39. Wu F, Park F, Cowley AW Jr, et al. Quantification of nitric oxide synthase activity in microdissected segments of the rat kidney. Am J Physiol 1999;276(6 Pt 2): F874–81.

40. Cowley AW Jr, Mori T, Mattson D, et al. Role of renal NO production in the regulation of medullary blood flow. Am J Physiol Regul Integr Comp Physiol 2003; 284(6):R1355–69.

41. Dickhout JG, Mori T, Cowley AW Jr. Tubulovascular nitric oxide crosstalk: buffering of angiotensin II-induced medullary vasoconstriction. Circ Res 2002; 91(6):487–93.

42. Mattson DL, Roman RJ, Cowley AW Jr. Role of nitric oxide in renal papillary blood flow and sodium excretion. Hypertension 1992;19(6 Pt 2):766–9.

43. Mori T, Cowley AW Jr. Angiotensin II-NAD(P)H oxidase-stimulated superoxide modifies tubulovascular nitric oxide cross-talk in renal outer medulla. Hypertension 2003;42(4):588–93.

44. Beltowski J, Marciniak A, Jamroz-Wisniewska A, et al. Nitric oxide – superoxide cooperation in the regulation of renal Na(+),K(+)-ATPase. Acta Biochim Pol 2004;51(4):933–42.

45. Silva GB, Ortiz PA, Hong NJ, et al. Superoxide stimulates NaCl absorption in the thick ascending limb via activation of protein kinase C. Hypertension 2006;48(3): 467–72.

46. Silva GB, Garvin JL. Angiotensin II-dependent hypertension increases Na transport-related oxygen consumption by the thick ascending limb. Hypertension 2008;52(6):1091–8.

47. Guyenet PG. The sympathetic control of blood pressure. Nat Rev Neurosci 2006; 7(5):335–46.

48. Gordon FJ, Haywood JR, Brody MJ, et al. Effect of lesions of the anteroventral third ventricle (AV3V) on the development of hypertension in spontaneously hypertensive rats. Hypertension 1982;4(3):387–93.

49. Brody MJ. Central nervous system and mechanisms of hypertension. Clin Physiol Biochem 1988;6(3–4):230–9.

50. Whyte DG, Johnson AK. Thermoregulatory role of periventricular tissue surrounding the anteroventral third ventricle (AV3V) during acute heat stress in the rat. Clin Exp Pharmacol Physiol 2005;32(5–6):457–61.

51. Brody M, Fink G, Buggy J, et al. Critical role of the AV3V region in development and maintenance of experimental hypertension. In: Perspectives in nephrology and hypertension. New York: Wiley and Flammarion; 1978. p. 76–84.

52. Peterson JR, Sharma RV, Davisson RL. Reactive oxygen species in the neuropathogenesis of hypertension. Curr Hypertens Rep 2006;8(3):232–41.

53. Zimmerman MC, Lazartigues E, Lang JA, et al. Superoxide mediates the actions of angiotensin II in the central nervous system. Circ Res 2002; 91(11):1038–45.

54. Zimmerman MC, Lazartigues E, Sharma RV, et al. Hypertension caused by angiotensin II infusion involves increased superoxide production in the central nervous system. Circ Res 2004;95(2):210–6.

55. Zimmerman MC, Sharma RV, Davisson RL. Superoxide mediates angiotensin II-induced influx of extracellular calcium in neural cells. Hypertension 2005;45(4):717–23.

56. Zimmerman MC, Dunlay RP, Lazartigues E, et al. Requirement for Rac1-dependent NADPH oxidase in the cardiovascular and dipsogenic actions of angiotensin II in the brain. Circ Res 2004;95(5):532–9.

57. Erdos B, Broxson CS, King MA, et al. Acute pressor effect of central angiotensin II is mediated by NAD(P)H-oxidase-dependent production of superoxide in the hypothalamic cardiovascular regulatory nuclei. J Hypertens 2006;24(1):109–16.

58. Luoh SH, Chan SH. Inhibition of baroreflex by angiotensin II via Fos expression in nucleus tractus solitarii of the rat. Hypertension 2001;38(1):130–5.

59. Wang G, Anrather J, Huang J, et al. NADPH oxidase contributes to angiotensin II signaling in the nucleus tractus solitarius. J Neurosci 2004;24(24):5516–24.

60. Nozoe M, Hirooka Y, Koga Y, et al. Inhibition of Rac1-derived reactive oxygen species in nucleus tractus solitarius decreases blood pressure and heart rate in stroke-prone spontaneously hypertensive rats. Hypertension 2007;50(1):62–8.

61. Guyenet PG, Darnall RA, Riley TA. Rostral ventrolateral medulla and sympathorespiratory integration in rats. Am J Physiol 1990;259(5 Pt 2):R1063–74.

62. Kishi T, Hirooka Y, Kimura Y, et al. Overexpression of eNOS in RVLM improves impaired baroreflex control of heart rate in SHRSP. Rostral ventrolateral medulla. Stroke-prone spontaneously hypertensive rats. Hypertension 2003;41(2):255–60.

63. Kishi T, Hirooka Y, Kimura Y, et al. Increased reactive oxygen species in rostral ventrolateral medulla contribute to neural mechanisms of hypertension in stroke-prone spontaneously hypertensive rats. Circulation 2004;109(19):2357–62.

64. Li Z, Mao HZ, Abboud FM, et al. Oxygen-derived free radicals contribute to baroreceptor dysfunction in atherosclerotic rabbits. Circ Res 1996;79(4):802–11.

65. Mohazzab KM, Kaminski PM, Wolin MS. NADH oxidoreductase is a major source of superoxide anion in bovine coronary artery endothelium. Am J Physiol 1994;266(6 Pt 2):H2568–72.

66. Pagano PJ, Ito Y, Tornheim K, et al. An NADPH oxidase superoxide-generating system in the rabbit aorta. Am J Physiol 1995;268(6 Pt 2):H2274–80.

67. Griendling KK, Minieri CA, Ollerenshaw JD, et al. Angiotensin II stimulates NADH and NADPH oxidase activity in cultured vascular smooth muscle cells. Circ Res 1994;74(6):1141–8.

68. Rajagopalan S, Kurz S, Munzel T, et al. Angiotensin II-mediated hypertension in the rat increases vascular superoxide production via membrane NADH/NADPH oxidase activation. Contribution to alterations of vasomotor tone. J Clin Invest 1996;97(8):1916–23.

69. Landmesser U, Dikalov S, Price SR, et al. Oxidation of tetrahydrobiopterin leads to uncoupling of endothelial cell nitric oxide synthase in hypertension. J Clin Invest 2003;111(8):1201–9.

70. Schnackenberg CG, Wilcox CS. The SOD mimetic tempol restores vasodilation in afferent arterioles of experimental diabetes. Kidney Int 2001;59(5):1859–64.

71. Gongora MC, Qin Z, Laude K, et al. Role of extracellular superoxide dismutase in hypertension. Hypertension 2006;48(3):473–81.

72. Didion SP, Ryan MJ, Didion LA, et al. Increased superoxide and vascular dysfunction in CuZnSOD-deficient mice. Circ Res 2002;91(10):938–44.

73. Taddei S, Virdis A, Ghiadoni L, et al. Vitamin C improves endothelium-dependent vasodilation by restoring nitric oxide activity in essential hypertension. Circulation 1998;97(22):2222–9.

74. Zafari AM, Ushio-Fukai M, Akers M, et al. Role of NADH/NADPH oxidase-derived H2O2 in angiotensin II-induced vascular hypertrophy. Hypertension 1998;32(3): 488–95.

75. Weber DS, Rocic P, Mellis AM, et al. Angiotensin II-induced hypertrophy is potentiated in mice overexpressing p22phox in vascular smooth muscle. Am J Physiol Heart Circ Physiol 2005;288(1):37–42.

76. Folkow B, Grimby G, Thulesius O. Adaptive structural changes of the vascular walls in hypertension and their relation to the control of the peripheral resistance. Acta Physiol Scand 1958;44(3–4):255–72.

77. Pu Q, Neves MF, Virdis A, et al. Endothelin antagonism on aldosterone-induced oxidative stress and vascular remodeling. Hypertension 2003;42(1):49–55.

78. Patel R, Cardneau JD, Colles SM, et al. Synthetic smooth muscle cell phenotype is associated with increased nicotinamide adenine dinucleotide phosphate oxidase activity: effect on collagen secretion. J Vasc Surg 2006;43(2):364–71.

79. Virdis A, Neves MF, Amiri F, et al. Role of NAD(P)H oxidase on vascular alterations in angiotensin II-infused mice. J Hypertens 2004;22(3):535–42.

80. Landmesser U, Harrison DG. Oxidative stress and vascular damage in hypertension. Coron Artery Dis 2001;12(6):455–61.

81. Manning AM, Bell FP, Rosenbloom CL, et al. NF-kappa B is activated during acute inflammation in vivo in association with elevated endothelial cell adhesion molecule gene expression and leukocyte recruitment. J Inflamm 1995;45(4):283–96.

82. Theuer J, Dechend R, Muller DN, et al. Angiotensin II induced inflammation in the kidney and in the heart of double transgenic rats. BMC Cardiovasc Disord 2002; 2(3).

83. Liu J, Yang F, Yang XP, et al. NAD(P)H oxidase mediates angiotensin II-induced vascular macrophage infiltration and medial hypertrophy. Arterioscler Thromb Vasc Biol 2003;23(5):776–82.

84. Vaziri ND, Rodriguez-Iturbe B. Mechanisms of disease: oxidative stress and inflammation in the pathogenesis of hypertension. Nat Clin Pract Nephrol 2006; 2(10):582–93.

85. Liao TD, Yang XP, Liu YH, et al. Role of inflammation in the development of renal damage and dysfunction in angiotensin II-induced hypertension. Hypertension 2008;52(2):256–63.

86. Sesso HD, Buring JE, Rifai N, et al. C-reactive protein and the risk of developing hypertension. JAMA 2003;290(22):2945–51.

87. Preston RA, Ledford M, Materson BJ, et al. Effects of severe, uncontrolled hypertension on endothelial activation: soluble vascular cell adhesion molecule-1, soluble intercellular adhesion molecule-1 and von Willebrand factor. J Hypertens 2002;20(5):871–7.

88. Guzik TJ, Hoch NE, Brown KA, et al. Role of the T cell in the genesis of angiotensin II induced hypertension and vascular dysfunction. J Exp Med 2007; 204(10):2449–60.

89. Ganta CK, Lu N, Helwig BG, et al. Central angiotensin II-enhanced splenic cytokine gene expression is mediated by the sympathetic nervous system. Am J Physiol Heart Circ Physiol 2005;289(4):H1683–91.

90. Hoch NE, Guzik TJ, Chen W, et al. Regulation of T-cell function by endogenously produced angiotensin II. Am J Physiol Regul Integr Comp Physiol 2009;296(2): R208–16.

Towards a New Paradigm About Hypertensive Heart Disease

Javier Díez, MD, PhD[a,b,c],*

KEYWORDS

- Hypertensive heart disease • Left ventricular hypertrophy
- Myocardial remodeling • Apoptosis • Fibrosis
- Biochemical markers • Myocardial repair

A new paradigm is emerging related to the impact of chronic hypertension on the cardiac parenchyma. In fact, although macroscopic left ventricular hypertrophy (LVH) is the hallmark of hypertensive heart disease (HHD), a number of changes in the cardiomyocyte and the noncardiomyocyte components of the myocardium also develop in hypertension that alter the composition and structure of the myocardium.[1] The occurrence of these alterations may explain why the presence of LVH is independently associated with increased risk of cardiac complications, namely heart failure (HF), in hypertensive patients. Whereas LVH may be detected early and accurately in hypertensive patients by electrocardiography and echocardiography, newer cardiac imaging methods and the monitoring of several circulating biomarkers holds promise as a noninvasive tool for the diagnosis of myocardial remodeling. A large number of clinical studies have shown that long-term antihypertensive treatment may be associated with regression of LVH, and this is associated with the decrease of the risk of cardiovascular morbidity and mortality. However, because the remaining risk is unacceptably high, new therapeutic strategies aimed not just to decrease left

This work was partially funded through the Red Temática de Investigación Cooperativa en Enfermedades Cardiovasculares from the Instituto de Salud Carlos III, Ministry of Health, Spain (Grant RD06/0014/0008), and the Network of Excellence on Integrated Genomics, Clinical Research and Care in Hypertension, Ingenious HyperCare, financed by the European Commission (contract No. LSHM-CT-2006-037093).
a Cardiovascular Medicine, School of Medicine, Spain
b Division of Cardiovascular Sciences, Centre for Applied Medical Research, Spain
c Molecular Cardiology Unit, Department of Cardiology and Cardiovascular Surgery, University Clinic, University of Navarra, 55, 31008 Pamplona, Spain
* Área de Ciencias Cardiovasculares, Centro de Investigación Médica Aplicada, Avda/ Pío XII, 55, 31008 Pamplona, Spain.
E-mail address: jadimar@unav.es

Med Clin N Am 93 (2009) 637–645
doi:10.1016/j.mcna.2009.02.002
0025-7125/09/$ – see front matter

ventricular mass, but also to repair myocardial remodeling are necessary. All these aspects are reviewed in brief in this article.

CHANGING THE PATHOPHYSIOLOGIC VIEW OF HHD

The essential criterion in defining HHD is the presence of LVH in the absence of a cause other than arterial hypertension. Beyond macroscopic hypertrophy, however, complex changes in myocardial composition, which are responsible for the structural remodeling of the myocardium, develop in arterial hypertension. Whereas cardiomyocyte hypertrophy leading to LVH provides the adaptive response of the heart to pressure overload in an attempt to normalize systolic wall stress, pathologic remodeling develops as the consequence of a number of pathologic processes, mediated by hormones, growth factors, and cytokines acting on the cardiomyocyte and other cells of the myocardium (**Fig. 1**).[1]

Cardiomyocyte Hypertrophy

Hypertrophic growth of cardiomyocytes is the primary mechanism by which the heart reduces stress on the ventricular wall imposed by pressure overload. It entails stimulation of intracellular signaling cascades that activate gene expression and promote protein synthesis, protein stability, or both, with consequent increases in protein content and in the size and organization of force-generating units (sarcomeres) that, in turn, will lead to increased size of individual cardiomyocytes.[2]

The long-held views are that these morphologic and genetic changes, in response to pressure overload, serve to restore cardiac muscle economy back to normal and counteract myocardial dysfunction. However, evidence exists that a blunting of cardiomyocyte hypertrophy and an attenuation of the fetal gene re-expression did not result in dysfunction or failure, despite pressure overload. Therefore, a shift in paradigm is occurring in the sense that genetic reprogramming associated with cardiomyocyte hypertrophy is no longer considered as an adaptive process.[3] In fact, a detailed analysis of the genetic changes that accompany cardiomyocyte hypertrophy allows us to conclude that they will translate into derangements in energy metabolism, contractile cycle and excitation-contraction coupling, cytoskeleton and

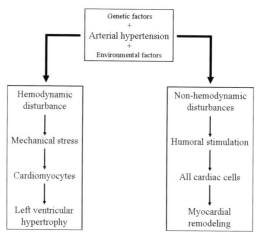

Fig. 1. General pathways involved in the development of LVH and myocardial remodeling in HHD.

membrane properties, and autocrine functions that, in turn, will provide the basis for the cardiomyocyte malfunctioning that is associated with LVH and that predisposes to diastolic and systolic dysfunction and HF.[4]

Myocardial Remodeling

Hypertensive myocardial remodeling involves increased rates of cardiomyocyte cell death, myocardial fibrosis, and alterations of the coronary microcirculation (**Fig. 2**).[1] Two types of findings suggest that nonhemodynamic factors also contribute to these lesions in human hypertension. First, they have been identified in the left and right ventricles, the interventricular septa, and the left atria of patients with HHD. Second, it has been shown that the ability of antihypertensive treatment to reverse these lesions in hypertensive patients is independent of its antihypertensive efficacy. Thus, myocardial remodeling could be the consequence of the loss of reciprocal regulation that normally exists between proremodeling and antiremodeling molecules (**Box 1**).[1]

Historically, there are three types of cell death: apoptosis, autophagy, and necrosis. Although the three types of cardiomyocyte death have been observed simultaneously in failing human hearts as a consequence of pressure overload, apoptosis is the most thoroughly characterized form of cell death in the hypertensive myocardium.[5]

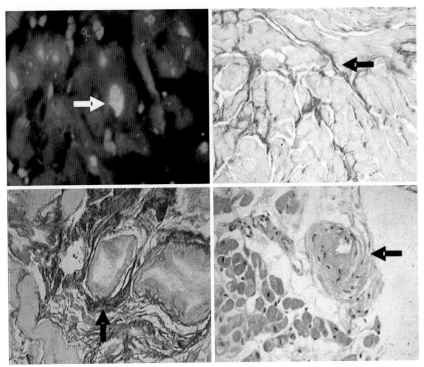

Fig. 2. Components of myocardial remodeling: cardiomyocyte apoptosis (*upper left panel, arrow*, FITC stain, magnification ×20), interstitial fibrosis (*upper right panel, arrow*, picro-sirius red stain, magnification ×20), perivascular fibrosis (*lower left panel, arrow*, picro-sirius red stain, magnification ×20), and intramyocardial artery wall thickening and lumen narrowing (*lower right panel, arrow*, hematoxylin-eosin stain, magnification ×20).

Box 1

Main molecules that participate in the process of myocardial remodeling in arterial hypertension

Excess of proremodeling molecules

Vasoactive substances (norepinephrine, angiotensin II)

Hormones (thyroid hormone, aldosterone)

Growth factors (transforming growth factor-β)

Cytokines (cardiotrophin-1)

Other (reactive oxygen species)

Deficit of antiremodeling molecules

Vasoactive substances (nitric oxide, prostacyclin)

Hormones (glucocorticoids)

Growth factors (insulin-like growth factor-1)

Cytokines (tumor necrosis factor-α)

Other (endogenous PPARα ligands)

Several observations suggest that apoptosis of cardiomyocytes may contribute to the development of left ventricular dysfunction or failure through different pathways.[6] First, an association of increased cardiomyocyte apoptosis with diminished cardiomyocyte number has been found in the failing heart of hypertensive patients. Thus, apoptosis may be one of the mechanisms involved in the loss of contractile mass and function in HHD. Second, impaired myocardial contractile function may reflect not only a decrease in the number of viable, fully functional cardiomyocytes, but also a decrement in the function of viable cardiomyocytes, or a combination of these mechanisms. It has been recently reported that caspase-3 cleaves cardiac myofibrillar proteins, resulting in an impaired force/Ca^{2+} relationship and myofibrillar adenosine triphosphatase (ATPase) activity. Finally, cytochrome C plays a major role in ATP production through mitochondrial oxidative phosphorylation. Thus, it has been hypothesized that release of cytochrome C from mitochondria during the occurrence of the apoptotic process could interfere with cardiomyocyte energy production and lead to functional impairment.

Myocardial fibrosis secondary to an exaggerated accumulation of collagen type I and type III fibers within the interstitium and surrounding intramural coronary arteries and arterioles is one of the key features of structural remodeling of the hypertensive hypertrophied left ventricle. Excess of myocardial collagen present in LVH is suggested to be the result of both increased collagen synthesis by fibroblasts and phenotypically transformed fibroblast-like cells, or myofibroblasts, and unchanged or decreased collagen degradation by matrix metalloproteinases.[7]

Fibrosis might contribute to the increased risk of adverse cardiac events in hypertensive patients with LVH through different pathways.[8] First, a linkage between fibrosis and left ventricular dysfunction or failure may be established. Initially, the accumulation of collagen fibers compromises the rate of relaxation, diastolic suction, and passive stiffness, contributing to impaired diastolic function. Continued accumulation of fibrotic tissue, accompanied by changes in the spatial orientation of collagen fibers, further impairs diastolic filling and compromises transduction of cardiomyocyte contraction into myocardial force development, thus impairing systolic performance. Second, impaired coronary flow reserve associated with LVH might be related to several factors, including perivascular fibrosis. In fact, it has been demonstrated that the amount of perivascular collagen correlated inversely with coronary flow reserve in hypertensive patients with LVH. Third, fibrosis may also contribute to ventricular arrhythmias in hypertensive LVH. It has been reported that patients with arrhythmias exhibited higher values of left ventricular mass and myocardial collagen than patients without arrhythmias, the ejection fraction and the frequency of coronary vessels with significant stenosis being similar in the two groups of patients. Fibrosis would induce conduction abnormalities, as promoters of local re-entry, and thereby arrhythmias.

Hypertensive LVH is characterized by different structural alterations in the small intramyocardial vessels.[9] On the one hand, hyperplasia and hypertrophy, and altered alignment of vascular smooth muscle cells leading to encroachment of the tunica media into the lumen, cause both an increase in the medial thickness/lumen ratio and a reduction in the maximal cross-sectional area of intramyocardial arteries. On the other hand, if the density of arterioles and capillaries is estimated as the vessel number per unit area, there is a relative decrease in arteriolar and capillary density in LVH. This can be caused by both capillary rarefaction (ie, the vessels are actually missing or temporarily not perfused or "recruited") and inadequate vascular growth (ie, impaired angiogenesis) in response to increasing muscle mass.

These structural alterations of microcirculation, together with increased arteriolar tone, endothelial dysfunction, and extravascular systolic compression account for the decrease in coronary vasodilator response present hypertensive patients with LVH.[10]

BUILDING A NEW CLINICAL APPROACH TO HHD

The time has come to revisit the current management of HHD simply focused on detecting and treating LVH. It is necessary to develop new approaches aimed at early identification of hypertensive patients highly exposed to develop LVH, more accurate measurement of left ventricular anatomy and function, assessment of those pathologic changes responsible for myocardial remodeling, and repair of the molecular and cellular alterations of the myocardium that compromise its structure and function (**Box 2**). In so doing, the adverse risk associated with HHD will be reduced in a more-effective manner.

Early Detection

Although in most studies and meta-analyses the relationship between changes in office blood pressure and left ventricular mass was relatively weak (correlation coefficient <0.50), emerging evidence indicates that 24-hour monitoring of blood pressure may help to identify those hypertensive patients highly exposed to developing LVH (ie, patients with an early morning rise in blood pressure and patients with a nondipping profile) and more prone to benefit from the ability of some antihypertensive drugs to prevent it.[11]

Left ventricular mass is a complex phenotype influenced by the interacting effects of multiple genetic and environmental (ie, nutritional and hygienic) factors. Genetic variation probably contributes to interindividual differences in left ventricular mass by virtue of effects on blood-pressure level, as well as via pathways that are not captured by measurements of blood pressure. It is possible that identification of genes that influence the mass of the left ventricle may enhance the ability to detect those patients who deserve early treatment to prevent the development of LVH. In this regard, a recent meta-analysis of case-controlled studies and association studies has shown

---

Box 2
Potential novel tools for the clinical handling of HHD

Aimed to identify patients prone to develop LVH

24-hour monitoring of blood pressure

Insertion/deletion polymorphism of angiotensin-converting enzyme gene

Circulating cardiotrophin-1

Aimed to optimize the diagnosis of left ventricular hypertrophy

Three-dimensional echocardiography

Magnetic resonance imaging

Aimed to detect noninvasive myocardial remodeling

Special ultrasound techniques

Magnetic resonance imaging

Nuclear molecular imaging techniques

ELISA of circulating biochemical markers

Aimed to provide therapeutic benefit beyond reduction of left ventricular mass

Antihypertensive agents that protect cardiac function and electrical activity

Antihypertensive agents that improve intramyocardial perfusion

Antihypertensive agents that repair myocardial remodeling

Novel compounds that target events inside the cardiac cells

---

that the D allele of the insertion/deletion polymorphism of the angiotensin-converting enzyme gene behaved as a marker for LVH in untreated hypertensive patients.[12]

Plasma concentration of cardiotrophin-1, a cytokine that induces cardiomyocyte hypertrophy, has been found to be abnormally increased in hypertensive patients, in particular in those with echocardiographic LVH.[13] It is interesting to point out that 31% of hypertensive patients without echocardiographic LVH already exhibited concentrations of cardiotrophin-1 abnormally elevated, suggesting that the circulating levels of this cytokine increase early during the evolution of arterial hypertension, and thus may be useful to identify those patients prone to developing LVH.

Optimized Diagnosis

New three-dimensional techniques for imaging the heart, including MRI and three-dimensional echocardiography, can measure left ventricular mass and dimensions more accurately than conventional echocardiographic techniques, and may thus offer an advantage.[14] Being largely used for research purposes, the diffusion of these techniques for the routine assessment of hypertensive LVH is still hampered by practical and economic reasons.

On the other hand, special ultrasound methodologies (ie, analysis of backscatter) aimed to assess myocardial texture may be useful for the detection of myocardial remodeling as well, and in particular, fibrosis.[15] MRI is another promising technique for characterizing the composition of the myocardium; in particular, the presence of late gadolinium enhancement areas in the myocardium probably represent regions characterized by fibrosis.[16]

Nuclear imaging techniques, especially single-photon emission tomography and positron emission tomography are well suited for cardiac molecular imaging because of the large number of potentially available molecular targets, relatively high intrinsic sensitivity, and excellent depth of penetration. MRI is also rapidly evolving within the field of cardiac molecular imaging, with the introduction of an increasing number of high-affinity molecular probes imaged at exceptionally high spatial resolution. Within the field of myocardial remodeling, molecular imaging is rapidly expanding to involve imaging and monitoring of apoptotic cell loss and collagen matrix turnover.[17]

The identification of biochemical markers of potential usefulness for the clinical handling of cardiac diseases evolving to HF has been a prolific field in recent years. However, for a circulating molecule to be considered a biochemical marker of hypertensive LVH and myocardial remodeling, it must fulfill several criteria.[18] Up to now, two molecules have been characterized as biochemical markers of hypertensive myocardial remodeling: Annexin A5 as a marker of cardiomyocyte apoptosis, and the carboxy-terminal propeptide of procollagen type I as a biochemical marker of myocardial fibrosis.

Global Treatment

In the treatment of patients with HHD, beyond controlling blood pressure and reducing left ventricular mass, it is necessary to pay attention also to the correction of alterations in left ventricular function and electrical activity, and coronary microcirculation that associate with LVH. Although several trials have been performed to analyze these aspects, methodologic problems of design and the confounding influence of factors, such as the antihypertensive and antihypertrophic effects of treatment, make evaluating the available information difficult. Nevertheless, from the reported findings it appears that the use of pharmacologic agents interfering with the production and actions of angiotensin II provides a higher benefit than the use of other agents.[19,20]

There is no doubt that all classes of antihypertensive drugs posses the ability to reduce the quantity of left ventricular mass in patients with LVH. However, as mentioned above, it is not so clear if they also restore the structural quality of the remodeled myocardium. For example, it has been shown that despite similar antihypertensive and antihypertrophic efficacy, the angiotensin type 1 receptor antagonist losartan, but not the calcium channel blocker amlodipine, was able to reduce cardiomyocyte apoptosis and myocardial fibrosis in patients with HHD.[21,22] Of interest, the reduction of myocardial fibrosis by losartan is associated with the decrease in left ventricular chamber stiffness and the improvement of diastolic filling.[23] From these data it seems that the goal of repairing myocardial remodeling is achievable in patients with HHD using specific antihypertensive agents. Furthermore, this preliminary information sets the stage for large and long-term clinical trials aimed at determining whether the reversal of myocardial remodeling in HHD is associated with higher beneficial effects on the patient's cardiac function and prognosis than just the regression of LVH.

On the other hand, most of the antihypertensive agents that have antihypertrophic effects target outside-in signaling cardiac cells, but their effectiveness seems limited, and so attention has recently turned to the potential of targeting intracellular events. Hypothetically, these novel therapeutic interventions could be directed to the following aspects:[24–26] (*i*) to block the detrimental intracellular mechanisms activated in mechanical stress-based cardiomyocyte hypertrophic response (eg, inhibiting oxidative stress, kinases such as Rho-kinase, and phosphatases such as calcineurin); (*ii*) to prevent inhibition of negative-signaling modulators and negative-interacting proteins that are repressed in the mechanical stress-based cardiomyocyte hypertrophic response (eg, increasing the availability and actions of cyclic guanosine monophosphate); (*iii*) to take advantage of beneficial mechanisms inherent in mechanical stress-based cardiomyocyte hypertrophic response (eg, via enhancement of important aspects of the IGF1/PI3K/Akt pathway, such as angiogenesis); (*iv*) to block the deleterious modulation that pathologic stresses impose on protein synthesis (eg, through inhibition of histone deacetylases or sets of microRNAs); (*v*) to preserve functioning cardiomyocytes (eg, through the inhibition of the process of apoptosis or preservation of cell-survival mechanisms); (*vi*) to regenerate lost cardiomyocytes (eg, using stem cell therapy); and (*vii*) to restore the normal turnover of collagen network (eg, restoring the balance between fibrillar collagen synthesis/deposition and collagen fiber degradation/removal).

SUMMARY

A new pathophysiologic paradigm on HHD is emerging. This entity is the result of the pathologic structural remodeling of the myocardium in response to a mosaic of hemodynamic and nonhemodynamic factors altered in hypertension more than just the adaptive hypertrophy of the left ventricular wall to increased pressure. The potential clinical relevance of this paradigm is given by the fact that it entails a new approach to HHD in terms of more detailed diagnosis and more demanding treatment. But this novel view of HHD may also have epidemiologic importance. In fact, the possibility that myocardial individuals prone to develop HHD may be detected before the appearance of clinical detectable LVH opens a new way to the prevention of cardiac complications associated with hypertension and its impact on the heart, namely heart failure.[27]

REFERENCES

1. Díez J, Gonzalez A, López B, et al. Mechanisms of disease: pathologic structural remodeling is more than adaptive hypertrophy in hypertensive heart disease. Nat Clin Pract Cardiovasc Med 2005;2(4):209–16.
2. LeWinter MM, VanBuren P. Sarcomeric proteins in hypertrophied and failing myocardium: an overview. Heart Fail Rev 2005;10(3):173–4.
3. Samuel JL, Swynghedauw B. Is cardiac hypertrophy a required compensatory mechanism in pressure-overloaded heart? J Hypertens 2008;26(5):857–8.
4. Sadoshima J, Izumo S. The cellular and molecular response of cardiac myocytes to mechanical stress. Annu Rev Physiol 1997;59:551–71.
5. González A, Fortuño MA, Querejeta R, et al. Cardiomyocyte apoptosis in hypertensive cardiomyopathy. Cardiovasc Res 2003;59(3):549–62.
6. González A, Ravassa S, López B, et al. Apoptosis in hypertensive heart disease: a clinical approach. Curr Opin Cardiol 2006;21(4):288–94.
7. Díez J. Mechanisms of cardiac fibrosis in hypertension. J Clin Hypertens 2007; 9(7):546–50.
8. Díez J, López B, González A, et al. Clinical aspects of hypertensive myocardial fibrosis. Curr Opin Cardiol 2001;16(6):328–35.
9. Feihl F, Liaudet L, Waeber B, et al. Hypertension and microvascular remodelling. Cardiovasc Res 2008;78(2):274–85.
10. Kelm M, Strauer BE. Coronary flow reserve measurements in hypertension. Med Clin North Am 2004;88(1):99–113.
11. Kawano Y, Horio T, Matayoshi T, et al. Masked hypertension: subtypes and target organ damage. Clin Exp Hypertens 2008;30(3):289–96.

12. Kuznetsova T, Staessen JA, Wang JG, et al. Antihypertensive treatment modulates the association between the D/I ACE gene polymorphism and left ventricular hypertrophy: a meta-analysis. J Hum Hypertens 2000;14(7):447–54.
13. López B, González A, Lasarte JJ, et al. Is plasma cardiotrophin-1 a marker of hypertensive heart disease? J Hypertens 2005;23(3):625–32.
14. Alfakih K, Reid S, Hall A, et al. The assessment of left ventricular hypertrophy in hypertension. J Hypertens 2006;24(7):1223–30.
15. Kerut EK, Given M, Giles TD. Review of methods for texture analysis of myocardium from echocardiographic images: a means of tissue characterization. Echocardiography 2003;20(8):727–36.
16. Iles L, Pfluger H, Phrommintikul A, et al. Evaluation of diffuse myocardial fibrosis in heart failure with cardiac magnetic resonance contrast-enhanced T1 mapping. J Am Coll Cardiol 2008;52(19):1574–80.
17. Chun HJ, Narula J, Hofstra L, et al. Intracellular and extracellular targets of molecular imaging in the myocardium. Nat Clin Pract Cardiovasc Med 2008;5(Suppl 2): S33–41.
18. González A, López B, Ravassa S, et al. Biochemical markers of myocardial remodelling in hypertensive heart disease. Cardiovasc Res 2009;81:509–18.
19. Wright JW, Mizutani S, Harding JW. Pathways involved in the transition from hypertension to hypertrophy to heart failure. Treatment strategies. Heart Fail Rev 2008;13(3):367–75.
20. Prisant LM. Management of hypertension in patients with cardiac disease: use of renin-angiotensin blocking agents. Am J Med 2008;121(Suppl 8):S8–15.
21. González A, López B, Ravassa S, et al. Stimulation of cardiac apoptosis in essential hypertension: potential role of angiotensin II. Hypertension 2002;39(1):75–80.
22. López B, Querejeta R, Varo N, et al. Usefulness of serum carboxy-terminal propeptide of procollagen type I in assessment of the cardioreparative ability of antihypertensive treatment in hypertensive patients. Circulation 2001;104(3):286–91.
23. Díez J, Querejeta R, López B, et al. Losartan-dependent regression of myocardial fibrosis is associated with reduction of left ventricular chamber stiffness in hypertensive patients. Circulation 2002;105(21):2512–7.
24. Luedde M, Katus HA, Frey N. Novel molecular targets in the treatment of cardiac hypertrophy. Recent Pat Cardiovasc Drug Discov 2006;1(1):1–20.
25. González A, López B, Díez J. New directions in the assessment and treatment of hypertensive heart disease. Curr Opin Nephrol Hypertens 2005;14(5):428–34.
26. Díez J. Diagnosis and treatment of myocardial fibrosis in hypertensive heart disease. Circ J 2008;72(Suppl A):A8–12.
27. Schocken DD, Benjamin EJ, Fonarow GC, et al. Prevention of heart failure: a scientific statement from the American Heart Association Councils on Epidemiology and Prevention, Clinical Cardiology, Cardiovascular Nursing, and High Blood Pressure Research; Quality of Care and Outcomes Research Interdisciplinary Working Group; and Functional Genomics and Translational Biology Interdisciplinary Working Group. Circulation 2008;117(19):2544–65.

Diastolic Dysfunction as a Link Between Hypertension and Heart Failure

Anil Verma, MD[a], Scott D. Solomon, MD[b],*

KEYWORDS

- Hypertension • Diastolic dysfunction • Heart failure
- Heart failure with preserved ejection fraction
- Diastolic heart failure • Left ventricular hypertrophy

Left ventricular diastolic dysfunction (DD) is characterized by abnormalities in left ventricular (LV) filling, including decreased diastolic distensibility and impaired relaxation, and it may represent an important pathophysiologic link between hypertension and heart failure, in particular in patients who have heart failure with normal or preserved ejection fraction. LVDD has been found to be commonly prevalent in the community setting, with isolated DD as common as systolic dysfunction, and worsening diastolic function of the left ventricle has been associated with an increased frequency of heart failure development.[1] Hypertension significantly contributes to cardiovascular (CV) morbidity and mortality by causing substantial structural and functional adaptations, including DD, LV hypertrophy (LVH), ventricular and vascular stiffness, and progressive renal dysfunction. Heart failure with preserved ejection fraction (HFPEF) is now recognized as a major public health problem because nearly one half of the patients presenting with heart failure syndrome have preserved LV ejection fraction (LVEF).[2,3] The prevalence of HFPEF has increased over the past decade, with unchanged rates of death.[3] Although various therapies, including inhibition of renin angiotensin and aldosterone system (RAAS), have been shown to improve survival in patients who have heart failure with LV systolic dysfunction, no pharmacologic therapy has been shown to be effective in improving outcomes in patients who have heart failure with a preserved LVEF. These trends underscore the importance of this growing public health problem and a need to understand the potential mechanisms primarily responsible for this clinical syndrome and its relationship to hypertension and DD.

[a] Ochsner Clinic Foundation, 1514 Jefferson Highway, New Orleans, LA 70121, USA
[b] Non-Invasive Cardiology, Harvard Medical School, Brigham and Women's Hospital, 75 Francis Street, Boston, MA 02115, USA
* Corresponding author.
E-mail address: ssolomon@rics.bwh.harvard.edu (S.D. Solomon).

Med Clin N Am 93 (2009) 647–664
doi:10.1016/j.mcna.2009.02.013
0025-7125/09/$ – see front matter © 2009 Elsevier Inc. All rights reserved.

medical.theclinics.com

EPIDEMIOLOGIC ASPECTS OF DIASTOLIC DYSFUNCTION AND HEART FAILURE WITH PRESERVED EJECTION FRACTION

Hypertension and aging contribute significantly to adverse cardiac morphology and poor outcomes. Advancing age and female gender are associated with increases in vascular and ventricular systolic and diastolic stiffness, even in the absence of CV disease.[4] The Strong Heart Study, which was a population-based cohort study of cardiac risk factors and prevalent and incident cardiac disease, used mitral inflow patterns to characterize diastolic function. Its investigators reported that simple Doppler evidence of grade I DD was present in 16% of the cohort group and that evidence of Grade II to IV DD was present in 3% of the cohort group. DD is more common with advancing age and in people with hypertension, coronary artery disease, or risk factors for coronary artery disease.[5] Similarly, Redfield and colleagues,[1] using Doppler parameters, graded DD as mild in subjects with impaired relaxation but without evidence of increased filling pressures, as moderate in subjects with impaired relaxation and a moderate elevation of filling pressures or a pseudo-normal pattern, and as severe in subjects with advanced reduction in compliance and reversible or fixed restrictive filling. They found that 20.8% of the subjects had mild DD, 6.6% had moderate DD, and 0.7% had severe DD, with 5.6% of the population having moderate or severe DD with normal ejection fraction. The presence of any DD imparted an eightfold to 10 fold increased mortality risk in their population.

The proportion of patients who have HFPEF increases with age, from 46% in patients younger than 45 years to 59% in patients older than 85 years.[6] In epidemiologic studies and clinical trial settings, patients presenting with HFPEF were more likely to be older, of female gender, have a higher mean body-mass index, and have higher rates of hypertension and atrial fibrillation but lower prevalence rates of coronary artery disease and any valvular disorders.[3] Owan and colleagues[3] reported a higher survival rate among patients who had preserved ejection fraction than among those who had reduced ejection fraction, although the difference was small (29% versus 32% at one year and 65% and 68% at five years, respectively). Bhatia and colleagues[7] reported similar mortality rates among patients who had HFPEF and heart failure with reduced ejection fraction, at 25.5% and 22.2%, respectively, after one year.[8] Clinical presentation of HFPEF is indistinguishable from that of heart failure with reduced ejection fraction, with echocardiography providing the only reliable discriminator.[8] Thus, among patients hospitalized for heart failure, approximately 50% will have LVEF greater than 50%, with mortality rates similar to those of patients who have reduced ejection fraction heart failure.

PHYSIOLOGIC ASPECTS OF THE DIASTOLE

The diastole of the cardiac cycle occurs during the period of time from the aortic valve closure to the mitral valve closure, with the rest of the cardiac cycle being defined as the systole. There are four distinct phases to the diastole: (1) isovolumetric relaxation, (2) early LV filling, (3) diastasis, and (4) filling at atrial contraction. Isovolumetric relaxation begins with aortic valve closure and ends with mitral valve opening. The LV pressure decreases without a change in volume during this phase. Isovolumetric relaxation ends when the LV pressure decreases to less than the left atrial pressure. LV relaxation is an energy-dependent process that starts with sodium/calcium exchanger–induced extrusion of calcium from the cytosol and sarcoplasmic reticulum calcium ATPase (SERCA2a)–induced calcium sequestration into the sarcoplasmic/endoplasmic reticulum, which in turn inactivates the troponin-tropomyosin complex, detaching the actin-myosin cross-bridge and bringing the sarcomere to its resting length.[9–11] The concentration of the products of ATP hydrolysis (ADP and inorganic phosphate) must remain low and produce the appropriate relative ADP/ATP ratio to maintain this energy-dependent phase of LV relaxation and thus maintain normal diastolic function.[12]

The time constant of LV relaxation (τ), estimated from the rate of intracavitary pressure decay during isovolumetric relaxation, is the time that it takes the LV pressure to fall to approximately two-thirds of its peak value, and it provides a quantitative assessment of global LV relaxation.[11,13] Measurement of the end systolic pressure and fiber stretch, coronary flow, and stored energy (elastic recoil) helps determine the rate of myocardial relaxation. The near-simultaneous and rapid relaxation of the left ventricle decreases the LV intracavitary pressure during the early diastole and creates a pressure gradient across the mitral valve, drawing blood from the left atrium and rapidly filling the left ventricle. The ensuing rapid LV filling is followed by a fall in the transmitral pressure gradient and a phase of passive LV filling (diastasis) that is dependent on the LV chamber stiffness. Late in the diastole, atrial contraction increases, re-establishing the transmitral pressure gradient and LV filling. Diastolic function can be impaired at any point in this sequence as a result of changes in the passive stiffness of the myocardium or in the process of active myocardial relaxation, which is indicated as a shift upward and to the left in a graph of the end diastolic pressure volume relationship **(Fig. 1)**, reflecting enhanced sensitivity of intraventricular filling pressures to even small changes in filling volume. The consequential limitations on myocardial reserve narrow the window for clinical compensation, enhancing vulnerability to the development of heart failure symptoms as a consequence of rapid changes in afterload (eg, during bouts of uncontrolled hypertension), dietary sodium indiscretion, onset of new arrhythmias, or development of myocardial ischemia.[14]

PATHOPHYSIOLOGIC ASPECTS OF DIASTOLIC DYSFUNCTION AND DEVELOPMENT OF HEART FAILURE WITH PRESERVED EJECTION FRACTION

In the Valsartan in Diastolic Dysfunction (VALIDD) trial, the authors demonstrated that the mean lateral mitral relaxation velocity (a measurement of LV diastolic function performed using tissue Doppler imaging) in patients who had hypertension and underwent screening was substantially reduced and was inversely related to age. Notably, LVH was only present in 15 (3%) of the screened patients, despite their

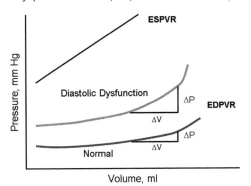

Fig. 1. Graph of the end-diastolic pressure volume relationship in patients who have normal filling and DD (end systolic pressure volume relationship [ESPVR] is also included as part of the pressure volume curve). In patients who have DD, increased ventricular stiffness in the diastole is expressed as an increase in the slope of the end diastolic pressure volume relationship (EDPVR), such that any given filling volume occurs only at the expense of higher filling pressures.

histories of hypertension.[15] Thus, abnormalities of ventricular relaxation and the consequences of DD may signify an early measure of myocardial end-organ damage in patients who have hypertension that might precede ventricular hypertrophy[15,16] Thus, DD could represent a potential mechanism by which treating hypertension might attenuate progression to heart failure.

Hypertension and Aging

The prevalence of hypertension increases with advancing age, to the point at which more than one half of the people between 60 and 69 years of age and approximately three fourths of those 70 years of age and older are affected.[17] Hypertension and aging are closely linked and interact with each other to cause various morphologic changes in the CV system, such as increased vascular stiffness, coronary insufficiency, and LVH. It is systolic blood pressure and not diastolic pressure in patients who have hypertension that represents the greatest blood pressure–related risk for adults older than 50 years of age who have cardiac and cerebrovascular diseases.[18] Aging is associated with increased blood pressure sensitivity to dietary sodium intake, and advancing age could exacerbate the adverse CV effects of high salt consumption because an increase in dietary salt intake raises arterial pressure and increases arterial stiffness in elderly patients who have systolic hypertension.[19] A study by Gates and colleagues[20] showed that large elastic artery compliance in humans improved with dietary sodium restriction and that rapid improvements in central arterial compliance with dietary sodium restriction were strongly related to corresponding reductions in systolic blood pressure. Structural changes involving ECM proteins in the arterial wall are believed to play a major role in the reductions in central arterial compliance and consequent increases in systolic blood pressure associated with human aging.[20,21] Increased salt load could result in activation of local tissue renin–angiotensin systems, increased production of tissue ouabain-like substances, endothelial dysfunction, and elevated secretion of marinobufagenin (a potent inhibitor of the sodium–potassium pump) that could accelerate ventricular fibrosis and dysfunction.[19] Increased collagen deposition and cross-linking, and increased interstitial fibrosis with disturbance of calcium homeostasis are associated with aging, as is decreased coronary reserve and increased oxidative stress,[22] which combined with hypertension could contribute to DD and a predisposition to heart failure development.

Extracellular Matrix and Cytoskeleton in Hypertension

Extracellular matrix

Under ideal physiologic conditions, collagen synthesis and degradation are maintained in equilibrium in the extracellular matrix (ECM). Among structural alterations, changes in the cardiac myocyte cytoskeleton and ECM have been implicated as potential underlying causes of DD.[23–25] The myocardial ECM is composed of three important constituents:[26] (1) fibrillar protein, such as collagen type I, collagen type III, and elastin; (2) proteoglycans; and (3) basement membrane proteins, such as collagen type IV, laminin, and fibronectin. Alterations in ECM fibrillar collagen, including the amount, geometry, distribution, degree of cross-linking, and ratio of collagen type I versus collagen type III, contribute to the development and reversal of DD. Major regulators of collagen synthesis include those that are mechanical (eg, relating to ventricular load, including preload and afterload) and neurohumoral (eg, the RAAS and the sympathetic nervous system) as well as numerous growth factors and cytokines (eg, transforming growth factor, connective tissue growth factor, platelet-derived growth factor, epidermal growth factor, basic fibroblast growth factor, insulin-like growth factor, interleukin 1, and tumor necrosis factor).[19,27] Collagen degradation is under the control of proteolytic enzymes, which include a family of zinc-dependent enzymes, the matrix metalloproteinases.[26,28] In hypertension and aging, the rate of collagen turnover increases greatly, and although both synthesis and degradation are increased, the disequilibrium primarily is the result of a rapid increase in collagen synthesis.[19] These structural changes in the ECM result in fibrosis of the myocardium, leading to increased ventricular stiffness, impaired relaxation, and DD.

Age-related formation of advanced glycation end products results in increased collagen cross-linking, which is further aggravated by hypertension and diabetes, resulting in increases of ventricular and vascular stiffness.[19] The advanced glycation end products have been shown to be responsible for increases in proinflammatory activity, increased production of superoxide anions and oxidative stress, and the inducement of premature senescence of endothelial cells,[29] contributing to increased ventricular fibrosis and DD.

Cytoskeleton and cardiac myocyte
Restoration of diastolic calcium ion levels in the cytosol governs the active phase of diastolic relaxation of the cardiac myocyte. Abnormalities of calcium reuptake in the cardiac myocyte may cause LV diastolic abnormalities and impaired relaxation. Phosphorylation of phospholamban, a sarcoplasmic/endoplasmic reticulum calcium ATPase (SERCA2a) inhibitor, by protein kinase A or Ca^{2+}/calmodulin-dependent kinase attenuates inhibition of SERCA2a, thus accelerating relaxation. The energy-dependent reuptake of the cytosolic calcium back into the sarcoplasmic reticulum may explain why DD develops earlier than myocardial contraction abnormality. Abnormal sarcoplasmic reticulum calcium reuptake can be caused by a decrease in SERCA2a, abnormalities in the sarcolemmal channels, and changes in the phosphorylation state of the proteins that modify SERCA2a function.[26] Interference with the rapid uptake of the cytosolic calcium results in a slower rate of LV relaxation as the result of decreased elastic recoil from the energy stored during systole,[9] leading to delayed mitral valve opening, a lower early transmitral gradient, and a shift to a LV filling pattern that has a greater proportion of filling at atrial contraction, causing increased left atrial pressure.[30] With aging, SERCA2a receptor concentration declines[31] and hypertension causes a predisposition to prolonged calcium-decay time, elevated diastolic calcium ion levels in response to force-frequency stimulation, and decreased SERCA2a receptor concentration, as shown in animal models with DD, causing excessively slow diastolic relaxation time.[32] Excessively slow diastolic relaxation causes a predisposition to elevated diastolic pressures, more so at high heart rates and with exercise.

Changes in the cytoskeletal proteins may alter diastolic function.[33,34] These changes could be in the microtubule architecture, and increased network density and distribution could contribute to altered viscosity and increased myocardial and cardiomyocyte stiffness.[35] Similarly, changes in the titin isotypes could alter relaxation and viscoelastic stiffness in pressure overload situations.[26] An increased collagen volume fraction, higher cardiomyocyte diameter, and higher resting cardiomyocyte tension have been correlated with LV diastolic stiffness and HFPEF.[36,37] Administration of protein kinase A to cardiomyocytes from subjects in a diastolic heart failure group lowered resting cardiomyocyte tension to control values, suggesting that reduced phosphorylation of sarcomeric proteins is involved in HFPEF.[36,37]

Endothelial and neurohormonal function
The endothelium plays a major role in the regulation of vascular tone, and disruption in the endothelial function and neurohormonal activation is present in people who have

hypertension before overt vascular changes.[38] Endothelial dysfunction has been shown to adversely impact coronary reserve flow and ventricular diastolic and systolic function.[38,39] Acute activation or inhibition of neurohumoral and cardiac endothelial systems has been shown to alter relaxation and stiffness.[39] Chronic activation of the RAAS increases ECM fibrillar collagen content, promotes hypertrophy of the cardiac myocytes, causes a marked increase in tissue aldosterone, causes an increase in perivascular interstitial fibrosis,[40] and has been associated with increased ventricular stiffness.[26] Inhibition of the RAAS prevents or reverses this increase in fibrillar collagen and generally but not consistently reduces myocardial stiffness.[26] Aldosterone may be a mediator of adverse vascular and myocardial remodeling and contribute to increased inhibition of nitric oxide synthesis, endothelial dysfunction, and myocardial stiffness. A high level of angiotensin II in cardiac tissue activates an increase in local cardiac endothelin-1 synthesis, which via ETB receptors stimulates aldosterone release, and this in turn may increase collagen production.[41] Administration of spironolactone, an aldosterone blocker and inhibitor of the rennin angiotensin and aldosterone system, to patients who have HFPEF has been shown to relieve symptoms and decrease left atrial area (size), suggesting a beneficial effect on diastolic function.[42]

Left Ventricular Hypertrophy and Cardiac Remodeling in Hypertension

The prevalence of LVH is closely associated with advancing age and the severity of hypertension, ranging from 6% in people younger than 30 years of age to 43% in those older than age 69,[43] and from 20% to 50% in people who have mild to severe hypertension.[44] An increase in protein synthesis and deposition by protein and collagen in the ECM and an increase in the size and heightened organization of force-generating units (sarcomeres) within individual myocytes are the hallmarks of LVH in hypertensive hearts.[45] Pathologic hypertrophy occurs in response not only to increased hemodynamic load but also to neurohumoral activation and altered genotypes, leading to an increase in cardiac myocyte size and heightened organization of the sarcomeres (indicated by bold, parallel bands of sarcomeric proteins on microscopic examination).[45] LVH undoubtedly reflects the progressive sequelae of hypertension on the heart and is associated with abnormalities of diastolic function.

Changes induced by volume and pressure overload or a combination of both cause different LV geometric adaptations in patients who have hypertension, including changes in normal geometry, concentric ventricular remodeling, or eccentric or concentric hypertrophy; these adaptations can be used to identify groups with distinctive pathophysiologic patterns (**Fig. 2**). Increased LV mass (LVM) and LVH are powerful and independent predictors of conditions that can cause CV morbidity and mortality, including sudden death, ventricular dysrhythmias, heart failure, and coronary artery disease.[46,47]

In the general population, left atrial enlargement is associated both with the duration of elevated blood pressure and with the level of systolic blood pressure that is present in severe hypertension,[48] and it is a finding that is frequently associated with hypertension and may signify LV dysfunction even before clinical evidence of LVH can be found.[49,50] Left atrial size increases with increasing LV filling pressure and correlates with Doppler evidence of DD and with increasing severity of DD as defined by invasive hemodynamic study.[51] Increased left atrial volumes are increasingly viewed as a chronic marker for DD, and atrial dilation frequently occurs with aging, which can contribute to alterations in left atrial pressure and therefore with reduced early diastolic filling.[52]

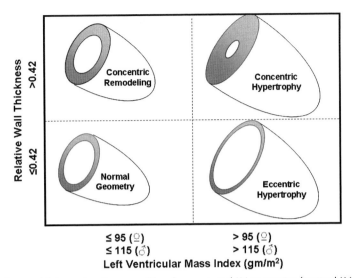

Fig. 2. Patients with hypertension can either have normal LV geometry (normal LV mass and relative wall thickness (RWT) ≤ 0.42), concentric remodeling (normal LV mass with RWT ≥ 0.42), increased LV mass with either concentric (RWT ≥ 0.42) or eccentric (RWT ≤ 0.42) hypertrophy.

Vascular and Ventricular Interaction in the Pathogenesis of Diastolic Dysfunction and Heart Failure With Preserved Ejection Fraction

Ventricular and vascular stiffness increase with advancing age, and they are further amplified by the presence of hypertension and diabetes. Vascular stiffening results secondary to arterial remodeling from collagen cross-linking, from geometric changes, and from alterations in endothelial function, structural protein composition, and neurohumoral signaling.[53] Increased central arterial stiffness contributes directly to the generation of wide pulse pressure and elevated systolic pressure. With widening pulse pressure and increased central arterial stiffness, the primary reflected waves arrive back at the aortic root during the late systole, where they interact with the incident wave and add to the central pulse pressure and the LV afterload. An increase in the net and late-systolic afterload alters ventricular systolic and diastolic function, increasing the myocardial work load and myocardial oxygen consumption, which leads to impairment of CV reserve function and labile systemic blood pressures, diminished coronary flow reserve, impaired diastolic relaxation, and increased diastolic filling pressures.[54,55] Recently, investigators demonstrated that early myocardial velocities as assessed using Doppler tissue imaging were inversely related to vascular stiffness and net afterload and directly related to total arterial compliance and that myocardial relaxation was strongly related to the pulsatile component, particularly late-systolic load.[54,56] Parallel increases in ventricular and vascular stiffening associated with advancing age and female gender may contribute to the enhanced prevalence of DD and HFPEF among the elderly, and elderly women in particular.[4]

ASSESSMENT OF DIASTOLIC FUNCTION

DD is characterized by impairment of isovolumetric ventricular relaxation, decreased ventricular compliance, and an abnormally increased LV end diastolic pressure. Impaired relaxation can be assessed by measurement of the peak instantaneous rate of LV pressure decline (–dP/dt) using a high-fidelity micromanometer catheter, increased τ (time constant of relaxation), or prolonged isovolumetric relaxation time (IVRT), which is the period of time between aortic valve closure and mitral valve opening. LV end diastolic pressure can be reliably estimated during cardiac catheterization and has been considered as a gold standard for assessment of LV filling pressure.[57] Given that cardiac catheterization is invasive and impractical for daily practice, echocardiography is the most commonly used tool to assess diastolic function and LV filling pressure noninvasively and to differentiate between systolic and diastolic LV dysfunction.

Images showing mitral inflow velocities produced on pulse wave Doppler (**Fig. 3**) are used to initially characterize LV filling. The early mitral inflow (E wave) velocity represents the dynamics of the pressure gradient between the left atrium and the left ventricle and is influenced by LV compliance and left atrial pressure at the end of the LV systole. The second part of the mitral inflow velocity (A wave) is impacted by atrial contractility and LV compliance. The deceleration time of the E wave velocity correlates with the length of time it takes to reach a point of equal pressure between the left atrium and left ventricle, and the IVRT is the time interval between aortic valve closure and mitral valve opening. In young people who do not have cardiac disorders of any kind, most of the inflow occurs in the early diastole, with an E/A ratio greater than 1.5, along with a short E-wave deceleration time of <180 milliseconds and an IVRT of<80 milliseconds. Early DD (grade I DD) is characterized by delayed LV relaxation, increased early diastolic pressures, and a reduced transmitral pressure gradient; it is accompanied by vigorous atrial contraction, and accordingly the E/A ratio becomes less than 0.9, with prolongation of the deceleration time (>240 ms) and IVRT (>90 ms).[58] With further worsening of diastolic function and impedance to atrial emptying (grade II DD), the left atrial pressure increases, leading to a higher E velocity and E/A ratio (0.9–1.5), a deceleration time of 160 to 240 milliseconds, and an IVRT of less than 90 milliseconds; this state has sometimes been referred to a pseudonormal filling pattern. With a restrictive filling pattern (grade III DD), the E/A ratio becomes greater than 2, with a reduction in deceleration time to less than 150 milliseconds, and an IVRT of less than 70 milliseconds. Patients who have a restrictive filling pattern but show improvement using maneuvers that reduce preload, such as using the Valsalva maneuver for impaired relaxation, have less severe DD and a better prognosis than those who have an irreversible restrictive pattern (grade IV DD).[58] These

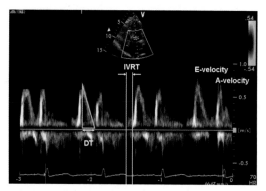

Fig. 3. Mitral inflow velocities profile on pulse wave Doppler. A-velocity, atrial component of mitral filling; DT, deceleration time; E-velocity, early diastolic mitral inflow velocity.

measures are limited by higher heart rates and atrial fibrillation. and they are highly preload dependent.

Pulmonary venous flow Doppler images recorded in the apical four-chamber view can provide an estimate of late diastolic LV pressure but are difficult to obtain.[59] An increase in early diastolic LV filling pressure is associated with a decrease in forward systolic flow (S velocity) and a more prominent diastolic velocity (D velocity). As left atrial afterload increases, there is more resistance to forward flow across the mitral valve, and flow reversal into the pulmonary veins (Ar velocity) increases both in duration (usually >35 ms) and amplitude (Ar velocity >30 cm/s).[59]

Using the color M mode in Doppler imaging, the flow propagation velocity (Vp) in the early diastole can be readily recorded using high temporal and spatial resolution.[58] The Vp (normal >50 cm/s) has a significant correlation with the intraventricular pressure gradient and LV relaxation.[60] The Vp was shown in earlier studies to be insensitive to preload changes; the ratio of mitral E velocity to Vp was used to correct for the influence of LV relaxation on E velocity, and thus to predict filling pressures, with an E/Vp ratio greater than 1.5 suggestive of a pulmonary capillary wedge pressure of greater than 15 mm Hg.[58,61] Again, these measures are highly preload dependent.

Given the limitations of the above measures, impaired LV relaxation may be better characterized through the evaluation of mitral annular motion using pulsed-wave tissue Doppler imaging (TDI). Pulsed-wave TDI is used to measure peak myocardial velocities and is particularly well suited to the measurement of long-axis ventricular motion because the longitudinally oriented endocardial fibers are most parallel to the ultrasound beam in the apical views and are less load dependent.[62] Because the apex remains relatively stationary throughout the cardiac cycle, mitral annular motion is a good surrogate measure of overall longitudinal LV contraction and relaxation.[62] During the diastole in patients with sinus rhythm, velocities can be recorded during the isovolumetric relaxation period and the early (Ea) and late (Aa) diastole (**Fig. 4**). When validated against invasive hemodynamic measures, TDI can be correlated with the time constant of isovolumetric relaxation. In adults older than 30 years of age, a lateral Ea velocity greater than 12 cm/s is associated with normal LV diastolic function. Reductions in lateral Ea velocity to 8 cm/s in middle-aged to older adults indicate impaired LV relaxation and can assist in differentiating a normal from a pseudonormal mitral inflow pattern.[58,62] A ratio of Ea velocity to mitral E velocity (E/Ea) can be used to reliably predict left ventricular filling pressure and has been shown to correlate to LV filling pressure obtained at cardiac catheterization.[63,64]

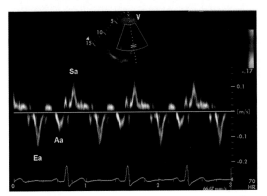

Fig. 4. Pulsed-wave TDI of the mitral annulus. Aa, atrial contraction; Ea, early diastolic motion; Sa, systolic myocardial motion.

The use of two-dimensional speckle tracking technology is a relatively new echocardiographic technique that can characterize myocardial function in terms of deformation or strain and by the rate of deformation or strain, and unlike velocity, it is not affected by tethering and translation. The global diastolic strain rate during the isovolumetric relaxation phase of the cardiac cycle (SRivr) behaves as a load-independent index of LV relaxation, relates well with the time constant of LV relaxation, and is less influenced by annular and valvular pathology and by preload. The relationship of the mitral E-wave velocity to the SRivr appears to relate well to an elevation in mean pulmonary capillary wedge pressure when compared with the E/Ea ratio.[65]

In the evaluation for DD, an echocardiographic assessment of left atrial volume and the LV mass index is imperative and cannot be ignored. The left atrial volume provides insight into the chronicity of elevation of LV filling pressure and is regarded as a barometer of the chronicity of DD, and to make an analogy, left atrial volume is to diastolic function and to all forms of heart disease as HbA_{1c} is to diabetes.[58] During ventricular diastole, the left atrium is directly exposed to LV pressure through the open mitral valve, and as an adaptation to the decreased ventricular compliance, left atrial pressure rises, increasing left atrial wall tension and stretching the atrial myocardium. Thus, increased left atrial volume and enlargement usually reflect elevated ventricular filling pressure,[58] are common findings in hypertension,[49] and provide useful criteria for classifying functional impairment in hypertensive heart disease.[50]

CURRENT THERAPEUTIC STRATEGIES FOR DIASTOLIC DYSFUNCTION AND HEART FAILURE WITH PRESERVED EJECTION FRACTION

Currently, the best evidence for improving structural abnormalities comes from clinical trials to date that have focused exclusively on patients who have systolic heart failure, postmyocardial infarction, or hypertension in which pharmacologic therapy using beta-blockers and inhibitors of RAAS has been shown to improve morbidity and mortality. Above all, DD has not been defined as a therapeutic target for prevention or treatment of HFPEF. Thus, the treatment recommendations are based upon empiric therapies and expert opinions.

Regular exercise and endurance training has been shown to reduce arterial pressure, improve endothelial function[39,66] in the vasculature, reduce ventricular and vascular stiffness, and even to prevent age-related increases in ventricular stiffness and development of DD,[67] which in turn could prevent increases in LV filling pressure during exercise and subsequent development of heart failure. Reduction in dietary salt lowers arterial pressure and could reduce arterial stiffness, improve diastolic function, and attenuate adverse CV effects of aging in patients who have hypertension.[20] Thus, lifestyle modification with regular exercise and dietary salt restriction should be encouraged in patients who have hypertension.

Optimal blood pressure reduction using agents such as diuretics, calcium antagonists, and RAAS antagonists can reduce CV-related morbidity and mortality and is associated with enhanced myocardial relaxation,[15,68] reduced central aortic stiffness,[69] and a dramatic reduction in the incidence of heart failure.[70] Blood pressure reduction using a combination of the angiotensin-converting enzyme inhibitor (ACEI) benazepril and the calcium-channel blocker amlodipine was found to be superior to the combination of the ACEI benazepril and the thiazide diuretic hydrochlorothiazide in reducing CV events (hazard ratio, 0.80 for the benazepril–amlodipine combination; 95% confidence interval, 0.72 to 0.90; $P<.001$) in the recently concluded Avoiding CV Events through Combination Therapy in Patients Living with Systolic Hypertension (ACCOMPLISH) trial.[71] The reduction in the central arterial systolic pressure is believed to account for the greater effectiveness of the ACEI, angiotensin receptor blockers (ARBs), and calcium blocker compared with conventional diuretics and beta-blocking drugs in reducing adverse CV events in people who have hypertension.[69,72] The ACEI and ARBs inhibit the RAAS and prevent neurohormonal activation, reducing fibrillar collagen deposition[73] and myocardial stiffness and reversing LVH.[74] Some of these actions are thought to be load-independent mechanisms related to a blockade of angiotensin II-mediated myocyte hypertrophy, a reduction in the cardiac extracellular collagen matrix, and decreases in aldosterone release and bradykinin-mediated actions.[75,76] Long-term therapy with the ACEI ramipril in the Heart Outcomes Prevention Evaluation (HOPE)[77] study revealed favorable effects on LV structure and function by reducing LVM and LV volumes and the reduction loss in LVEF in high-risk patients who had vascular disease while controlling blood pressure and reducing CV mortality, myocardial infarction, and stroke.[78] Similarly, the Losartan Intervention For Endpoint Reduction in Hypertension (LIFE) study demonstrated that treatment with the ARB losartan was associated with greater reduction in LV mass compared with the use of β-beta-blocker therapy, with a significant reduction in CV mortality and the number of heart failure–relatedhospitalizations.[74,79]

The Candesartan in Heart Failure: Assessment of Reduction in Mortality and Morbidity (CHARM)-Preserved trial did not show any beneficial effect for the ARB candesartan on CV death in patients who had heart failure and LVEF above 40%, but it showed a significantly reduced number of hospitalizations for heart failure (230 versus 279, $P = .017$), and there was a nonsignificant trend to reduction in the composite primary endpoint of CV death or heart failure–related hospitalizations (covariate-adjusted hazard ratio 0.86 for candesartan versus placebo, $P = .051$).[80] Similarly, in the Perindopril in Elderly People with Chronic Heart Failure (PEP-CHF) trial,[81] the ACEI perindopril failed to show any beneficial impact on the primary outcome, with a composite of all-cause mortality and unplanned heart failure–related hospitalizations secondary to insufficient power, but at the end of the first year, patients treated with perindopril were less likely to experienced the primary outcome (10.8% versus 15.3%, hazard ratio, 0.69; 95% CI, 0.47–1.01; $P = .055$) and hospitalization for heart failure (hazard ratio, 0.63; 95% CI, 0.41–0.97; $P = .03$) and they showed an improvement in functional class and a six-minute walk distance. Thus, there is a growing rational for use of inhibitors of the RAAS for the treatment of DD and the prevention of heart failure due to the additional cardioprotection achieved from these agents in patients who have a variety of CV disorders.

Despite evidence from the above studies, the recently published Irbesartan in Heart Failure with Preserved Ejection Fraction (I-PRESERVE) study,[82] which was designed to evaluate the effect of the ARB irbesartan in patients who have HFPEF, failed to demonstrate a beneficial effect for irbesartan in reducing the primary outcome of death from any cause or hospitalization for a CV cause (heart failure, myocardial infarction, unstable angina, arrhythmia, or stroke) (hazard ratio, 0.95; 95% CI, 0.86 to 1.05; $P = .35$).[82]

Even though no pharmacologic therapy has been shown to be effective in improving outcomes in patients who have HFPEF, reduction in arterial pressure has proven to be effective in improving diastolic function. The VALIDD trial was designed to test the hypothesis that lowering blood pressure using the ARB valsartan would improve diastolic function to a greater extent than lowering blood pressure using non-RAAS approaches in patients who have Stage 1 or 2 hypertension.[15] At the primary end point of the trial, diastolic function was evaluated using TDI of mitral annular relaxation velocities at baseline and after 38 weeks of therapy. The difference in blood pressure reduction between the two groups was not significant. The diastolic relaxation velocity increased by 0.60 cm/s from baseline in the valsartan group ($P<0.0001$) and by

0.44 cm/s from baseline in the placebo group ($P<0\cdot0001$) by week 38 (**Fig. 5**). However, there was no significant difference in the change in diastolic relaxation velocity between the groups ($P = 0.29$).[15] Reduction in blood pressure was associated with increases in annular relaxation velocity, even after adjusting for baseline relaxation velocity, blood pressure, age, and study treatment group ($P = 0\cdot01$), with a blood pressure reduction of 10 mm Hg or greater demonstrating the greatest degree of improvement in relaxation velocity (**Fig. 6**).[15] The investigators in the Antihypertensive and Lipid-Lowering Treatment to Prevent Heart Attack Trial (ALLHAT), in their analysis on the effect of the initial drug used to treat hypertension on the subsequent risk of heart failure requiring hospitalization stratified by ejection fraction, concluded that treatment of hypertension with the thiazide diuretic chlorthalidone reduced the risk of HFPEF compared with other therapies using amlodipine, lisinopril, or doxazosin; the hazard ratios were 0.69 (95% CI, 0.53 to 0.91; $P = .009$), 0.74 (95% CI, 0.56 to 0.97; $P = .032$), and 0.53 (95% CI, 0.38 to 0.73; $P<.001$), respectively.[83] Lowering arterial pressure and treating hypertension could be effective in improving diastolic function and reducing the risk of developing heart failure irrespective of the type of antihypertensive agent used, as supported by analysis of the VALIDD and ALLHAT studies.

In addition to adequate control of hypertension, therapies should be directed at controlling the heart rate and restoring the sinus rhythm in patients who have supraventricular tachyarrhythmias, reducing the congestive state, and avoiding coronary ischemia.[84] There are several ongoing studies of DD that may further add to our understanding of the pathophysiology and treatment of diastolic dysfunction. The EXforge Aggressive Control of Hypertension to Evaluate Efficacy in Diastolic Dysfunction trial is an investigator-initiated, randomized, open-label, blinded endpoint–design trial to test the effects of standard versus intensive blood pressure lowering using a combination of the calcium-channel blocker amlodipine plus the ARB valsartan on diastolic function and vascular stiffness in patients who have uncontrolled type II hypertension with preserved systolic function and echocardiographic evidence of DD. The National Institutes of Health–sponsored Treatment of Preserved Systolic Function Heart Failure with an Aldosterone Antagonist (TOPCAT) trial, which is based on the observation that aldosterone-related myocardial fibrosis may play a similar role in the pathogenesis of age- and hypertension-related DD, is evaluating the effectiveness of aldosterone

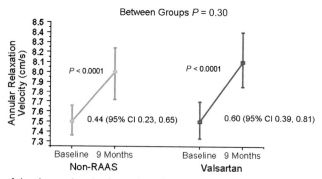

Fig. 5. Graph of the change in mitral annular relaxation velocity from baseline to follow-up in the VALIDD trial (non-RAAS, non–renin-angiotensin-aldosterone system). (*From* Solomon SD, Janardhanan R, Verma A, et al. Effect of angiotensin receptor blockade and antihypertensive drugs on diastolic function in patients with hypertension and diastolic dysfunction: a randomised trial. Lancet 2007;369:2079–87; with permission.)

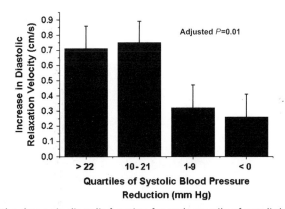

Fig. 6. Graph of the change in diastolic function for each quartile of systolic blood pressure reduction in the VALIDD trial. Error bars are standard error. (*From* Solomon SD, Janardhanan R, Verma A, et al. Effect of angiotensin receptor blockade and antihypertensive drugs on diastolic function in patients with hypertension and diastolic dysfunction: a randomised trial. Lancet 2007;369:2079–87; with permission.)

antagonist therapy in reducing all-cause mortality in patients who have HFPEF. The ongoing Effect of Losartan and Amlodipine on Left Ventricular Diastolic Function in Patients with Mild-to-Moderate Hypertension (J-ELAN) study is a multicenter, prospective, randomized trial designed to assess the effects of losartan and amlodipine on LV diastolic function in patients who have hypertension and DD in the absence of systolic dysfunction.[85] Novel therapeutic targets focusing on disease mechanism that have been identified and are under investigation include regression of hypertrophy by inhibition of rho-kinase[86] and phase II trials evaluating MCC-135 (Mitsubishi Pharma Corp. Compound, or Caldaret) in subjects who have chronic heart failure.[87]

SUMMARY

LVDD as an early measure of myocardial end-organ damage is commonly associated with hypertension and may well precede development of LVH in hypertension. About half of the patients presenting with heart failure have a normal ejection fraction, a clinical syndrome that is commonly referred to as HFPEF or diastolic heart failure and is commonly associated with impaired LV relaxation and increased diastolic stiffness. DD and HFPEF are commonly associated with advancing age and hypertension and increase in prevalence in association with these conditions, but there is a paucity of data on any specific therapeutic regimen. Hypertension control appears to be the most effective strategy in improving diastolic function and possibly for reducing the morbidity and mortality associated with HFPEF.

REFERENCES

1. Redfiled MM, Jacobsen SJ, Burnett JC Jr, et al. Burden of systolic and diastolic ventricular dysfunction in the community: appreciating the scope of the heart failure epidemic. JAMA 2003;289:194–202.
2. Yancy CW, Lopatin M, Stevenson LW, et al. Clinical presentation, management, and in-hospital outcomes of patients admitted with acute decompensated heart failure with preserved systolic function: a report from the Acute Decompensated

Heart Failure National Registry (ADHERE) database. J Am Coll Cardiol 2006;47: 76–84.

3. Owan TE, Hodge DO, Herges RM, et al. Trends in prevalence and outcome of heart failure with preserved ejection fraction. N Engl J Med 2006;355:251–9.

4. Redfiled Steven J, Jacobsen, Borlaug BA, et al. Age- and gender-related ventricular-vascular stiffening: a community-based study. Circulation 2005;112: 2254–62.

5. Bella JN, Palmieri V, Roman MJ, et al. Mitral ratio of peak early to late diastolic filling velocity as a predictor of mortality in middle-aged and elderly adults: the strong heart study. Circulation 2002;105:1928–33.

6. Chinnaiyan KM, Alexander D, Maddens M, et al. Curriculum in cardiology: integrated diagnosis and management of diastolic heart failure. Am Heart J 2007; 153:189–200.

7. Bhatia RS, Tu JV, Lee DS, et al. Outcome of heart failure with preserved ejection fraction in a population-based study. N Engl J Med 2006;355:260–9.

8. Solomon SD, Anavekar N, Skali H, et al. Candesartan in Heart Failure Reduction in Mortality (CHARM) Investigators [2005]. Influence of ejection fraction on cardiovascular outcomes in a broad spectrum of heart failure patients. Circulation 2005;112:3738–44.

9. Morgan JP. Abnormal intracellular modulation of calcium as a major cause of cardiac contractile dysfunction. N Engl J Med 1991;325(9):625–32.

10. Slama M, Susic D, Varagic J, et al. Diastolic dysfunction in hypertension. Curr Opin Cardiol 2002;17:368–73.

11. Zile M, Brutsaert D. New concepts in diastolic dysfunction and diastolic heart failure: Part I: diagnosis, prognosis, and measurements of diastolic function. Circulation 2002;105:1387–93.

12. Tian R, Nascimben L, Ingwall JS, et al. Failure to maintain a low ADP concentration impairs diastolic function in hypertrophied rat hearts. Circulation 1997;96:1313–9.

13. Garcia M. Left ventricular filling. Heart Fail Clin 2008;4:47–56.

14. Desai A. Current understanding of heart failure with preserved ejection fraction. Curr Opin Cardiol 2007;22:578–85.

15. Solomon SD, Janardhanan R, Verma A, et al. Effect of angiotensin receptor blockade and antihypertensive drugs on diastolic function in patients with hypertension and diastolic dysfunction: a randomised trial. Lancet 2007;369:2079–87.

16. Aeschbacher BC, Hutter D, Fuhrer J, et al. Diastolic dysfunction precedes myocardial hypertrophy in the development of hypertension. Am J Hypertens 2001;14:106–13.

17. Chobanian AV, Bakris GL, Black HR, et al. and the National High Blood Pressure Education Program Coordinating Committee. Seventh report of the joint national committee on prevention, detection, evaluation, and treatment of high blood pressure. Hypertension 2003;42:1206–52.

18. Izzo JL Jr, Levy D, Black HR. Clinical advisory statement. Importance of systolic blood pressure in older Americans. Hypertension 2000;35:1021–4.

19. Susic D, Frohlich ED. The aging hypertensive heart: a brief update. Nat Clin Pract Cardiovasc Med 2008;5(2):104–10.

20. Gates PE, Tanaka H, Hiatt WR, et al. Dietary sodium restriction rapidly improves large elastic artery compliance in older adults with systolic hypertension. Hypertension 2004;44:35–41.

21. O'Rourke M. Arterial stiffness, systolic blood pressure, and logical treatment of arterial hypertension. Hypertension 1990;15:339–47.

22. Ouzounian M, Lee DS, Liu P. Diastolic heart failure: mechanism and controversies. Nat Clin Pract Cardiovasc Med 2008;5(7):375–86.
23. Bronzwaer JG, Paulus WJ. Matrix, cytoskeleton, or myofilaments: which one to blame for diastolic left ventricular dysfunction? Prog Cardiovasc Dis 2005; 47(4):276–84.
24. Norton GR, Tsotetsi J, Trifunovic B, et al. Myocardial stiffness is attributed to alterations in cross-linked collagen rather than total collagen or phenotypes in spontaneously hypertensive rats. Circulation 1997;96(6):1991–8.
25. Weber KT, Brilla CG. Pathological hypertrophy and cardiac interstitium: fibrosis and renin–angiotensin–aldosterone system. Circulation 1991;83:1849–65.
26. Zile MR, Brutsaert DL. New concepts in diastolic dysfunction and diastolic heart failure: part II: causal mechanisms and treatment. Circulation 2002;105: 1503–8.
27. Weber KT. Cardiac interstitium in health and disease: the fibrillar collagen network. J Am Coll Cardiol 1989;13:1637–52.
28. Spinale FS, Coker ML, Bond BR, et al. Myocardial matrix degradation and metalloproteinase activation in the failing heart: a potential therapeutic target. Cardiovasc Res 2000;46:225–38.
29. Susic D, Varagic J, Ahn J, et al. Crosslink breakers: a new approach to cardiovascular therapy. Curr Opin Cardiol 2004;19:336–40.
30. Zhao W, Choi JH, Hong G, et al. Left ventricular relaxation. Heart Fail Clin 2008;4: 37–46.
31. Cain BS, Meldrum DR, Joo KS, et al. Human SERCA2a levels correlate inversely with age in senescent human myocardium. J Am Coll Cardiol 1998; 32:458–67.
32. Flesch M, Schiffer F, Zolk O, et al. Contractile systolic and diastolic dysfunction in renin-induced hypertensive cardiomyopathy. Hypertension 1997;30:383–91.
33. Cooper G IV. Cardiocyte cytoskeleton in hypertrophied myocardium. Heart Fail Rev 2000;5:187–201.
34. Tagawa H, Wang N, Narishige T, et al. Cytoskeletal mechanics in pressure overload cardiac hypertrophy. Circ Res 1997;80:281–9.
35. Zile MR, Green GR, Schuyler GT, et al. Cardiocyte cytoskeleton in patients with left ventricular pressure overload hypertrophy. J Am Coll Cardiol 2001;37(4): 1080–4.
36. Borbely A, van der Velden J, Papp Z, et al. Cardiomyocyte stiffness in diastolic heart failure. Circulation 2005;111:774–81.
37. van Heerebeek L, Borbély A, Nissen HWM, et al. Myocardial structure and function differ in systolic and diastolic heart failure. Circulation 2006;113:1966–73.
38. Brutsaert DL, Fransen P, Andries LJ, et al. Cardiac endothelium and myocardial function. Cardiovasc Res 1998;38:281–90.
39. Taddei S, Virdis A, Ghiadoni L, et al. Endothelium, aging, and hypertension. Curr Hypertens Rep 2006;8:84–9.
40. Struthers AD. Aldosterone blockade in cardiovascular disease. Heart 2004;90: 1229–34.
41. Hahn AW, Resink TJ, Scott Burden T, et al. Stimulation of endothelin mRNA and secretion in rat vascular smooth muscle cells: a novel autocrine function. Cell Regul 1990;1:649–59.
42. Mottram PM, Haluska B, Leano R, et al. Effect of aldosterone antagonism on myocardial dysfunction in hypertensive patients with diastolic heart failure. Circulation 2004;110:558–65.

43. Levy D, Savage DD, Garrison RJ, et al. Echocardiographic criteria for left ventricular hypertrophy: the Framingham Heart Study. Am J Cardiol 1987;59:956–60.
44. Levy D, Garrison RJ, Savage DD, et al. Prognostic implications of echocardiographically determined left ventricular mass in the Framingham Heart Study. N Engl J Med 1990;322:1561–6.
45. Hill JA, Olson E. Cardiac plasticity. N Engl J Med 2008;358:1370–80.
46. Vakili BA, Okin PM, Devereux RB. Prognostic implications of left ventricular hypertrophy. Am Heart J 2001;141(3):334–41.
47. Klapholz M, Maurer M, Lowe AM, et al. Hospitalization for heart failure in the presence of a normal left ventricular ejection fraction: results of the New York Heart Failure Registry. J Am Coll Cardiol 2004;43(8):1432–8.
48. Vaziri SM, Larson MG, Lauer MS, et al. Influence of blood pressure on left atrial size: the Framingham Heart Study. Hypertension 1995;25:1155–60.
49. Tarazi RC, Miller A, Frohlich ED, et al. Electrocardiographic changes reflecting left atrial abnormality in hypertension. Circulation 1966;34(5):818–22.
50. Frohlich ED, Tarazi R, Dustan HP. Clinical-physiological correlations in the development of hypertensive heart disease. Circulation 1971;44(3):446–55.
51. Matsuda M, Matsuda Y. Mechanism of left atrial enlargement related to ventricular diastolic impairment in hypertension. Clin Cardiol 1996;19:954–9.
52. Pritchett AM, Mahoney DW, Jacobsen SJ, et al. Diastolic dysfunction and left atrial volume: a population-based study. J Am Coll Cardiol 2005;45:87–92.
53. Safar ME, Levy BI, Struijker-Boudier H. Current perspectives on arterial stiffness and pulse pressure in hypertension and cardiovascular diseases. Circulation 2003;107:2864–9.
54. Borlaug BA, Kass DA. Ventricular–vascular interaction in heart failure. Heart Fail Clin 2008;4:23–36.
55. Izzo JL. Arterial stiffness and the systolic hypertension syndrome. Curr Opin Cardiol 2004;19:341–52.
56. Borlaug BA, Melenovsky V, Redfield MM, et al. The impact of arterial load and loading sequence on left ventricular tissue velocities in humans. J Am Coll Cardiol 2007;50(16):1570–7.
57. Yamamoto K, Nishimura RA, Redfield MM. Assessment of mean left atrial pressure from the left ventricular pressure tracing in patients with cardiomyopathies. Am J Cardiol 1996;78:107–10.
58. Lester SJ, Tajik J, Nishimura RA, et al. Unlocking the mysteries of diastolic function: deciphering the Rosetta Stone 10 years later. J Am Coll Cardiol 2008;51:679–89.
59. Rossvoll O, Hatle LK. Pulmonary venous flow velocities recorded by transthoracic Doppler ultrasound: relation to left ventricular diastolic pressures. J Am Coll Cardiol 1993;21:1687–96.
60. Brun P, Tribouilloy C, Duval AM, et al. Left ventricular flow propagation during early filling is related to wall relaxation: a color M-mode Doppler analysis. J Am Coll Cardiol 1992;20:420–32.
61. Firstenberg MS, Levine BD, Garcia MJ, et al. Relationship of echocardiographic indices to pulmonary capillary wedge pressures in healthy volunteers. J Am Coll Cardiol 2000;36:1664–9.
62. Ho CY, Solomon SD. A clinician's guide to tissue Doppler imaging. Circulation 2006;113:e396–8.
63. Nagueh SF, Middleton KJ, Kopelen HA, et al. Doppler tissue imaging: a noninvasive technique for evaluation of left ventricular relaxation and estimation of filling pressures. J Am Coll Cardiol 1997;30:1527–33.

64. Ommen SR, Nishimura RA, Appleton CP, et al. Clinical utility of Doppler echocardiography and tissue Doppler imaging in the estimation of left ventricular filling pressures: a comparative simultaneous Doppler–catheterization study. Circulation 2000;102:1788–94.
65. Wang J, Khoury DS, Thohan V, et al. Global diastolic strain rate for the assessment of left ventricular relaxation and filling pressures. Circulation 2007;115:1376–83.
66. McGuire DK, Levine BD, Williamson JW, et al. A 30-year follow-up of the Dallas Bedrest and Training Study: II. Effect of age on cardiovascular adaptation to exercise training. Circulation 2001;104:1358–66.
67. Arbab-Zadeh A, Dijk E, Prasad A, et al. Effect of aging and physical activity on left ventricular compliance. Circulation 2004;110:1799–805.
68. Wachtell K, Bella JN, Rokkedal J, et al. Change in diastolic left ventricular filling after one year of antihypertensive treatment: The Losartan Intervention for Endpoint Reduction in Hypertension (LIFE) Study. Circulation 2002;105(9):1071–6.
69. Williams B, Lacy PS, Thom SM, et al. Differential impact of blood pressure-lowering drugs on central aortic pressure and clinical outcomes: principal results of the Conduit Artery Function Evaluation (CAFE) study. Circulation 2006;113(9):1213–25.
70. Kostis JB, Davis BR, Cutler J, et al. Prevention of heart failure by antihypertensive drug treatment in older persons with isolated systolic hypertension. SHEP Cooperative Research Group. JAMA 1997;278(3):212–6.
71. Jamerson K, Weber MA, Bakris GL, et al. ACCOMPLISH trial investigators. Benazepril plus amlodipine or hydrochlorothiazide for hypertension in high-risk patients. N Engl J Med 2008;359(23):2417–28.
72. Rg Asmar, London GM, O'Rourke MF, et al. Improvement in blood pressure, arterial stiffness, and wave reflections with a very-low-dose perindopril/indapamide combination in hypertensive patients: comparison with atenolol. Hypertension 2001;38:922–6.
73. Brilla CG, Funck RC, Rupp H. Lisinopril-mediated regression of myocardial fibrosis in patients with hypertensive heart disease. Circulation 2000;102:1388–93.
74. Devereux RB, Dahlöf B, Gerdts E, et al. Regression of hypertensive left ventricular hypertrophy by losartan compared with atenolol: the Losartan Intervention For Endpoint Reduction in Hypertension (LIFE) trial. Circulation 2004;110:1456–62.
75. Dzau VJ. Tissue angiotensin and pathobiology of vascular disease: a unifying hypothesis. Hypertension 2001;37:1047–52.
76. Lonn EM, Yusuf S, Jha P, et al. Emerging role of angiotensin-converting enzyme inhibitors in cardiac and vascular protection. Circulation 1994;90:2056–69.
77. Lonn E, Shaikholeslami R, Yi Q, et al. Effects of ramipril on left ventricular mass and function in cardiovascular patients with controlled blood pressure and with preserved left ventricular ejection fraction: a substudy of the Heart Outcomes Prevention Evaluation (HOPE) Trial. J Am Coll Cardiol 2004;43(12):2200–6.
78. Yusuf S, Sleight P, Pogue J, et al. The Heart Outcomes Prevention Evaluation Study investigators. Effects of an angiotensin-converting-enzyme inhibitor, ramipril, on cardiovascular events in high-risk patients. N Engl J Med 2000;342:145–53.
79. Wachtell K, Dahlöf B, Rokkedal J, et al. Change in left ventricular geometric pattern after 1 year of antihypertensive treatment: the Losartan Intervention For Endpoint reduction in hypertension (LIFE) study. Am Heart J 2002;144:1057–64.

80. Yusuf S, Pfeffer MA, Swedberg K, et al. Effects of candesartan in patients with chronic heart failure and preserved left-ventricular ejection fraction: the CHARM-Preserved trial. Lancet 2003;362(9386):777–81.
81. Cleland JGF, Tendera M, Adamus J, et al. On behalf of PEP-CHF Investigators. The Perindopril in Elderly People with Chronic Heart Failure (PEP-CHF) study. Eur Heart J 2006;27:2338–45.
82. Massie BM, Carson PE, McMurray JJ, et al. The I-PRESERVE Investigators. Irbesartan in heart failure with preserved ejection fraction. N Engl J Med 2008;359(23):2456–67.
83. Davis BR, Kostis JB, Simpson LM, et al. Heart failure with preserved and reduced left ventricular ejection fraction in the Antihypertensive and Lipid-Lowering Treatment to Prevent Heart Attack trial. Circulation 2008;118:2259–67.
84. Aurigemma GP, Gaasch WH. Clinical practice. Diastolic heart failure. N Engl J Med 2004;351(11):1097–105.
85. The J-ELAN Investigators. Effect of losartan and amlodipine on left ventricular diastolic function in patients with mild-to-moderate hypertension (J-ELAN): rationale and design. Circ J 2006;70:124–8.
86. Higashi M, et al. Long-term inhibition of Rho-kinase suppresses angiotensin II-induced cardiovascular hypertrophy in rats in vivo: effect on endothelial NAD(P)H oxidase system. Circ Res 2003;93:767–75.
87. Zile M, Gaasch W, Little W, et al. MCC-135 GO1 Investigators. A phase II, double-blind, randomized, placebo-controlled, dose comparative study of the efficacy, tolerability, and safety of MCC-135 in subjects with chronic heart failure, NYHA class II/III (MCC-135-GO1 study): rationale and design. J Card Fail 2004;10: 193–9.

Hypertension and Cardiac Failure in its Various Forms

Krishna K. Gaddam, MD, Anil Verma, MD, Mark Thompson, MD, Rohit Amin, MD, Hector Ventura, MD*

KEYWORDS

- Hypertension • Left ventricular hypertrophy
- Hypertensive heart disease • Systolic heart failure
- Diastolic heart failure

Hypertension leads to the development of left ventricular hypertrophy (LVH), atherosclerotic heart disease, and heart failure (with reduced systolic function or preserved systolic function), which are often collectively referred to as hypertensive heart disease and may represent a continuum. More than 75% of patients who have heart failure have antecedent hypertension.[1,2] Besides heart failure with systolic dysfunction, diastolic dysfunction with preserved ejection fraction (EF) is being recognized as an increasingly prevalent condition and is associated with significant morbidity and mortality.[3,4] This association underscores the importance of early and aggressive intervention in patients who have hypertension in order to prevent progression to clinical heart failure. This article reviews the interrelation between various components of hypertensive heart disease: epidemiology, pathophysiology, diagnosis, and treatment.

EPIDEMIOLOGY

An estimated 550,000 new cases of heart failure occur each year in the United States and more than five million Americans have heart failure.[2] The prevalence of heart failure continues to increase, largely due to an aging population and modern therapies leading to prolonged survival of cardiac patients. Hypertension increases the risk for heart failure in all age groups. Data from the Framingham Heart Study and from the Center for Disease Control and Prevention (CDC) suggest that 1 in 5 adults aged 40 will develop heart failure during their lifetime. Besides the overall lifetime risk, it has also been shown that 1 in 9 men and 1 in 6 women among patients with hypertension and without antecedent myocardial infarction develop heart failure, highlighting the

Department of Medicine, Division of Cardiovascular Diseases, Ochsner Clinic Foundation, 1514 Jefferson Highway, New Orleans, LA 70121, USA
* Corresponding author.
E-mail address: hventura@ochsner.org (H. Ventura).

Med Clin N Am 93 (2009) 665–680
doi:10.1016/j.mcna.2009.02.005
0025-7125/09/$ – see front matter © 2009 Elsevier Inc. All rights reserved.

medical.theclinics.com

risk attributable to hypertension alone. In those individuals aged 40 years or older whose blood pressure is greater than or equal to 160/100 mm Hg, the lifetime risk for developing heart failure may be twice as high as that for their age-matched counterparts with blood pressure less than 140/90 mm Hg.[2,5] The impact of hypertension on the progress of heart failure has been described in the literature by the population attributable risk (PAR) that takes into account both the hazard ratio and the prevalence of the predisposing condition in the population. The First National Health and Nutrition Examination Survey (NHANES I) of 13,643 men and women found that of the risk factors for heart failure, the PAR for hypertension was 10% and that for coronary heart disease was 62%.[6]

Cross-sectional studies show that among subjects with clinical heart failure, half of them have reduced ejection fraction, and half have preserved ejection fraction.[3,4] In addition, heart failure in either form is associated with high mortality. In a study including 2671 participants from the Cardiovascular Health Study who had no prior history of coronary heart disease, heart failure, or atrial fibrillation at baseline, 170 participants (6.4% of the cohort) developed heart failure defined as a constellation of symptoms (shortness of breath, fatigue, orthopnea and paroxysmal nocturnal dyspnea) and signs (edema, rales, tachycardia, a gallop rhythm, and a displaced apical impulse) at a mean follow up of 5.2 years.[7] Forty-seven percent of the participants who developed heart failure had hypertension at baseline compared with 28% (P = .0001) in subjects who did not develop heart failure (mean blood pressure at baseline was 145 $\pm$ 22/73 $\pm$ 13 vs. 134 $\pm$ 21/70 $\pm$ 11 mm Hg; P = .0001/0.0006). Among the participants who developed heart failure, 57% of the subjects had a normal ($\geq$ 55%) or borderline (> 45% but < 55%) ejection fraction. In multivariate modeling, besides markers of systolic function, peak Doppler peak E independently predicted incident heart failure. Both high and low Doppler E/A ratios were predictive of incident heart failure, thus indicating that diastolic dysfunction is an independent predictor for future development of heart failure. Similarly, data from the Strong Heart Study indicated that low (<0.6) or high E/A (1.5) ratio is associated with increased all-cause mortality and cardiac mortality, highlighting the importance of diastolic dysfunction as a potential target of treatment to improve cardiac morbidity and mortality.[8] Overall, heart failure in either form is a major global health problem contributing to a significant morbidity and mortality and requiring a significant portion of health care spending.

PATHOPHYSIOLOGY OF HYPERTENSIVE HEART DISEASE

The mechanisms by which hypertension predisposes to heart failure is not clearly understood. Within the normal heart, the framework of the cardiac structure is determined in part by a balance of collagen synthesis and degradation. This balance is held in check by several mediators having either profibrotic (such as growth factors, cytokines, and renin-angiotensin-aldosterone system [RAAS]) or collagenolytic (nitric oxide, bradykinins, natriuretic peptides) effects.[9] Various conditions, including hypertension, diabetes mellitus, obesity, smoking, valvular heart disease, and coronary heart disease, derail the balance, leading to systolic and diastolic dysfunction.[6,10] Antecedent hypertension in survivors of acute myocardial infarction has been shown to be strongly associated with left ventricular (LV) dysfunction, heart failure, or both.[11–13] Patients who have hypertension demonstrated greater neurohormonal activation compared with those without hypertension following an acute myocardial infarction, suggesting a neurohormonal-mediated deterioration of LV function in patients who have hypertension.[11] Persistent hypertension promotes neurohumoral (RAAS and sympathetic nervous system) activation, which results in a profibrotic milieu leading to alterations in extracellular matrix (amount, geometry, distribution, degree of crosslinking, and ratio of collagen subtypes).[14,15] In addition to myocardial fibrosis, hypertrophy of the cardiac myocytes (secondary to increased afterload) increase their circumferential diameter, leading to concentric ventricular hypertrophy, impaired ventricular performance (either systolic or diastolic), and clinical heart failure.[16] Recent observation studies have also indicated that cardiomyocyte apoptosis is stimulated in the hypertrophied left ventricle of patients with essential hypertension, no angiographic evidence of coronary artery disease and normal cardiac function, suggesting that cardiomyocyte apoptosis precedes the impairment of ventricular function.[17] Pharmacologic strategies to inhibit and/or counteract the apoptotic process with an aim to protect the cardiomyocyte and prevent the progression to heart failure in patients with hypertensive heart disease are being carried out. Hypertension further promotes atherosclerosis and myocardial infarction with resultant ischemic heart disease and heart failure, which are not necessarily always separate pathways but may often overlap (**Fig. 1**).[18]

Two recent studies demonstrate subtle systolic dysfunction suggested by a reduction in long axis strain rate, peak systolic strain, cyclic variation in subjects without a prior history of hypertension but with a hypertensive response to exercise,[19] and regional differences in end systolic strain and peak systolic strain in subjects who have mild hypertension even in the absence of LVH and standard functional indices of LV dysfunction.[20] A growing body of evidence also suggests that diastolic dysfunction can be present in hypertensive patients even in the absence of LVH.[21] These studies underscore the role of hypertension as an important contributor to the development of either form of heart failure.

IDENTIFICATION OF HYPERTENSIVE HEART DISEASE

Echocardiography is the most commonly used imaging modality to assess for LVH, systolic, and diastolic function. Left ventricular hypertrophy can be detected using specific electrocardiographic (ECG) criteria, most commonly the Sokolow-Lyon index (sum of SV1 + RV5 or V6 > 3.5 mV) or the Cornell voltage criteria (men: RaVL + SV3 > 2.8 mV; women: RaVL + SV3 > 2.0 mV).[22–24] Estimates of LV mass are conventionally indexed to body surface area (grams/meter^2) or height (grams/meter) to correct for body size. The American Society of Echocardiography defines LVH as LV mass index of greater than 95 g/m^2 in women or greater than 115 g/m^2 in men using 2D echocardiography (**Fig. 2**) (**Table 1**).[25]

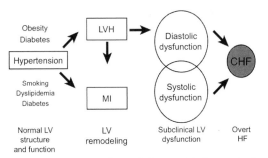

Fig. 1. Progression from hypertension to heart failure. LV, left ventricular; LVH, left ventricular hypertrophy; MI, myocardial infarction; CHF, congestive heart failure; HF, heart failure. (*Reprinted from* Vasan RS, et al. The role of hypertension in the pathogenesis of heart failure. A clinical mechanistic overview. Arch Intern Med 1996;156(16):1789–96; with permission. Copyright © 1996, American Medical Association.)

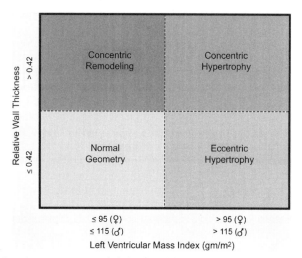

Fig. 2. Distinction between normal left ventricular geometry, concentric remodeling, concentric left ventricular hypertrophy and eccentric left ventricular hypertrophy based on left ventricular mass index and relative wall thickness. (*Reprinted from* Lang RM, et al. Recommendations for chamber quantification: a report from the American Society of Echocardiography's Guidelines and Standards Committee and the Chamber Quantification Writing Group, developed in conjunction with the European Association of Echocardiography, a branch of the European Society of Cardiology. J Am Soc Echo 2005;18(12):1440–63; with permission.)

LV ejection fraction less than 50% (in some studies < 40%) is usually considered as systolic dysfunction. Echocardiographic markers of diastolic dysfunction include a ratio of early mitral valve flow (E) to early diastolic lengthening (E′) velocities (E/E′) >15, a ratio of peak early (E) to peak late (A) Doppler mitral valve flow velocity (E/A) <0.5, a deceleration time of early Doppler mitral valve flow greater than 280 ms, a left atrial volume indexed to body surface area greater than 40 mL/m^2, and LV mass index greater than 122 g/m^2 for women and greater than 149 g/m^2 for men.[26] Diastolic dysfunction is further categorized as mild, moderate, or severe, based on tissue Doppler findings (**Fig. 3**). Cardiac magnetic resonance imaging is increasingly being used for the same and is highly accurate and reproducible for the assessment of cardiac volumes, global function, myocardial thickness, myocardial mass, and cardiac valves.[27,28]

Another useful tool in the diagnosis of heart failure is the measurement of plasma B-type natriuretic peptide (BNP). The ventricles respond to stress by activating BNP transcription and subsequent release of this peptide in patients who have both systolic and diastolic dysfunction. Although, the diagnostic potential of natriuretic peptides has not been clearly established, a low–normal concentration in an untreated patient makes heart failure unlikely as the cause of symptoms.[29,30] In patients who have symptoms of heart failure and preserved LV systolic function, a plasma BNP level of greater than 57 pg/mL had a positive predictive value of 100% for diastolic abnormalities as defined by the aforementioned echocardiographic modalities.[31]

PREVENTION OF HEART FAILURE

Lifestyle modifications have been shown to reduce overall cardiovascular risk, including risk of heart failure. Current guidelines and a recent AHA Scientific Statement

Table 1
Reference limits and partition values of left ventricular mass and geometry

	Women				Men			
	Reference Range	Mildly Abnormal	Moderately Abnormal	Severely Abnormal	Reference Range	Mildly Abnormal	Moderately Abnormal	Severely Abnormal
Lineas method								
LV mass, g	67–162	163–186	187–210	≥211	88–224	225–258	259–292	≥293
LV mass/BSA, g/m²	43–95	96–108	109–121	≥122	49–115	116–131	132–148	≥149
LV mass/height, g/m	41–99	100–115	116–128	≥129	52–126	127–144	145–162	≥163
LV mass/height, g/m²·⁷	18–44	45–51	52–58	≥59	20–48	49–55	56–63	≥64
Relative wall thickness, cm	0.22–0.42	0.43–0.47	0.48–0.52	≥0.53	0.24–0.42	0.43–0.46	0.47–0.51	≥0.52
Septal thickness, cm	0.6–0.9	1.0–1.2	1.3–1.5	≥1.6	0.6–1.0	1.1–1.3	1.4–1.6	≥1.7
Posterior wall thickness, cm	0.6–0.9	1.0–1.2	1.3–1.5	≥1.6	0.6–1.0	1.1–1.3	1.4–1.6	≥1.7
2D method								
LV mass, g	66–150	151–171	172–182	≥193	96–200	201–227	228–254	≥255
LV mass/BSA, g/m²	44–88	89–100	101–112	≥113	50–102	103–116	117–130	≥131

Abbreviations: BSA, Body surface area; LV, Left ventricular; 2D, 2-dimensional.

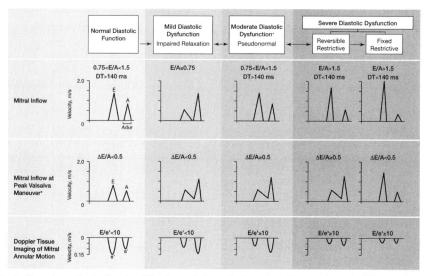

Fig. 3. Doppler criteria for classification of diastolic function. E = peak early filling velocity; A = velocity of atrial contraction; e′ = velocity of mitral annulus early diastolic motion; a′ = velocity of mitral annulus motion with atrial systole; DT = mitral E velocity deceleration time. (*Reprinted from* Redfield MM, et al. Burden of systolic and diastolic ventricular dysfunction in the community: appreciating the scope of the heart failure epidemic. JAMA 2003;289(2):194–202; with permission. Copyright © 2003, American Medical Association.)

recommend lifestyle modifications (ie, smoking cessation, reduction in alcohol consumption, cessation of illicit drug use, regular physical activity, and weight reduction) for prevention of heart failure.[30,32–34]

Studies including hypertensive subjects have demonstrated an association between LVH and the risk of heart failure.[35,36] Randomized controlled trials have established that antihypertensive treatment results in regression of LVH and reduces the risk of developing heart failure by about 50%.[1,37,38] Antihypertensive treatment with drugs from all classes except direct vasodilators is effective in reversing LVH.[38,39]

The Losartan Intervention for Endpoint Reduction in Hypertension (LIFE) study is a randomized controlled trial of antihypertensive treatment that enrolled subjects with LVH based on electrocardiographic criteria.[40] LIFE tested the hypothesis that selective blockade of angiotensin II action with an ARB would improve LVH beyond reducing blood pressure and consequently would decrease the risk of cardiovascular morbidity and death. LIFE randomized 9193 participants to once-daily losartan-based or atenolol-based antihypertensive treatment in a double-blind, randomized, parallel-group study design. The primary composite endpoint (cardiovascular mortality, myocardial infarction, or stroke) was decreased significantly (508 vs. 588 events; relative risk 0.87; 95% CI, 0.77–0.98; P = .021) with losartan-based treatment despite similar blood pressure reductions in both study arms. In a recent analysis of data from the LIFE study, it was shown that during a mean follow-up of 4.7 years, decrease in electrocardiographic LVH during treatment in hypertensive subjects was associated with fewer hospitalizations for new–onset heart failure.[41] On the contrary, absence of reduction in LVH was associated with a higher rate of new–onset heart failure. This relationship was independent of the degree of blood pressure reduction, treatment method, and other risk factors for heart failure.

Diuretics, β-blockers, and RAAS inhibitors have been shown to be highly effective in preventing heart failure and are recommended for that indication by the Seventh Report of the Joint National Committee on Prevention, Detection, Evaluation, and Treatment.[42–49] However, most of the outcome studies that examined this issue did not distinguish heart failure with systolic dysfunction from that with diastolic dysfunction. The Antihypertensive and Lipid-Lowering Treatment to Prevent Heart Attack Trial (ALLHAT) demonstrated that treatment with the thiazide-like diuretic chlorthalidone was more effective than either ACE inhibitor, CCB, or α-blocker treatment in preventing heart failure in high-risk, older hypertensive patients.[44–47]

In the recent study including ALLHAT participants who were hospitalized for a first episode of heart failure and had ejection fraction estimated by echocardiography, contrast ventriculography, or radionuclide study (n = 910), it was shown that 56% had systolic dysfunction (EF < 50%) and 44% had heart failure with preserved systolic function (EF > 50%).[47] Cox regression models unadjusted and adjusted for baseline characteristics of age, race, gender, prior hypertension treatment, systolic blood pressure, diastolic blood pressure, heart rate, smoking, diabetes mellitus, LVH, history of coronary disease, estimated glomerular filtration rate, body mass index, and high density lipoprotein levels demonstrated that chlorthalidone significantly reduced the overall risk of hospitalized heart failure. Chlorthalidone also significantly reduced the incidence of new–onset heart failure with reduced or preserved ejection fraction compared with amlodipine and doxazosin but had an effect similar to lisinopril.

In the Hypertension in the Very Elderly Trial (HYVET), 3845 subjects who were 80 years of age or older and had a sustained systolic blood pressure of 160 mm Hg or more were randomly assigned to receive active treatment (a diuretic indapamide 1.5 mg) (n = 1933) or matching placebo (n = 1912) and then had the ACE inhibitor perindopril (2 or 4 mg) or matching placebo added in the respective groups if necessary to achieve the target blood pressure of 150/80 mm Hg.[48] Following 2 years of treatment, active treatment resulted in a fall in seated blood pressure by a mean of 29.5/12.9 mm Hg versus 14.5/6.8 mm Hg in the placebo group. In addition to a significant decrease in the primary endpoints of fatal or nonfatal stroke, active treatment was associated with a 64% reduction in the rate of heart failure (95% CI, 42 to 78; $P<.001$).

TREATMENT OF HEART FAILURE

All of the major classes of antihypertensive drugs with the exception of calcium antagonists, particularly β-blockers and RAS antagonists, have been shown to improve survival in patients who have LV systolic dysfunction (**Table 2**).[50–60] The Studies of Left Ventricular Dysfunction (SOLVD) trial was the first clinical trial to demonstrate that in subjects (n = 2569) with chronic heart failure and LV systolic dysfunction, addition of enalapril to conventional therapy compared with placebo decreased mortality and hospitalization.[55] The TRandalopril Cardiac Evaluation (TRACE)[61] and Survival and Ventricular Enlargement (SAVE) trials demonstrated that treatment with an ACE inhibitor resulted in significant long-term survival benefits in subjects who have LV dysfunction following an acute myocardial infarction. Similarly, the efficacy of ARBs in reducing cardiovascular morbidity and mortality in subjects who have heart failure was demonstarted in the Candesartan in Heart Failure: Assessment of Reduction in Mortality and Morbidity (CHARM) study,[57] the Valsartan Heart Failure Trial (Val-HeFT)[62] and the Valsartan in Acute Myocardial Infarction trial (VALIANT).[60]

Several beta blockers, including carvedilol, metoprolol, bisoprolol, and nebivolol, have been proven to be effective in decreasing cardiovascular mortality in patients

Table 2
Summary of clinical trials in the utility of various antihypertensive agents in heart failure

				Results	
Trial (n)	Intervention	Follow-up	Inclusion Criteria	Primary Outcome	Secondary Outcome
CIBIS II (n = 2647)[51]	Bisoprolol versus placebo	15 mo (mean)	NYHA class III-IV HF and LVEF ≤ 35%	32% reduction in all-cause mortality (P<.0001)	14% reduction in all-cause hospitalizations (P = .0006); 32% reduction in heart failure admissions (P = .0001); 45% reduction in sudden cardiac death (P<.0011); 26% reduction in cardiovascular deaths (P = .0049)
United States Carvedilol Heart Failure Study[50] (n = 1094)	Carvedilol versus placebo	6.5 mo (median)	Patients who had symptoms of HF and LVEF ≤ 35%	65% reduction in death (P<.001)	38% reduction in combined risk of death or hospitalization (P<.001)
MERIT-HF (n = 3991)[52]	Metoprolol CR/XL versus placebo	12 mo (mean)	NYHA class II-IV HF and LVEF ≤ 40%	34% reduction in all-cause mortality (P = .00009)	40% fewer sudden deaths (P = .0002) and 48% fewer deaths from heart failure (P = .0023)
SENIORS (n = 2128)[53]	Nebivolol versus placebo	21 mo (mean)	Hospital admission for HF regardless of ejection fraction in patients ≥ 70 years	12% reduction in composite of all-cause mortality or cardiovascular hospital admission (P = .039)	No differences were noted in secondary outcomes
SOLVD (n = 2569)[55]	Enalapril versus placebo	41.4 mo (mean)	NYHA class II-III HF and LVEF ≤ 35%	16% reduction in mortality (P = .0036)	26% fewer admissions or deaths from heart failure (P<.0001)
SAVE (n = 2231)[56]	Captopril versus placebo	42 mo (mean)	Postmyocardial infarction with LVEF < 40%	20% reduction in all-cause mortality	Development of severe heart failure was 37% less and 22% fewer heart failure hospitalizations

Trial	Comparison	Duration	Inclusion criteria	Outcome	Additional findings
CHARM (n = 7601)[57]	Candesartan versus placebo	37.7 mo (median)	NYHA class II–IV HF and LVEF ≤ 40% who are being treated with an ACE inhibitor or who are ACE intolerant	Significant reduction in covariate adjusted all cause mortality; significantly lower cardiovascular deaths and HF admissions	Significant reduction in each component of the primary outcome
Val-HeFT (n = 5010)[62]	Valsartan versus placebo	23 mo (mean)	NYHA class II–IV HF and LVEF < 40%	No difference in overall mortality, but the combined endpoint of mortality and morbidity was 13.2% lower (P = .009)	27.5% reduction of hospitalization with heart failure (P<.001) + significant improvement in NYHA class and fewer worsenings
VALIANT (n = 14,808)[60]	Valsartan versus valsartan + captopril versus captopril	24.7 mo (median)	Recent myocardial infarction (within 0.5 to 10 days) + clinical or radiological signs of heart failure + LVEF ≤ 35% by echo or angiography or ≤ 40% on radionuclide ventriculography	Valsartan was noninferior to captopril in reducing the primary outcome of death from any cause	Combination of valsartan and captopril increased the frequency of adverse events without improving the survival
RALES (n = 1663)[58]	Spironolactone versus placebo	24 mo (mean)	NYHA class III–IV HF and LVEF ≤ 35%	30% reduction in risk of death (P<.001).	Frequency of hospitalization with worsening HF was 35% lower (P<.001)
EPHESUS (n = 6632)[59]	Eplerenone versus placebo	16 mo (mean)	HF with EF ≥45%, controlled SBP	15% reduction in all-cause death (P = .008) + fewer deaths and hospitalizations from cardiovascular causes	21% reduction in rate of sudden death (P = .03) + fewer deaths and hospitalizations from any cause

Abbreviations: HF, Heart failure; LVEF, Left ventricular ejection fraction; MI, Myocardial infarction; NYHA, New York Heart Association.

who have LV systolic dysfunction.[50–54] The United States Carvedilol Heart Failure Study included 1094 subjects who have chronic heart failure (LVEF ≤ 35%) who were treated with diuretics and ACE inhibitors.[50] Subjects were assigned to one of four treatment protocols (placebo or 6.25 mg, 12.5 mg or 25 mg of carvedilol twice daily). Carvedilol therapy resulted in a 65% reduction of overall mortality (P<.001) and a 27% reduction in the risk of hospitalization from cardiovascular causes (P = .036). Similarly, the Metoprolol CR/XL Randomized Intervention Trial in Heart Failure (MERIT-HF) clearly established that treatment with beta-1 selective antagonist metoprolol lowered all-cause mortality, sudden deaths, and deaths from heart failure compared with placebo when added to ongoing optimum therapy (diuretics + ACE inhibitors) in subjects with EF ≤ 40% and the New York Heart Association (NYHA) functional class II-IV.[52] The Study of the Effects of Nebivolol Intervention on Outcomes and Hospitalization in Seniors with Heart Failure (SENIORS) study, performed in 2128 elderly subjects who have heart failure, demonstrated that, compared with placebo, nebivolol decreased the composite risk of all-cause mortality and cardiovascular hospital admission in subjects who have either heart failure with reduced ejection fraction or preserved ejection fraction.[53,54]

Aldosterone is being increasingly associated with the severity of blood pressure. Cross-sectional and prospective studies have indicated that aldosterone contributes significantly both to the development and severity of hypertension as well as to resistance to antihypertensive treatment.[63–65] There is also increasing evidence of antihypertensive benefit of mineralocorticoid receptor antagonists in treating resistant hypertension.[66,67] Aldosterone also has an important role in the pathophysiology of heart failure[68–70] on the basis of which two large clinical trials were conducted in subjects who have advanced LV systolic heart failure[58] or myocardial infarction complicated with LV systolic dysfunction.[59] In the Randomized Aldactone Evaluation Study (RALES), 1663 subjects who have NYHA class III or IV heart failure, LVEF ≤ 35%, and who were being treated with diuretics and ACE inhibitors were randomized to spironolactone or placebo. Based on interim results, the trial was discontinued early. After a mean follow-up of 24 months, there was a 30% (P<.001) reduction in mortality from progressive heart failure or sudden cardiac death and a 35% (P<.001) reduction in hospitalization for worsening heart failure in subjects treated with spironolactone compared with the placebo-treated group. Comparable results were also seen in the Eplerenone Post-Acute Myocardial Infarction Heart Failure Efficacy and Survival Study (EPHESUS) in which eplerenone was compared with placebo.

Although the above discussed studies provide evidence for the preferred antihypertensive agents in patients who have LV systolic heart failure, blood pressure goals in systolic heart failure have not been specifically defined on the basis of clinical trial data. However, reducing systolic blood pressure to the range of 110 to 130 mm Hg appears to be beneficial. Some experts even advocate lowering systolic blood pressure to < 100 mm Hg or as low as tolerated, in part on the basis of results of the Carvedilol Prospective Randomized Cumulative Survival (COPERNICUS) trial.[50]

Unlike heart failure with reduced systolic function, there is no treatment proven to be useful in treatment of heart failure with preserved EF. Treatment is largely empiric, focusing on blood pressure control and treating or avoiding intravascular volume overload. Major regulators of collagen synthesis, LVH, and LV stiffness include physical forces (preload and afterload) and neurohumoral activation by the RAS and sympathetic nervous system. Inhibition of RAS prevents or reverses this increase in fibrillar collagen and reduces myocardial stiffness.[71] Given the increasing evidence of cardiac fibrosis and LVH as common contributors to heart failure with preserved ejection fraction and extensive evidence of the role of RAS antagonists in limiting or reversing cardiac fibrosis, these agents seem appropriate for prevention and treatment of diastolic dysfunction and heart failure with preserved ejection fraction. RAS modulators and some CCBs are the only antihypertensive classes shown to improve exercise tolerance in patients who have diastolic dysfunction.[72–74] Studies including subjects who have hypertension and heart failure with preserved ejection fraction and in animal models of diastolic dysfunction and heart failure with preserved ejection fraction have implicated aldosterone and mineralocorticoid receptors in the pathogenesis of those disorders.[75–79] Administration of spironolactone to patients who have heart failure with preserved ejection fraction has been shown to relieve symptoms and decrease left atrial area, suggesting a beneficial effect on diastolic function.[75] There is paucity of clinical trials including subjects who have heart failure with preserved ejection fraction. However, the available data does not definitively support the use of any specific agents in treating HFPEF, which is discussed in detail by Verma and colleagues elsewhere in this issue).[80–84]

SUMMARY

Hypertension clearly increases the risk of systolic or diastolic heart failure. With aging population and advancements in treatment of cardiovascular diseases, the prevalence of heart failure is ever-increasing and is a principal cause of cardiovascular morbidity and mortality. Treating hypertension has been shown to decrease the risk of development of heart failure and hence underscores the early recognition and treatment of hypertension and hypertensive heart disease. Antihypertensive treatment with drugs from all classes except direct vasodilators is effective in reversing LVH and preventing heart failure. Also, all of the major classes of antihypertensive drugs, particularly β-blockers and RAS antagonists, with the exception of calcium antagonists, have been shown to improve survival in patients who have LV systolic dysfunction. However, phenotyping and identifying the pathophysiology and appropriate treatments for patients who have diastolic dysfunction and heart failure with preserved ejection fraction has been a daunting task. At this time, treatment of these patients is largely empiric, focusing on BP control, and treating or avoiding intravascular volume overload.

REFERENCES

1. Levy D, Larson MG, Vasan RS, et al. The progression from hypertension to congestive heart failure. JAMA 1996;275(20):1557–62.
2. Rosamond W, Flegal K, Furie K, et al. Heart disease and stroke statistics–2008 update: a report from the American Heart Association Statistics Committee and Stroke Statistics Subcommittee. Circulation 2008;117(4):e25–146.
3. Redfield MM, Jacobsen SJ, Burnett JC Jr, et al. Burden of systolic and diastolic ventricular dysfunction in the community: appreciating the scope of the heart failure epidemic. JAMA 2003;289(2):194–202.
4. Bursi F, Weston SA, Redfield MM, et al. Systolic and diastolic heart failure in the community. JAMA 2006;296(18):2209–16.
5. Lloyd-Jones DM, Larson MG, Leip EP, et al. Lifetime risk for developing congestive heart failure: the Framingham Heart Study. Circulation 2002;106(24):3068–72.
6. He J, Ogden LG, Bazzano LA, et al. Risk factors for congestive heart failure in US men and women: NHANES I epidemiologic follow-up study. Arch Intern Med 2001;161(7):996–1002.

7. Aurigemma GP, Gottdiener JS, Shemanski L, et al. Predictive value of systolic and diastolic function for incident congestive heart failure in the elderly: the cardiovascular health study. J Am Coll Cardiol 2001;37(4):1042–8.

8. Bella JN, Palmieri V, Roman MJ, et al. Mitral ratio of peak early to late diastolic filling velocity as a predictor of mortality in middle-aged and elderly adults: the Strong Heart Study. Circulation 2002;105(16):1928–33.

9. Laurent GJ. Dynamic state of collagen: pathways of collagen degradation in vivo and their possible role in regulation of collagen mass. Am J Physiol 1987;252 (1 Pt 1):C1–9.

10. Zile MR, Brutsaert DL. New concepts in diastolic dysfunction and diastolic heart failure: part I: diagnosis, prognosis, and measurements of diastolic function. Circulation 2002;105(11):1387–93.

11. Richards AM, Nicholls MG, Troughton RW, et al. Antecedent hypertension and heart failure after myocardial infarction. J Am Coll Cardiol 2002;39(7):1182–8.

12. Lewis EF, Moye LA, Rouleau JL, et al. Predictors of late development of heart failure in stable survivors of myocardial infarction: the CARE study. J Am Coll Cardiol 2003;42(8):1446–53.

13. Thune JJ, Signorovitch J, Kober L, et al. Effect of antecedent hypertension and follow-up blood pressure on outcomes after high-risk myocardial infarction. Hypertension 2008;51(1):48–54.

14. Moncrieff J, Lindsay MM, Dunn FG. Hypertensive heart disease and fibrosis. Curr Opin Cardiol 2004;19(4):326–31.

15. Ahmed SH, Clark LL, Pennington WR, et al. Matrix metalloproteinases/tissue inhibitors of metalloproteinases: relationship between changes in proteolytic determinants of matrix composition and structural, functional, and clinical manifestations of hypertensive heart disease. Circulation 2006;113(17):2089–96.

16. Frohlich ED. State of the art lecture. Risk mechanisms in hypertensive heart disease. Hypertension 1999;34:782–9.

17. Gonzalez A, Susana R, Lopez B, et al. Apoptosis in hypertensive heart disease: a clinical approach. Curr Opin Cardiol 2006;21:288–94.

18. Vasan RS, Levy D, et al. The role of hypertension in the pathogenesis of heart failure. A clinical mechanistic overview. Arch Intern Med 1996;156(16):1789–96.

19. Mottram PM, Haluska B, Yuda S, et al. Patients with a hypertensive response to exercise have impaired systolic function without diastolic dysfunction or left ventricular hypertrophy. J Am Coll Cardiol 2004;43(5):848–53.

20. Baltabaeva A, Marciniak M, Bijnens B, et al. Regional left ventricular deformation and geometry analysis provides insights in myocardial remodelling in mild to moderate hypertension. Eur J Echocardiogr 2008;9(4):501–8.

21. Aeschbacher BC, Hutter D, Fuhrer J, et al. Diastolic dysfunction precedes myocardial hypertrophy in the development of hypertension. Am J Hypertens 2001;14(2):106–13.

22. Sokolow M, Lyon TP. The ventricular complex in left ventricular hypertrophy as obtained by unipolar precordial and limb leads. Am Heart J 1949;37(2):161–86.

23. Casale PN, Devereux RB, Kligfield P, et al. Electrocardiographic detection of left ventricular hypertrophy: development and prospective validation of improved criteria. J Am Coll Cardiol 1985;6(3):572–80.

24. Casale PN, Devereux RB, Kligfield P, et al. Improved sex-specific criteria of left ventricular hypertrophy for clinical and computer interpretation of electrocardiograms: validation with autopsy findings. Circulation 1987;75(3):565–72.

25. Lang RM, Bierig M, Devereux RB, et al. Recommendations for chamber quantification: a report from the American Society of Echocardiography's Guidelines and

Standards Committee and the Chamber Quantification Writing Group, developed in conjunction with the European Association of Echocardiography, a branch of the European Society of Cardiology. J Am Soc Echocardiogr 2005;18(12): 1440–63.

26. Paulus WJ, Tschope C, Sanderson JE, et al. How to diagnose diastolic heart failure: a consensus statement on the diagnosis of heart failure with normal left ventricular ejection fraction by the Heart Failure and Echocardiography Associations of the European Society of Cardiology. Eur Heart J 2007;28(20):2539–50.

27. Bellenger NG, Francis JM, Davies CL, et al. Establishment and performance of a magnetic resonance cardiac function clinic. J Cardiovasc Magn Reson 2000; 2(1):15–22.

28. Grothues F, Moon JC, Bellenger NG, et al. Interstudy reproducibility of right ventricular volumes, function, and mass with cardiovascular magnetic resonance. Am Heart J 2004;147(2):218–23.

29. Swedberg K, Cleland J, Dargie H, et al. Guidelines for the diagnosis and treatment of chronic heart failure: executive summary (update 2005): The Task Force for the Diagnosis and Treatment of Chronic Heart Failure of the European Society of Cardiology. Eur Heart J 2005;26(11):1115–40.

30. Hunt SA, Abraham WT, Chin MH, et al. ACC/AHA 2005 Guideline Update for the Diagnosis and Management of Chronic Heart Failure in the Adult: a report of the American College of Cardiology/American Heart Association Task Force on Practice Guidelines (Writing Committee to Update the 2001 Guidelines for the Evaluation and Management of Heart Failure): developed in collaboration with the American College of Chest Physicians and the International Society for Heart and Lung Transplantation: endorsed by the Heart Rhythm Society. Circulation 2005;112(12):e154–235.

31. Krishnaswamy P, Lubien E, Clopton P, et al. Utility of B-natriuretic peptide levels in identifying patients with left ventricular systolic or diastolic dysfunction. Am J Med 2001;111(4):274–9.

32. Levine BD, Lane LD, Buckey JC, et al. Left ventricular pressure-volume and Frank-Starling relations in endurance athletes. Implications for orthostatic tolerance and exercise performance. Circulation 1991;84(3):1016–23.

33. Meyer TE, Kovacs SJ, Ehsani AA, et al. Long-term caloric restriction ameliorates the decline in diastolic function in humans. J Am Coll Cardiol 2006;47(2): 398–402.

34. Schocken DD, Benjamin EJ, Fonarow GC, et al. Prevention of heart failure: a scientific statement from the American Heart Association Councils on Epidemiology and Prevention, Clinical Cardiology, Cardiovascular Nursing, and High Blood Pressure Research; Quality of Care and Outcomes Research Interdisciplinary Working Group; and Functional Genomics and Translational Biology Interdisciplinary Working Group. Circulation 2008;117(19):2544–65.

35. Aronow WS, Ahn C, Kronzon I, et al. Congestive heart failure, coronary events and atherothrombotic brain infarction in elderly blacks and whites with systemic hypertension and with and without echocardiographic and electrocardiographic evidence of left ventricular hypertrophy. Am J Cardiol 1991;67(4):295–9.

36. Aronow WS, Ahn C. Association of electrocardiographic left ventricular hypertrophy with the incidence of new congestive heart failure. J Am Geriatr Soc 1998;46(10):1280–1.

37. Moser M, Hebert PR. Prevention of disease progression, left ventricular hypertrophy and congestive heart failure in hypertension treatment trials. J Am Coll Cardiol 1996;27(5):1214–8.

38. Klingbeil AU, Schneider M, Martus P, et al. A meta-analysis of the effects of treatment on left ventricular mass in essential hypertension. Am J Med 2003;115(1): 41–6.

39. Schmieder RE, Martus P, Klingbeil A. Reversal of left ventricular hypertrophy in essential hypertension. A meta-analysis of randomized double-blind studies. JAMA 1996;275(19):1507–13.

40. Dahlof B, Devereux RB, Kjeldsen SE, et al. Cardiovascular morbidity and mortality in the losartan intervention for endpoint reduction in hypertension study (LIFE): a randomised trial against atenolol. Lancet 2002;359(9311):995–1003.

41. Okin PM, Devereux RB, Harris KE, et al. Regression of electrocardiographic left ventricular hypertrophy is associated with less hospitalization for heart failure in hypertensive patients. Ann Intern Med 2007;147(5):311–9.

42. Chobanian AV, Bakris GL, Black HR, et al. Seventh report of the Joint National Committee on prevention, detection, evaluation, and treatment of high blood pressure. Hypertension 2003;42(6):1206–52.

43. Kostis JB, Davis BR, Cutler J, et al. Prevention of heart failure by antihypertensive drug treatment in older persons with isolated systolic hypertension. SHEP Cooperative Research Group. JAMA 1997;278(3):212–6.

44. Major cardiovascular events in hypertensive patients randomized to doxazosin vs chlorthalidone: the Antihypertensive and Lipid-Lowering Treatment to Prevent Heart Attack Trial (ALLHAT). ALLHAT Collaborative Research Group. JAMA 2000;283(15):1967–75.

45. Major outcomes in high-risk hypertensive patients randomized to angiotensin-converting enzyme inhibitor or calcium channel blocker vs diuretic: the antihypertensive and lipid-lowering treatment to prevent heart attack trial (ALLHAT). JAMA 2002;288(23):2981–97.

46. Davis BR, Piller LB, Cutler JA, et al. Role of diuretics in the prevention of heart failure: the antihypertensive and lipid-lowering treatment to prevent heart attack trial. Circulation 2006;113(18):2201–10.

47. Davis BR, Kostis JB, Simpson LM, et al. Heart failure with preserved and reduced left ventricular ejection fraction in the antihypertensive and lipid-lowering treatment to prevent heart attack trial. Circulation 2008;118(22):2259–67.

48. Beckett NS, Peters R, Fletcher AE, et al. Treatment of hypertension in patients 80 years of age or older. N Engl J Med 2008;358(18):1887–98.

49. Bangalore S, Wild D, Parkar S, et al. Beta-blockers for primary prevention of heart failure in patients with hypertension insights from a meta-analysis. J Am Coll Cardiol 2008;52(13):1062–72.

50. Packer M, Bristow MR, Cohn JN, et al. The effect of carvedilol on morbidity and mortality in patients with chronic heart failure. U.S. Carvedilol Heart Failure Study Group. N Engl J Med 1996;334(21):1349–55.

51. The Cardiac Insufficiency Bisoprolol Study II (CIBIS-II): a randomised trial. Lancet 1999;353(9146):9–13.

52. Effect of metoprolol CR/XL in chronic heart failure: Metoprolol CR/XL Randomised Intervention Trial in Congestive Heart Failure (MERIT-HF). Lancet 1999;353(9169): 2001–7.

53. Flather MD, Shibata MC, Coats AJ, et al. Randomized trial to determine the effect of nebivolol on mortality and cardiovascular hospital admission in elderly patients with heart failure (SENIORS). Eur Heart J 2005;26(3):215–25.

54. Ghio S, Magrini G, Serio A, et al. Effects of nebivolol in elderly heart failure patients with or without systolic left ventricular dysfunction: results of the SENIORS echocardiographic substudy. Eur Heart J 2006;27(5):562–8.

55. Effect of enalapril on survival in patients with reduced left ventricular ejection fractions and congestive heart failure. The SOLVD Investigators. N Engl J Med 1991; 325(5):293–302.
56. Pfeffer MA, Braunwald E, Moye LA, et al. Effect of captopril on mortality and morbidity in patients with left ventricular dysfunction after myocardial infarction. Results of the survival and ventricular enlargement trial. The SAVE Investigators. N Engl J Med 1992;327(10):669–77.
57. Pfeffer MA, Swedberg K, Granger CB, et al. Effects of candesartan on mortality and morbidity in patients with chronic heart failure: the CHARM-Overall programme. Lancet 2003;327(9386):759–66.
58. Pitt B, Zannad F, Remme WJ, et al. The effect of spironolactone on morbidity and mortality in patients with severe heart failure. Randomized Aldactone Evaluation Study Investigators. N Engl J Med 1999;341(10):709–17.
59. Pitt B, Remme W, Zannad F, et al. Eplerenone, a selective aldosterone blocker, in patients with left ventricular dysfunction after myocardial infarction. N Engl J Med 2003;348(14):1309–21.
60. Pfeffer MA, McMurray JJ, Velazquez EJ, et al. Valsartan, captopril, or both in myocardial infarction complicated by heart failure, left ventricular dysfunction, or both. N Engl J Med 2003;349(20):1893–906.
61. Kober L, Torp-Pederson C. Clinical characteristics and mortality of patients screened for entry into the Trandalapril Cardiac Evaluation (TRACE) study. Am J Cardiol 1995;76:1–5.
62. Cohn JN, Tognoni G. A randomized trial of the angiotensin-receptor blocker valsartan in chronic heart failure. N Engl J Med 2001;345:1667–75.
63. Vasan RS, Evans JC, Larson MG, et al. Serum aldosterone and the incidence of hypertension in nonhypertensive persons. N Engl J Med 2004;351(1):33–41.
64. Calhoun DA, Nishizaka MK, Zaman MA, et al. Hyperaldosteronism among black and white subjects with resistant hypertension. Hypertension 2002; 40(6):892–6.
65. Gaddam KK, Nishizaka MK, Pratt-Ubunama MN, et al. Characterization of resistant hypertension: association between resistant hypertension, aldosterone, and persistent intravascular volume expansion. Arch Intern Med 2008;168(11): 1159–64.
66. Nishizaka MK, Zaman MA, Calhoun DA. Efficacy of low-dose spironolactone in subjects with resistant hypertension. Am J Hypertens 2003;16(11 Pt 1): 925–30.
67. Chapman N, Dobson J, Wilson S, et al. Effect of spironolactone on blood pressure in subjects with resistant hypertension. Hypertension 2007;49(4):839–45.
68. Dzau VJ, Colucci WS, Hollenberg NK, et al. Relation of the renin-angiotensin-aldosterone system to clinical state in congestive heart failure. Circulation 1981;63(3):645–51.
69. Swedberg K, Eneroth P, Kjekshus J, et al. Hormones regulating cardiovascular function in patients with severe congestive heart failure and their relation to mortality. CONSENSUS Trial Study Group. Circulation 1990;82(5):1730–6.
70. Weber KT, Villarreal D. Aldosterone and antialdosterone therapy in congestive heart failure. Am J Cardiol 1993;71(3):3A–11A.
71. Brilla CG, Funck RC, Rupp H. Lisinopril-mediated regression of myocardial fibrosis in patients with hypertensive heart disease. Circulation 2000;102(12): 1388–93.
72. Bonow RO, Dilsizian V, Rosing DR, et al. Verapamil-induced improvement in left ventricular diastolic filling and increased exercise tolerance in patients with

hypertrophic cardiomyopathy: short- and long-term effects. Circulation 1985; 72(4):853–64.

73. Setaro JF, Zaret BL, Schulman DS, et al. Usefulness of verapamil for congestive heart failure associated with abnormal left ventricular diastolic filling and normal left ventricular systolic performance. Am J Cardiol 1990;66(12):981–6.

74. Warner JG Jr, Metzger DC, Kitzman DW, et al. Losartan improves exercise tolerance in patients with diastolic dysfunction and a hypertensive response to exercise. J Am Coll Cardiol 1999;33(6):1567–72.

75. Mottram PM, Haluska B, Leano R, et al. Effect of aldosterone antagonism on myocardial dysfunction in hypertensive patients with diastolic heart failure. Circulation 2004;110(5):558–65.

76. Ohtani T, Ohta M, Yamamoto K, et al. Elevated cardiac tissue level of aldosterone and mineralocorticoid receptor in diastolic heart failure: beneficial effects of mineralocorticoid receptor blocker. Am J Physiol Regul Integr Comp Physiol 2007;292(2):R946–54.

77. Nagata K, Obata K, Xu J, et al. Mineralocorticoid receptor antagonism attenuates cardiac hypertrophy and failure in low-aldosterone hypertensive rats. Hypertension 2006;47(4):656–64.

78. Masson S, Staszewsky L, Annoni G, et al. Eplerenone, a selective aldosterone blocker, improves diastolic function in aged rats with small-to-moderate myocardial infarction. J Card Fail 2004;10(5):433–41.

79. Shapiro BP, Owan TE, Mohammed S, et al. Mineralocorticoid signaling in transition to heart failure with normal ejection fraction. Hypertension 2008;51(2): 289–95.

80. Yusuf S, Pfeffer MA, Swedberg K, et al. Effects of candesartan in patients with chronic heart failure and preserved left-ventricular ejection fraction: the CHARM-Preserved Trial. Lancet 2003;362(9386):777–81.

81. Cleland JG, Tendera M, Adamus J, et al. The perindopril in elderly people with chronic heart failure (PEP-CHF) study. Eur Heart J 2006;27(19):2338–45.

82. Janardhanan R, Daley WL, Naqvi TZ, et al. Rationale and design: the VALsartan In Diastolic Dysfunction (VALIDD) trial: evolving the management of diastolic dysfunction in hypertension. Am Heart J 2006;152(2):246–52.

83. Massie BM, Carson PE, McMurray JJ, et al. Irbesartan in patients with heart failure and preserved ejection fraction. N Engl J Med 2008;359(23):2456–67.

84. Solomon SD, Janardhanan R, Verma A, et al. Effect of angiotensin receptor blockade and antihypertensive drugs on diastolic function in patients with hypertension and diastolic dysfunction: a randomised trial. Lancet 2007;369(9579): 2079–87.

Hypertension and Myocardial Ischemia

Brian P. Murphy, MBChB, MRCP[a], Tony Stanton, PhD, MBChB, MRCP[b],
Francis G. Dunn, MBChB, FRCP, FACC[a],*

KEYWORDS

- Hypertension • Ischemia • Perfusion
- Mechanisms • Management

Hypertension is an established major risk factor for the clinical syndromes associated with CAD, and therefore has dominated thinking in regard to its known association with myocardial ischemia. Its importance as a risk factor is proven by an impressive epidemiologic base[1] and applies to angina, myocardial infarction, and sudden death. The relationship strengthens with higher blood pressure levels and when left ventricular hypertrophy (LVH) coexists as identified by ECG[2,3] or by echocardiography (ECHO).[4] The cause of these clinical events is often presumed to be obstructive epicardial CAD, but this may not always be the case because there are many factors in hypertension that contribute to these clinical events. This article explores the various ways in which hypertension can produce or contribute to myocardial ischemia (**Fig. 1**).

PATHOPHYSIOLOGY

The heart is a remarkable organ and a more efficient and effective pump than anything human engineering could invent. Oxidative metabolic pathways provide the energy to drive this pump. The successful functioning of the heart requires adequate oxygen supply to the myocardium. Ischemia results from an imbalance in this supply-and-demand relationship.

Increased Myocardial Oxygen Demand

The myocardium relies on aerobic metabolism. The main determinants of myocardial oxygen demand (MVO_2) are heart rate, contractility, and wall tension, which is dependent on aortic pressure, left ventricular (LV) volume, and myocardial fibril length.

[a] Cardiac Department, Stobhill Hospital, 133 Balornock Road, Glasgow G21 3UW, Scotland, UK
[b] Department of Medicine, University of Queensland, Level 4, Princess Alexandra Hospital, Ipswich Road, Brisbane Q4102, Australia
* Corresponding author.
E-mail address: frank.dunn@ggc.scot.nhs.uk (F.G. Dunn).

Med Clin N Am 93 (2009) 681–695
doi:10.1016/j.mcna.2009.02.003
0025-7125/09/$ – see front matter © 2009 Elsevier Inc. All rights reserved.

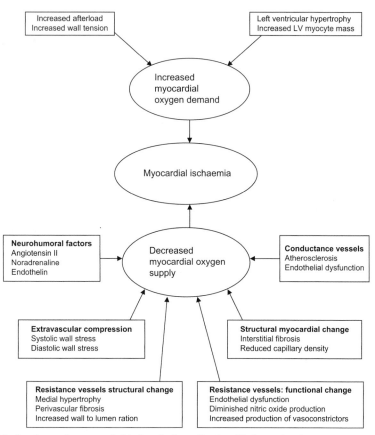

Fig. 1. Mechanisms of myocardial ischemia in patients with hypertension.

Sarnoff and colleagues[5] demonstrated in classic experiments that systolic arterial pressure is a key determinant of MVO_2 through its influence on LV wall tension. Therefore, a sudden or constant increase in systolic blood pressure will result in an increase in oxygen requirement for the heart and, potentially, in myocardial ischemia. LVH, although a compensatory mechanism to counteract the increased wall tension, also leads to increased oxygen demand through an increase in myocyte mass.

Decreased Myocardial Oxygen Supply

Decreased myocardial oxygen supply is principally dependent on coronary blood flow (CBF): myocardial oxygen extraction is near maximal at rest, so any increase in demand can only be met by increasing CBF, which primarily occurs during diastole due to high ventricular pressure and compression of intramyocardial vessels in systole. It is also dependent upon aortic driving pressure, intramyocardial pressure, and coronary vascular resistance.

The *epicardial arteries* are vessels that do not contribute greatly to coronary vascular resistance in the absence of obstructive CAD. The vessel conductance diameter, and hence CBF, can be affected by flow-mediated dilatation (increased shear stress on the vessel wall induces the production of nitric oxide from the arterial endothelium, causing vasodilatation), endothelial dysfunction, circulating vasoactive factors, and neurogenic stimuli.

The *prearterioles* are the principal controllers of CBF and contribute 25%–35% of total coronary vascular resistance. They maintain CBF at the origin of the precapillary arterioles over a preset autoregulatory range. This is dependent on myogenic tone responsive to distending pressure and flow-mediated dilatation in response to shear stress. Although not subject to atherosclerosis, endothelial dysfunction does occur that can affect the prearterioles' ability to control CBF.

The *precapillary arterioles* contribute 40%–50% of the total coronary resistance. They are principally responsive to metabolic stress. In ischemic myocardium, the ability of the myocyte to phosphorylate Adenosine Monophospate is saturated, so it is broken down to adenosine, a potent vasodilator of small arterioles. They are also responsive to neurogenic stimuli and locally active vasoactive substances.

MECHANISMS
Coronary Atherosclerosis

Hypertension has been shown to have both a role in the genesis of atherosclerosis and in the extent and instability of the atherosclerotic plaque.[6–8] The mechanisms by which elevated systemic arterial pressure promotes atherosclerosis are complex. Endothelial dysfunction is the key initiator in the development of atherosclerosis. Rather than stimulating vasodilation and inhibiting platelet aggregation, it becomes procoagulant, produces vasoconstrictor substances, and promotes leukocyte and platelet adhesion and migration. Left unchecked, particularly in the presence of hypercholesterolemia, this leads to smooth muscle hypertrophy and the accumulation of lipid-rich plaque.[9] The stages of atherosclerosis have been demonstrated in a mouse model of hypertension induced by aortic banding.[10] The first coronary arterial changes found 3 days after aortic banding were intense endothelial staining for intracellular adhesion molecules, and macrophage and neutrophil infiltration of the intima. These are the same initiating changes in human atherosclerotic lesions and can be induced by different coronary risk factors.

The direct mechanical effect of hypertension on the coronary arteries causes increased shear stress, transmural pressure, and increased wall stress (stretch stress on endothelial cells). This stimulates nitric oxide production from endothelial cells, but also increases the production of growth factors for vascular smooth muscle cells such as angiotensin II, and increases the surface expression of cellular adhesion molecules that permit leukocyte migration into the intima.[11] The transmural pressure stimulates vascular smooth muscle cell growth, and the stretching effect on endothelial cells leads to the release of factors that increase DNA and protein synthesis in vascular smooth muscle cells and augment endothelial cell angiotensin, converting enzyme activity and increasing angiotensin II production. All of these processes contribute to the development of atherosclerosis.[11]

A number of other neurohumoral factors that are activated in hypertension contribute to endothelial dysfunction and atherogenesis. Sympathetic activation results in structural, hormonal, and biochemical changes that increase the risk of coronary disease events.[12] Elevated angiotensin II levels, particularly in the vessel wall itself, produce several effects, including the promotion of vascular smooth muscle cell growth and stimulating atherosclerosis.[11] Insulin resistance is an important cause of atherosclerosis, and may indeed contribute to the development of hypertension. Through effects on vascular smooth muscle cell calcium handling, it can cause enhanced contractility that can lead to or worsen hypertension.[13] Lower adiponectin levels have been found in hypertensive subjects with CAD than in normal controls.[14] Adiponectin exhibits anti-inflammatory and anti-atherogenic effects, so lower levels may contribute to atherogenesis. Urotensin II, a powerful vasoconstrictor implicated in the etiology of hypertension, may also promote atherogenesis.[15]

Microcirculatory Dysfunction

Hypertension is frequently associated with chest pain and normal coronary arteries, and is often accompanied by evidence of ischemia on exercise stress testing or myocardial perfusion imaging.[16] Asymptomatic ischemia is also common.[17] Myocardial ischemia has been demonstrated on dipyridamole-stress sestamibi single-photon emission computed tomography in more than 1 in 4 subjects with hypertension but no CAD,[18] and it is more prevalent if LVH is present.[19,20] Vogt and colleagues,[21] demonstrated that there was no relationship between diastolic wall stress or extent of LVH and coronary flow reserve (CFR), strongly suggesting that the coronary microvascular abnormalities were of more importance than hemodynamic factors.

Resting CBF is normal in subjects who have hypertension with LVH, but CFR is severely impaired.[22,23] A reduced CFR has been demonstrated in subjects with LVH and angina,[24] and in patients with LVH, the reduction in CFR is more marked in those with evidence of ischemia on myocardial perfusion imaging.[25,26]

The association between impaired CFR and myocardial ischemia is not confined to subjects with LVH.[27] CFR in response to ergonovine and rapid atrial pacing was markedly reduced in subjects who have hypertension with angina and no LVH, compared with normal controls.

Structural Vascular Changes

Chronic systemic hypertension is associated with changes in the vascular wall of small resistance arteries and arterioles with an increased wall-to-lumen ratio, medial hypertrophy and perivascular fibrosis.[10,28,29] These changes are important in the reduced coronary vascular resistance found in hypertension. In subjects who have hypertension with angina and normal epicardial arteries, the reduction in CFR compared with normal controls correlated with the extent of medial hypertrophy and perivascular fibrosis, but not with LV mass index or end–diastolic pressure.[29]

Medial hypertrophy
Medial hypertrophy can be seen as a protective response to exposure to high arterial pressures. The elevated pressure stimulates vascular smooth muscle cell hypertrophy and hyperplasia to maintain the necessary resistance to prevent capillary hyperperfusion and myocyte damage. This protective response has two potentially deleterious effects: (1) the increased wall-to-lumen ratio and increased vascular tone impairs vasodilation in response to increased metabolic demand and may precipitate ischemia; (2) the increased vascular tone causes a shift of the CBF autoregulatory range to the right, and at lower pressures the resistance vessels are no longer able to vasodilate sufficiently to maintain capillary perfusion pressure, again resulting in myocardial ischemia.[30] This may explain the J-shaped curve of cardiovascular outcomes in some hypertension treatment trials, with a suggested increase in adverse outcomes at lower diastolic pressures.[31]

There is ample evidence to suggest that medial hypertrophy is a direct response to elevated arterial pressure. The vascular changes are absent in subjects with aortic stenosis and normal systemic blood pressure compared with subjects who have hypertension, both with similar degrees of LVH.[32] In spontaneously hypertensive rats (SHR), treatment of hypertension with hydralazine, although having no effect on perivascular and interstitial fibrosis, caused regression of medial hypertrophy, presumably as a direct blood pressure– lowering effect, with an associated improvement in CFR.[33] Similarly, in SHR treated with lisinopril, low-dose lisinopril reduced interstitial fibrosis, but only high-doses lowered the blood pressure, regressed medial hypertrophy, and improved CFR.[34] Although medial hypertrophy seems directly associated with elevated arterial pressure, the way in which this occurs is not certain. There is some evidence of a link to endothelial dysfunction, because stimulation of nitric oxide synthase in rats ameliorates the effect of hypertension on medial hypertrophy and impaired CFR,[35] and blockade of nitric oxide synthase induces the expression of angiogenic growth factors that lead to medial hypertrophy.[36] Angiotensin II also appears to be important in stimulating medial hypertrophy, and blockade of the renin angiotensin system inhibits this effect.[37,38]

Perivascular fibrosis reduces vascular distensibility and so potentially contributes to the diminished CFR found in hypertension. Direct pressure effects can influence collagen production and lead to fibrosis.[39] In a rat model, the perivascular fibrosis could be reversed by a low dose of angiotensin-converting enzyme-I (ACE-I), which did not lower BP, but CFR only improved when there was BP lowering and regression of medial hypertrophy.[34] This would suggest that perivascular fibrosis is not as pressure-dependent, nor contributing as much to the diminished CFR, as medial hypertrophy. However, in rats with hypertension induced by aortic banding, relieving the obstruction caused regression of medial hypertrophy but did not improve CFR. This only improved after resolution of the perivascular fibrosis with β-aminopropionitrile.[40] Also, in human studies, total and perivascular collagen volume fraction has been correlated with impaired CFR.[29] Impaired CFR also correlates with a serum marker of fibrosis, serum carboxy-terminal propeptide of procollagen type I, further evidence that perivascular fibrosis may be an important determinant of CFR.[41]

Endothelial Dysfunction and Neurogenic Factors

It has been established that there is endothelial dysfunction in the epicardial arteries in patients who have hypertension.[42–44] Whereas that may not significantly affect CFR, it does indicate that these patients are at risk of progressive atherosclerosis. More pertinent to microcirculatory disturbance has been the demonstration of impaired endothelial- dependent vasodilatation of resistance arteries in response to acetylcholine.[45] These findings establish endothelial dysfunction as a potential mechanism for diminished CFR. There is a clear physiologic basis for this. In hypertension there is diminished basal and pharmacologically stimulated nitric oxide production,[46] which limits CFR. Direct inhibition of nitric oxide synthesis leads to production of angiogenic growth factors that stimulate fibrosis and medial hypertrophy, and impair CFR.[36] Endothelial dysfunction also leads to the production of vasoactive substances such as endothelin-1, which is a powerful vasoconstrictor. There is also increased release of procoagulant factors such as plasminogen activator inhibitor-1, which also contributes to adverse vascular remodeling.[47]

Inhibition of constitutive nitric oxide production in hypertensive subjects has been shown to cause myocardial ischemia.[48] Administration of L-arginine (the substrate for nitric oxide synthase) to patients who have hypertension and angina improves blood pressure, anginal symptoms, and endothelial function.[49] Endothelial dysfunction is clearly a very important mechanism in the impaired CFR in this group of patients.

There may be sympathetic hyperreactivity in hypertension. Overproduction of norepinephrine can lead to an imbalance of its vasodilatory and vasoconstrictor actions (especially in the presence of endothelial dysfunction), leading to increased vascular tone in resistance arteries and arterioles.[50]

CLINICAL ASPECTS AND INVESTIGATIONS

Because it is clear that hypertension can produce and provoke myocardial ischemia, clinical assessment should be directed toward identifying any clues as to its presence. A thorough history with specific questions on ischemia or ischemic-equivalent symptoms should be followed by an assessment of the patient's cardiovascular risk factors. Any other precipitants for ischemia such as anemia and aortic stenosis should be considered and other clinical evidence of atherosclerotic disease identified.

Resting Electrocardiography

ECG remains of key importance in identifying the presence of LVH with or without associated ST-T changes. The pathophysiologic basis for these repolarization abnormalities has not been completely elucidated, but ischemia induced by impaired microvascular coronary reserve and fibrosis has been postulated as a contributory factor.[51]

Increased QRS duration and QT prolongation have also been linked to all-cause and cardiovascular death in hypertensive patients.[52] Again, myocardial ischemia is thought to be one of the main factors in the origin of these changes.

Previously unsuspected MI or ischemic changes may also be seen as well as more subtle abnormalities such as left atrial abnormality. The importance of left atrial abnormality as both a early sign of LV involvement and hemodynamic changes was demonstrated almost 40 years ago[53] and is as relevant today with the ongoing interest in diastolic dysfunction and in atrial fibrillation in patients who have hypertension. Atrial fibrillation is often found for the first time on an ECG in patients presenting with hypertension and can precipitate myocardial ischemia in this already vulnerable group of patients.

Silent ischemia is also common in hypertensive patients and can be picked up by ambulatory Holter monitoring.[17] This manifests as ST-segment depression on Holter monitoring without accompanying angina pectoris. It is estimated to have a prevalence of 20%–26% in hypertensive patients.[54] The ST-segment depression appears to be triggered by variations in blood pressure, heart rate, and circadian rhythm.[55] The presence of silent ischemia brings an accompanying increase in cardiovascular risk.[56]

Exercise Electrocardiography

This investigation is mandatory in any patient who has hypertension and clinical evidence of ischemia. Prognostic information gathered includes ECG changes indicative of ischemia, exercise workload, and blood pressure response. Each of these can be affected by the hypertensive process.

Patients who have hypertension with LVH often have resting ECG abnormalities, making interpretation of stress ECG changes difficult. Even in the absence of resting ECG changes, exercise ECG changes have a low specificity for diagnosing CAD.[57] Hypertensive patients often have impaired exercise tolerance due to decreased CFR, diastolic dysfunction induced by the stiffened, fibrosed ventricle, and the associated abnormal responses of the pulmonary and peripheral circulations. Even in patients who are normotensive at rest, a hypertensive response to exercise is predictive of progression to LVH[58] and a hypertensive response to exercise has been demonstrated to have a significant prognostic adverse effect.[59]

In summary, a negative stress test in the hypertensive patient is reassuring due to its negative predictive value. However in those with an abnormal resting ECG, positive ECG changes with stress (reported to be 30%–40% in hypertensive patients),[60] or those unable to achieve an adequate exercise threshold, another stress test with combined noninvasive imaging is mandatory.

Echocardiography

There is no general agreement on the need to perform ECHO in all patients who have hypertension. Many approach this in a selective manner but the evidence that LVH can be more accurately diagnosed on ECHO is secure. In well-validated laboratories the best option is a combined ECG and ECHO approach. Transthoracic echocardiography is a proven investigation in the evaluation of cardiac mass and function. More recent applications include the estimation of CFR and evaluation of myocardial perfusion.

Coronary flow reserve

CFR can be calculated using either transthoracic or transesophageal echocardiography. Schäfer and colleagues[61] showed that there was a reduction in CFR even in subjects who have hypertension without LVH or concentric remodeling. Marks and colleagues[62] followed 186 subjects, many with hypertension, who had chest pain but normal epicardial coronary arteries on angiography for a mean of 8.5 years. Subjects with impaired CFR had an increased mortality over the course of follow-up.

Stress echocardiography

It is now well documented that stress ECHO is a more reliable test for diagnosing CAD in the patient who has hypertension due to the frequent presence of ST-segment changes both at rest and on stress.[63] Stress ECHO has a sensitivity similar to nuclear imaging (88% versus 98%) for the detection of CAD in patients who have hypertension with a previously positive exercise ECG but a much higher specificity (80% versus 36%).[64] This fact, coupled with the lack of radiation exposure, makes stress ECHO the investigation of choice for the diagnosis of CAD in the hypertensive patient.

One criticism of stress ECHO is that the diagnostic accuracy of the test is dependent on the skill and experience of the reading physician. Newer echocardiographic techniques have been investigated, such as the measurement of myocardial deformation (strain and strain rate) derived from either tissue Doppler or grey-scale images ("speckle tracking"). However, these measures are also affected by LV geometry.[65]

The detection of fibrosis in the hypertensive patient without CAD can also be performed using strain rate imaging.[66] The fiber orientation of the LV at this level suggests that changes in longitudinal deformation will be preferentially affected.[67]

Myocardial contract echocardiography

Myocardial contract echocardiography (MCE) uses gas-filled microbubbles injected intravenously to image the myocardium. Typically, these microbubbles, which are 3–5μm in diameter, pass through the myocardial microcirculation in a similar fashion to red blood cells. Application of high-energy ultrasound to the bubbles causes their destruction, and the rate of microbubble replenishment within the myocardium is used as a measure of microcirculatory perfusion.[68] Using this technique, abnormalities in microcirculation have been shown in hypertensive subjects compared with a healthy control population.[69]

Cardiac Magnetic Resonance Imaging

The emergence of cardiac magnetic resonance imaging (CMR) as a clinical tool has provided another means of imaging the hypertensive patient. Adenosine stress CMR is now accepted as a reliable means of detecting CAD in these patients. Recent work has focused on the detection of subendocardial ischemia and fibrosis by the detection of subendocardial delayed-contrast (normally gadolinium) enhancement.[70] A recent article by Andersen and colleagues[71] also showed a significant correlation between delayed contrast enhancement and ST-segment depression during exercise in a group of subjects who have hypertension with symptoms of ischemia but normal coronary angiograms.

Nuclear Imaging

Single-photon emission computed tomography (SPECT) using extractable tracers such as thallium-201 and technetium-99m (Tc-99m) provides a noninvasive evaluation of myocardial blood flow. However, SPECT is limited in its ability to identify balanced reductions in coronary territories as may happen in the hypertensive patient.

Positron emission tomography (PET) allows estimation of regional myocardial blood flow, CFR, and myocardial metabolism. Several studies have demonstrated decreased CFR in hypertensive patients[72] and the use of PET in these patients is preferable to SPECT. Other authors have shown that PET is able to distinguish subendocardial from subepicardial CFR, thus allowing the calculation of transmural CFR distribution.[73] Recent research has focused on the use of hybrid PET/CT scanners that are able to provide both anatomic (CT) and quantitative (PET) measures of coronary flow.[74]

How aggressively should latent ischemia be sought in patients who have hypertension? Considering the percentage of the population who have hypertension, it would be a formidable exercise to undertake even standard treadmill exercise testing in all patients who have this disorder. Clearly if the patient has any effort-related symptoms or ST-T changes on the ECG, then a detailed search for the presence, extent, and basis for the ischemia should be sought (**Fig. 2**). In patients who are asymptomatic, the potential and likely presence of ischemia should be recognized and treatment tailored accordingly.

MANAGEMENT
Cardiovascular Risk Factor Reduction

Cessation of smoking, regular exercise, and a healthy diet require emphasis at every available opportunity. Statin therapy should be considered based on positive evidence

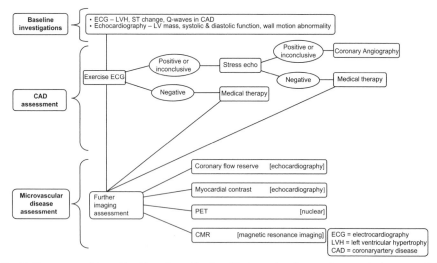

Fig. 2. Sequence of investigations in patients with hypertension and suspected myocardial ischemia.

from the ASCOT study.[75] The evidence for regular aspirin therapy is less clear-cut, but depending on the patient's risk this agent should be considered.

Target Blood Pressure

The recent American Heart Association guidelines on the treatment of hypertension amidst CAD have recommended a target BP of <130/<80 mmHg.[76] Although there is a good rationale to aim for a lower target than in patients who do not have coronary disease (<140/<90 mmHg), there is some concern about the effect of the excessive lowering of diastolic BP on cardiovascular events.

There is a clear relationship between increasing systolic and diastolic BP and cardiovascular risk. There is some evidence, however, that cardiovascular risk is raised at lower diastolic BPs, leading to a J-shaped curve of cardiovascular risk plotted against diastolic BP. This could also account for the increase in cardiovascular risk associated with increasing pulse pressure.[77] The microvascular changes induced by hypertension may alter the autoregulatory range of coronary blood flow. This may lead to diminished coronary flow at lower diastolic pressures due to a reduction in coronary perfusion pressure. Trial evidence in these areas provides conflicting data.[78–81]

Drug Selection

In terms of a reduction in cardiovascular events, the most important aspect in management appears to be the actual BP reduction rather than the agent used. In the ALLHAT trial there was no overall difference in outcome with diuretic-, amlodipine-, or lisinopril-based regimes.[82] In a recent meta-analysis including 190,617 subjects from 31 randomized controlled trials, no difference in outcome was found amongst men or women on the basis of the antihypertensive regime; the benefit was from BP lowering rather than the specific agent use.[83] If no specific agent is superior, one must consider the particular circumstances and tailor the antihypertensive therapy accordingly. With the combination of hypertension, myocardial ischemia, and normal coronary arteries, the main mechanism of ischemia, a reduced CFR, must be considered and those therapies targeted that can reverse the factors contributing to high BP, LV hypertrophy, and structural and functional vascular remodeling.

In humans, ACE-inhibitors have been shown to improve the vasodilatory response to flow-mediated dilatation[84] and cold pressor testing[85] in the conductance vessels of hypertensive subjects, with the likely method being through improvement in endothelial function. The combination of trandolapril and verapamil has been shown to reduce circulating soluble adhesion molecules.[86] Six-months treatment with verapamil significantly improves CFR compared with enalapril.[87] Treatment with nebivolol, a selective beta-1 antagonist with anti-oxidative properties, improves endothelial function in humans.[88]

In experimental models, ACE-inhibitors have been shown to reduce perivascular fibrosis and medial hypertrophy and normalize CFR.[34,38] These findings have been replicated with angiotensin receptor blockers.[37,38] Similarly spironolactone has been shown to reduce perivascular fibrosis, implicating aldosterone in this process.[89,90]

The dihydropyridine–calcium channel blocker benidipine appears to stimulate nitric oxide production in hypertensive rats, and thereby reduces the effect of hypertension on vascular remodeling and CFR.[35] Amlodipine (but not nifedipine or diltiazem) reversed perivascular fibrosis and prevented myocardial ischemia in nitric-oxide–deficient rats.[91] In humans, treatment with felodipine reduced asymptomatic ischemic episodes on Holter monitoring compared with a thiazide diuretic despite a similar reduction in BP and double product.[92]

The weight of evidence for improvement in endothelial function, reduction in oxidative stress, and beneficial vascular remodeling favors calcium channel blockers and ACE-inhibitors as first-line therapy for hypertension with associated myocardial ischemia and normal coronary arteries.[93] That is not to say that beta-blockers do not have a role, especially if there are ongoing anginal symptoms. Aldosterone antagonists also have a role in BP reduction and also specifically in reducing myocardial fibrosis, which can contribute to ischemia (perivascular fibrosis leads to increased distances that oxygen must diffuse and potentially lowers PaO_2).

SUMMARY

Detailed studies over the past 30 years have built up an impressive evidence base for the presence of myocardial ischemia in patients who have hypertension. This relationship ranges from the obvious association with obstructive coronary artery disease to mechanisms related to hemodynamic, microcirculatory, and neuroendocrine abnormalities. All of these factors serve to destabilize the critical balance between myocardial oxygen supply and demand. We have at our disposal a range of sophisticated investigations that allow us to demonstrate the presence and extent of the ischemia and therefore to target specific therapies to reduce the risk to these patients. Achieving target BP and managing all reversible components of the patient's cardiovascular risk status reduce to a minimum the clinical sequelae of myocardial ischemia in this vulnerable population.

REFERENCES

1. Kannel WB, Schwartz MJ, McNamara PM. Blood pressure and the risk of coronary heart disease: the Framingham study. Dis Chest 1969;56:43–52.
2. Kannel WB, Gordon T, Castelli WP, et al. Electrocardiographic left ventricular hypertrophy and risk coronary artery disease: the Framingham study. Ann Intern Med 1970;72:813–22.
3. Dunn FG, McLenachan J, Isles CG, et al. Left ventricular hypertrophy and mortality in hypertension: an analysis of data from the Glasgow Blood Pressure Clinic. J Hypertens 1990;8:775–82.
4. Casale PN, Devereux RB, Milner M, et al. Value of echocardiographic left ventricular mass in predicting cardiovascular morbid events in hypertensive men. Ann Intern Med 1986;105:1773–8.
5. Sarnoff SJ, Braunwald E, Welch GH Jr, et al. Hemodynamic determinants of oxygen consumption of the heart with special reference to tension-time index. Am J Phys 1958;192:148–56.
6. Davies MJ. Hypertension and atherosclerotic (ischaemic) heart disease. J Hum Hypertens 1991;5(Suppl 1):23–9.
7. Megnien JL, Simon A, Lemariey M, et al. Hypertension promotes coronary calcium deposit in asymptomatic men. Hypertension 1996;27:949–54.
8. Sipahi I, Tuzcu EM, Schoenhagen P, et al. Effects of normal, pre-hypertensive, and hypertensive blood pressure levels on progression of coronary atherosclerosis. J Am Coll Cardiol 2006;48:833–8.
9. Ross R. Atherosclerosis – an inflammatory disease. N Engl J Med 1999;340: 115–26.
10. Higashiyama H, Sugai M, Inoue H, et al. Histopathological study of time course changes in inter-renal aortic banding-induced left ventricular hypertrophy of mice. Int J Exp Pathol 2007;88:31–8.

11. Rakugi H, Yu H, Kamitani A, et al. Links between hypertension and myocardial infarction. Am Heart J 1996;132:213–21.

12. Julius S. Sympathetic hyperactivity and coronary risk in hypertension. Hypertension 1993;21:886–93.

13. Standicy PR, Zhang F, Ram JL, et al. Insulin attenuates vasopressin-induced calcium transients and a voltage-dependent calcium response in rat vascular smooth muscle cells. J Clin Invest 1991;88:1230–6.

14. Dzielinska Z, Januszewicz A, Wiecek A, et al. Decreased plasma concentration of a novel anti-inflammatory protein–adiponectin–in hypertensive men with coronary artery disease. Thromb Res 2003;110:365–9.

15. Watanabe T, Kanome T, Miyazaki A, et al. Human urotensin II as a link between hypertension and coronary artery disease. Hypertens Res 2006;29:375–87.

16. Picano E, Palinkas A, Amyot R. Diagnosis of myocardial ischemia in hypertensive patients. J Hypertens 2001;19:1177–83.

17. Pringle SD, Dunn FG, Tweddel AC, et al. Symptomatic and silent myocardial ischaemia in hypertensive patients with left ventricular hypertrophy. Br Heart J 1992;67:377–82.

18. Lacourciere Y, Cote C, Lefebvre J, et al. Identifying which treated hypertensive patients without known coronary artery disease should be tested for the presence of myocardial ischemia by perfusion imaging. J Clin Hypertens 2007;9:921–8.

19. Mansour P, Bostrom PA, Mattiasson I, et al. Low blood pressure levels and signs of myocardial ischaemia: importance of left ventricular hypertrophy. J Hum Hypertens 1993;7:13–8.

20. Stojanovic MM, O'Brien E, Lyons S, et al. Silent myocardial ischaemia in treated hypertensives with and without left ventricular hypertrophy. Blood Press Monit 2003;8:45–51.

21. Vogt M, Motz W, Strauer BE. Coronary haemodynamics in hypertensive heart disease. Eur Heart J 1992;13(Suppl D):44–9.

22. Stauer BE. Myocardial oxygen consumption in chronic heart disease: role of wall stress, hypertrophy and coronary reserve. Am J Cardiol 1979;44:730–40.

23. Pichard AD, Gorlin R, Smith H, et al. Coronary flow studies in patients with left ventricular hypertrophy of the hypertensive type: evidence for an impaired coronary vascular reserve. Am J Cardiol 1981;47:547–54.

24. Opherk D, Mall G, Zebe H, et al. Reduction of coronary reserve: a mechanism for angina pectoris in patients with arterial hypertension and normal coronary arteries. Circulation 1984;69:1–7.

25. Iriarte M, Caso R, Murga N, et al. Microvascular angina pectoris in hypertensive patients with left ventricular hypertrophy and diagnostic value of exercise thallium-201 scintigraphy. Am J Cardiol 1995;75:335–9.

26. Kataoka T, Hamasaki S, Ishida S, et al. Contribution of increased minimal coronary resistance and attenuated vascular adaptive remodeling to myocardial ischemia in patients with systemic hypertension and ventricular hypertrophy. Am J Cardiol 2004;94:484–7.

27. Brush JE Jr, Cannon RO, Schenke WH, et al. Angina due to coronary microvascular disease in hypertensive patients without left ventricular hypertrophy. N Engl J Med 1988;319:1302–7.

28. Tanaka M, Fujiwara H, Onodera T, et al. Quantitative analysis of narrowings of intramyocardial small arteries in normal hearts, hypertensive hearts, and hearts with hypertrophic cardiomyopathy. Circulation 1987;75:1130–9.

29. Schwartzkopff B, Motz W, Frenzel H, et al. Structural and functional alterations of the intramyocardial coronary arterioles in patients with arterial hypertension. Circulation 1993;88:993–1003.

30. Pepi M, Alimento M, Maltagliati A, et al. Electrocardiographic alterations sugges-tive of myocardial injury elicited by rapid pressure lowering in hypertension. Eur Heart J 1988;9:899–905.

31. Messerli FH, Mancia G, Conti CR, et al. Dogma disputed: can aggressively lowering blood pressure in hypertensive patients with coronary artery disease be dangerous? Ann Intern Med 2006;144:884–93.

32. Schwartzkopff B, Frenzel H, Dieckerhoff J, et al. Morphometric investigation of human myocardium in arterial hypertension and valvular aortic stenosis. Eur Heart J 1992;13(Suppl D):17–23.

33. Anderson PG, Bishop SP, Digerness SB. Vascular remodelling and improvement of coronary reserve after hydralazine treatment in spontaneously hypertensive rats. Circ Res 1989;64:1127–36.

34. Brilla CG, Janicki JS, Weber KT. Impaired diastolic function and coronary reserve in genetic hypertension. Role of interstitial fibrosis and medial thickening of intra-myocardial coronary arteries. Circ Res 1991;69:107–15.

35. Kobayashi N, Kobayashi K, Hara K, et al. Benidipine stimulates nitric oxide syn-thase and improves coronary circulation in hypertensive rats. Am J Hypertens 1993;12:483–91.

36. Goto D, Fujii S, Zaman AK, et al. Long-term blockade of nitric oxide synthesis in rats modulates coronary capillary network remodelling. Angiogenesis 1999;3: 137–46.

37. McEwan PE, Gray GA, Sherry L, et al. Differential effects of angiotensin II on cardiac cell proliferation and intramyocardial perivascular fibrosis in vivo. Circulation 1998;98:2765–73.

38. Ikeda Y, Nakamura T, Takano H, et al. Angiotensin II-induced cardiomyocyte hypertrophy and cardiac fibrosis in stroke-prone spontaneously hypertensive rats. J Lab Clin Med 2000;135:353–9.

39. González A, López B, Díez J. Fibrosis in hypertensive heart disease: role of the renin-angiotensin-aldosterone system. Med Clin North Am 2004;88:83–7.

40. Isoyama S, Ito N, Satoh U, et al. Collagen deposition and the reversal of coronary reserve in cardiac hypertrophy. Hypertension 1992;20:491–500.

41. Youn HJ, Ihm SH, Lee JM, et al. Relation between flow reserve capacity of pene-trating intramyocardial coronary arteries and myocardial fibrosis in hypertension: study using transthoracic Doppler echocardiography. J Am Soc Echocardiogr 2006;19:373–8.

42. Panza JA, Quyyumi AA, Brush JE, et al. Abnormal endothelium-dependent vascular relaxation in patients with hypertension. N Engl J Med 1990;323:22–7.

43. Antony I, Lerebours G, Nitenberg A. Loss of flow-dependent coronary artery dilatation in patients with hypertension. Circulation 1995;91:1624–8.

44. Nitenberg A, Antony I, Aptecar E, et al. Impairment of flow-dependent coronary dilation in hypertensive patients. Demonstration by cold pressor test induced flow velocity increase. Am J Hypertens 1995;8:13S–8S.

45. Houghton JL, Davison CA, Kuhner PA, et al. Heterogeneous vasomotor responses of coronary conduit and resistance vessels in hypertension. J Am Coll Cardiol 1998;31:374–82.

46. Quyyumi AA, Mulcahy D, Andrews NP, et al. Coronary vascular nitric oxide activity in hypertension and hypercholesterolemia. Comparison of acetylcholine and substance P. Circulation 1997;95:104–10.

47. Kaikita K, Fogo AB, Ma L, et al. Plasminogen activator inhibitor-1 deficiency prevents hypertension and vascular fibrosis in response to long-term nitric oxide synthase inhibition. Circulation 2001;104:839–44.

48. Mohri M, Ichiki T, Hirooka Y, et al. Endogenous nitric oxide prevents myocardial ischemia in patients with hypertension and left ventricular hypertrophy. Am Heart J 2002;143:684–9.
49. Palloshi A, Fragasso G, Piatti P, et al. Effect of oral L-arginine on blood pressure and symptoms and endothelial function in patients with systemic hypertension, positive exercise tests, and normal coronary arteries. Am J Cardiol 2004;93:933–5.
50. Kelm M, Strauer BE. Coronary flow reserve measurements in hypertension. Med Clin North Am 2004;88:99–113.
51. Houghton JL, Frank MJ, Carr AA, et al. Relations among impaired coronary flow reserve, left ventricular hypertrophy and thallium perfusion defects in hypertensive patients without obstructive coronary artery disease. J Am Coll Cardiol 1990;15(1):43–51.
52. Oikarinen L, Nieminen MS, Viitasalo M, et al. QRS duration and QT interval predict mortality in hypertensive patients with left ventricular hypertrophy: the Losartan Intervention for Endpoint Reduction in Hypertension Study. Hypertension 2004; 43(5):1029–34.
53. Tarazi RC, Miller A, Frohlich ED, et al. Electrocardiographic changes reflecting left atrial abnormality in hypertension. Circulation 1966;34(5):818–22.
54. Uen S, Un I, Fimmers R, et al. Myocardial ischemia during everyday life in patients with arterial hypertension: prevalence, risk factors, triggering mechanism and circadian variability. Blood Press Monit 2006;11(4):173–82.
55. Xanthos T, Ekmektzoglou KA, Papadimitriou L. Reviewing myocardial silent ischemia: specific patient subgroups. Int J Cardiol 2008;124(2):139–48.
56. Boon D, Piek JJ, van Montfrans GA. Silent ischaemia and hypertension. J Hypertens 2000;18(10):1355–64.
57. Smith RH, LePetri B, Moisa RB, et al. Association of increased left ventricular mass in the absence of electrocardiographic left ventricular hypertrophy with ST depression during exercise. Am J Cardiol 1995;76(12):973–4.
58. Kokkinos P, Pittaras A, Narayan P, et al. Exercise capacity and blood pressure associations with left ventricular mass in prehypertensive individuals. Hypertension 2007;49(1):55–61.
59. Allison TG, Cordeiro MA, Miller TD, et al. Prognostic significance of exercise-induced systemic hypertension in healthy subjects. Am J Cardiol 1999;83(3): 371–5.
60. Massie BM, Szlachcic Y, Tubau JF, et al. Scintigraphic and electrocardiographic evidence of silent coronary artery disease in asymptomatic hypertension: a case-control study. J Am Coll Cardiol 1993;22(6):1598–606.
61. Schäfer S, Kelm M, Mingers S, et al. Left ventricular remodeling impairs coronary flow reserve in hypertensive patients. J Hypertens 2002;20(7):1431–7.
62. Marks DS, Gudapati S, Prisant LM, et al. Mortality in patients with microvascular disease. J Clin Hypertens (Greenwich) 2004;6(6):304–9.
63. Cortigiani L, Paolini EA, Nannini E. Dipyridamole stress echocardiography for risk stratification in hypertensive patients with chest pain. Circulation 1998;98(25): 2855–9.
64. Fragasso G, Lu C, Dabrowski P, et al. Comparison of stress/rest myocardial perfusion tomography, dipyridamole and dobutamine stress echocardiography for the detection of coronary disease in hypertensive patients with chest pain and positive exercise test. J Am Coll Cardiol 1999;34(2):441–7.
65. Hare JL, Brown JK, Marwick TH. Association of myocardial strain with left ventricular geometry and progression of hypertensive heart disease. Am J Cardiol 2008; 102(1):87–91.

66. Park TH, Nagueh SF, Khoury DS, et al. Impact of myocardial structure and function postinfarction on diastolic strain measurements: implications for assessment of myocardial viability. Am J Physiol Heart Circ Physiol 2006; 290(2):H724–31.
67. Yuda S, Short L, Leano R, et al. Myocardial abnormalities in hypertensive patients with normal and abnormal left ventricular filling: a study of ultrasound tissue characterization and strain. Clin Sci (Lond) 2002;103(3):283–93.
68. Wei K, Jayaweera AR, Firoozan S, et al. Quantification of myocardial blood flow with ultrasound-induced destruction of microbubbles administered as a constant venous infusion. Circulation 1998;97(5):473–83.
69. Di Bello V, Pedrinelli R, Giorgi D, et al. Coronary microcirculation in essential hypertension: a quantitative myocardial contrast echocardiographic approach. Eur J Echocardiogr 2002;3(2):117–27.
70. Pilz G, Klos M, Ali E, et al. Angiographic correlations of patients with small vessel disease diagnosed by adenosine-stress cardiac magnetic resonance imaging. J Cardiovasc Magn Reson 2008;10(1):8.
71. Andersen K, Hennersdorf M, Cohnen M, et al. Myocardial delayed contrast enhancement in patients with arterial hypertension: initial results of cardiac MRI. Eur J Radiol 2008; doi:10.1016/j.ejrad.2008.03.009.
72. Masuda D, Nohara R, Tamaki N, et al. Evaluation of coronary blood flow reserve by 13N-NH3 positron emission computed tomography (PET) with dipyridamole in the treatment of hypertension with the ACE inhibitor (Cilazapril). Ann Nucl Med 2000;14(5):353–60.
73. Lorenzoni R, Gistri R, Cecchi F, et al. Coronary vasodilator reserve is impaired in patients with hypertrophic cardiomyopathy and left ventricular dysfunction. Am Heart J 1998;136(6):972–81.
74. Di Carli MF. Advances in positron emission tomography. J Nucl Cardiol 2004; 11(6):719–32.
75. Sever PS, Dahlof B, Poulter NR, et al. Prevention of coronary and stroke events with atorvastatin in hypertensive patients who have average or lower-than-average concentrations, in the Anglo-Scandinavian Cardiac Outcomes Trial–Lipid Lowering Arm (ASCOT-LLA): a multicentre randomised controlled trial. Lancet 2003;361:1149–58.
76. Rosendorff C, Black HR, Cannon CP, et al. Treatment of hypertension in the prevention and management of ischaemic heart diasease: a scientific statement from the American Heart Association Council for High Blood Pressure Research and the Councils on Clinical Cardiology and Epidemiology and Prevention. Circulation 2007;115:2761–88.
77. Narkiewicz K, Kjeldse SE, Hedner T. Hypertension and coronary artery disease: mechanistic insights and therapeutic challenges. Blood Press 2005; 14:260–1.
78. Cruickshank JM, Thorp JM, Zacharias FJ. Benefits and potential harm of lowering high blood pressure. Lancet 1987;1:581–4.
79. Nissen SE, Tuzcu EM, Libby P, et al. CAMELOT Investigators. Effect of antihypertensive agents on cardiovascular events in patients with coronary disease and normal blood pressure: the CAMELOT study: a randomized controlled trial. JAMA 2004;292:2217–26.
80. Pepine CJ, Handberg EM, Cooper-DeHoff RM, et al. INVEST Investigators. A calcium antagonist vs. a non-calcium antagonist treatment strategy for patients with coronary artery disease: the International Verapamil-Trandolapril study (INVEST): a randomized controlled trial. JAMA 2003;290:2805–16.

81. Hansson L, Zanchetti A, Carruthers SG, et al. Effects of intensive blood-pressure lowering and low-dose aspirin in patients with hypertension: principal results of the Hypertension Optimal Treatment (HOT) randomised trial. Lancet 1998;351: 1755–62.

82. ALLHAT-Officers and Coordinators for the ALLHAT Collaborative Research Group. Major outcomes in high-risk hypertensive patients randomized to angiotensin-converting enzyme inhibitor or calcium channel blocker vs diuretic: the Antihypertensive and Lipid-Lowering Treatment to Prevent Heart Attack Trial (ALLHAT). JAMA 2002;288:2981–97.

83. Turnbull F, Woodward M, Neal B, et al.Blood Pressure Lowering Treatment Trialists' Collaboration. Do men and women respond differently to blood pressure-lowering treatment? Results of prospectively designed overviews of randomized trials. Eur Heart J 2008;29:2669–80.

84. Antony I, Chemla D, Lerebours G, et al. Restoration of flow-dependent coronary dilation by ACE inhibition improves papaverine-induced maximal coronary blood flow in hypertensive patients: demonstration that large epicardial coronary arteries are more than conductance vessels. J Cardiovasc Pharmacol 2000;36: 570–6.

85. Antony I, Lerebours G, Nitenberg A. Angiotensin-converting enzyme inhibition restores flow-dependent and cold pressor test-induced dilations in coronary arteries of hypertensive patients. Circulation 1996;94:3115–22.

86. Rubio-Guerra AF, Vargas-Robles H, Vargas-Ayala G, et al. The effect of trandolapril and its fixed-dose combination with verapamil on circulating adhesion molecules levels in hypertensive patients with type 2 diabetes. Clin Exp Hypertens 2008;30:682–8.

87. Parodi O, Neglia D, Palombo C, et al. Comparative effects of enalapril and verapamil on myocardial blood flow in systemic hypertension. Circulation 1997;96: 864–73.

88. Pasini AF, Garbin U, Stranieri C, et al. Nebivolol treatment reduces serum levels of asymmetric dimethylarginine and improves endothelial dysfunction in essential hypertensive patients. Am J Hypertens 2008;21:1251–7.

89. Okada T, Nagai M, Taniguchi I, et al. Combined treatment with valsartan and spironolactone prevents cardiovascular remodeling in renovascular hypertensive rats. Int Heart J 2006;47:783–93.

90. Lal A, Veinot JP, Leenen FH. Prevention of high salt diet-induced cardiac hypertrophy and fibrosis by spironolactone. Am J Hypertens 2003;16:319–23.

91. de Oliveira CF, Nathan LP, Metze K, et al. Effect of Ca2+ channel blockers on arterial hypertension and heart ischaemic lesions induced by chronic blockade of nitric oxide in the rat. Eur J Pharmacol 1999;373:195–200.

92. Trenkwalder P, Dobrindt R, Aulehner R, et al. Antihypertensive treatment with felodipine but not with a diuretic reduces episodes of myocardial ischaemia in elderly patients with hypertension. Eur Heart J 1994;15:1673–80.

93. Mizuno Y, Jacob RF, Mason RP. Effects of calcium channel and renin-angiotensin system blockade on intravascular and neurohormonal mechanisms of hypertensive vascular disease. Am J Hypertens 2008;21:1076–85.

The Kidney, Hypertension, and Remaining Challenges

Nitin Khosla, MD[a], Rigas Kalaitzidis, MD[b], George L. Bakris, MD[b],*

KEYWORDS

- Kidney • Hypertension • Failure • Morbidity
- African-American

Chronic kidney disease (CKD) is a major worldwide public-health problem.[1] Eight million people in the United States had an estimated glomerular filtration rate (eGFR) less than 60 mL per minute per 1.73 m^2.[2] The estimated prevalence of CKD is about 14.8% of the general population.[3] Patients with CKD have significant morbidity, increased risk of cardiovascular disease,[4] progression to end-stage renal disease (ESRD), and death.[5] Furthermore, patients with CKD are 5 to 10 times more likely to die than to advance to ESRD;[3,6] among such patients, the rate of sudden death is three times higher.

A survey of the National Health and Nutrition Examination Survey database indicates that the prevalence of CKD has increased from 10.0% between 1994 and 1998 to 13.1% from 1999 to 2004.[2] In 2006, the estimated cost to treat hypertension and its comorbid conditions in the United States exceeded 55 billion dollars.[7] Similarly, the estimated cost for Medicare patients with CKD exceeded 49 billion dollars, nearly five times greater than costs in 1993. Overall Medicare expenditures, in contrast, have grown only 91% in the same period.[8]

One of the most difficult problems in managing patients with CKD is the achievement of blood pressure (BP) targets recommended by guidelines. The degree and duration of either systolic or diastolic BP elevation strongly influences cardiovascular (CV) outcomes in all patients. In the general population, risk of a CV event doubles for every increment of 20/10 mm Hg increase in BP over 115/75 mm Hg.[9] Not only is this risk amplified in patients with CKD, but hypertension accelerates the progression of CKD as well, especially when levels of proteinuria are greater than 300 mg/day.[10–14]

[a] Department of Medicine, Section of Nephrology and Hypertension, University of California at San Diego, San Diego, CA, USA
[b] Department of Medicine, Hypertensive Diseases Unit, Section of Endocrinology, Diabetes, and Metabolism, University of Chicago-Pritzker School of Medicine, 5841 South Maryland Avenue MC 1027, Chicago, IL 60637, USA
* Corresponding author.
E-mail address: gbakris@gmail.com (G.L. Bakris).

Med Clin N Am 93 (2009) 697–715
doi:10.1016/j.mcna.2009.02.001
0025-7125/09/$ – see front matter © 2009 Elsevier Inc. All rights reserved.
medical.theclinics.com

Post hoc analyses of randomized clinical trials in patients with greater than 300 mg/day of proteinuria have found that lower BP levels yield slower declines in kidney function. These observations have lead to the development of lower BP targets (ie, to <130/80 mm Hg) in those with CKD in an attempt to decrease the incidence of adverse CV and renal outcomes.[10,15]

This article focuses exclusively on management of hypertension in CKD and addresses the following issues: How good are the data to support a lower target BP in CKD? Are the data supporting a lower BP stronger in those with diabetes with CKD? Should reduction in proteinuria be a key element in choosing antihypertensive medications to prevent progression of CKD?

Before addressing these questions, however, some background information is pertinent. First, it has long been felt that management of hypertension in patients with advanced CKD (ie, eGFR <60 mL/min) will not be successful without using strategies that lower both BP and the spectrum of albuminuria. Microalbuminuria (MA) is defined as a protein excretion of greater than 30 mg to 299 mg per day or 20 μg to 200 μg per minute present on two different occasions.[16] MA is a marker of endothelial dysfunction and is an independent risk marker for CV events.[17–20] It is not, however, a marker of kidney disease,[21] but if measured with a simple spot urine, can provide as much if not more information as other inflammatory markers, such as highly sensitive C-reactive protein.[16] A guide to the evaluation of MA is presented in **Fig. 1**.[22] The best evidence demonstrating the association between MA reduction and reduction in CV events comes from a post hoc analysis of the Losartan Intervention for Endpoint trial, where an early reduction in MA was associated with a greater reduction in CV events that persisted over the 5-year follow-up.[23]

MA or proteinuria, defined as a protein excretion greater than 300 mg/day or greater than 200 μg/min,[22] is associated with a much higher CV risk and does indicate presence of CKD; there is a direct relationship between the degree of proteinuria and progression to ESRD.[24] Post hoc analyses of three appropriately powered CKD outcome trials demonstrate that reduction in MA (proteinuria) in those with advanced CKD delays CKD progression, an effect that could not be explained by BP lowering

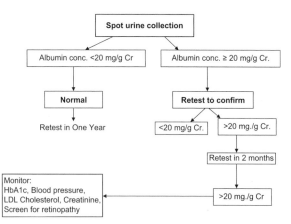

Fig. 1. Evaluation and Work-up of MA proposed by the National Kidney Foundation. (*Data from* Sarnak MJ, Levey AS, Schoolwerth AC, et al. Kidney disease as a risk factor for development of cardiovascular disease: a statement from the American Heart Association Councils on Kidney in Cardiovascular Disease, High Blood Pressure Research, Clinical Cardiology, and Epidemiology and Prevention. Hypertension 2003;42(5):1057.)

alone.[25] These studies demonstrate a reduction in proteinuria of more than 30% resulted in a 39% to 72% risk reduction for dialysis at 3 to 5 years (**Table 1**).[25–27]

Given this information, there have been numerous attempts to have the Food and Drug Administration approve changes in albuminuria as a surrogate marker for CKD progression. This effort has failed because the there is no randomized prospective trial that demonstrates a change in albuminuria alters CKD progression independent of BP reduction. Hence, albuminuria does not qualify as a surrogate marker.[28,29]

Finally, studies involving hypertension in CKD must be evaluated in the follow context: (a) BP actually achieved (independent of what target BP was) and time to achieve goal; (b) level of renal function at time of enrollment; and (c) amount of protein excretion present (MA versus proteinuria). The alpha blockade arm of the Antihypertensive and Lipid-Lowering Treatment to Prevent Heart Attack Trial (ALLHAT) illustrates the first point. Though this arm was terminated early because of a higher incidence of stroke and the combined outcome of stroke, angina treated outside the hospital, heart failure, and peripheral arterial disease, the alpha blocker arm had a consistently higher BP than the diuretic arm and this difference was greatest after the first year.[30] This likely contributed to the differences in outcome observed. Baseline kidney function and level of protein excretion are also key determinants of outcomes in CKD trials. The earlier a BP intervention occurs, the more likely it will stop kidney disease progression. Similarly, a late intervention will only slow progression already underway. In The Appropriate Blood Pressure Control in Diabetes (ABCD) trial, the average GFR was more than 80 mL/min at the start of the trial, whereas in most other diabetes trials, baseline GFR is generally less 50 mL/min.[31] Early and aggressive BP lowering (ie, <130/80 mmHg) in the ABCD trial was associated with GFR decline being slowed to rates seen in people with normal kidney function. Conversely, in other trials of more advanced CKD, GFR loss occurred at a rate of 2 mL to 7 mL per minute per year (see **Fig. 1**).[15,32] Thus, results of trials in patients with advanced CKD should not be extrapolated to patients with early CKD, as rates of decline in kidney function are not similar.

BP GOAL OF LESS THAN 130/80 MM HG: DOES THE EVIDENCE SUPPORT THIS BP IN CKD?

All published guidelines define goal BP as less than 130/80 mm Hg for those with diabetes or CKD (**Table 2**).[10,15] Data to support the goal of less than 130/80 mm Hg, among those with diabetic nephropathy, come from post hoc analyses of three different trials of patients with advanced (eGFR <60 mL/min) proteinuric (>300 mg/day) kidney disease. All these trials have a range of BPs at study end between 120 and 152/68 and 86 mm Hg; the mean is much higher than 130/80 mm Hg. Post hoc analyses of these diabetic nephropathy trials have also pointed to a J-shaped relationship, suggesting that a BP below 120/85 mm Hg may actually increase cardiovascular risk in these patients.[33] Thus, even in diabetic nephropathy where the data are somewhat more robust, the argument for a BP less than 130/80 mm Hg is weak.

Nondiabetic CKD trials are less robust with regard to BP goal, as only two such trials exist, the Modification of Diet in Renal Disease Study (MDRD) and the African American Study of Kidney Disease (AASK). These trials, like those in patients with diabetic nephropathy, were executed in patients with an eGFR less than 60 mL/min and with albuminuria.

The MDRD provides data that is instructive about advanced nephropathy progression. This is the first trial to randomize to two levels of BP and follow nephropathy progression, a mean arterial pressure (MAP) of less than 92 mm Hg versus one between 102 mm Hg and 107 mm Hg. When the trial ended, mean follow-up of 2.7 years, there was no advantage on CKD slowing in the lower BP group. However, after 8 additional years of follow-up, those with baseline proteinuria of more than 1 gm/day

Table 1
Outcomes studies with primary CKD progression endpoint

Study	Treatment Groups	Follow up (Mean in Years)	Achieved BP (mm Hg)	Change in Proteinuria	Relevant Outcomes
Captopril trial	Captopril or placebo	3 (median)	MAP 96 MAP 100	−30%	Captopril delays the progression of diabetic nephropathy
AASK[a]	Metoprolol, ramipril, or amlodipine and conventional or intensive blood pressure targets	4	128/78 for lowergroup 141/85 for usual group	−14% for metoprolol −20% for ramipril +58% for amlodipine at 6 months	Ramipril slowed the progression of renal disease when compared with the other groups
RENAAL[a]	Losartan or placebo	3.4	140/74 142/74	−35%	Losartan delayed the need for dialysis by 2 years when compared with placebo
IDNT[a]	Irbesartan or amlodipine or placebo	2.6	140/77 141/77 144/80	−33% −6% −10%	Irbesartan reduced proteinuria to a greater extent and lead to slower progression of renal disease when compared with the other groups

Abbreviations: AASK, African American Study of Kidney Disease; IDNT, Irbesartan in Diabetic Nephropathy Trail; RENAAL, Reduction of Endpoints in Non-insulin dependent diabetes mellitus with the Angiotensin II Antagonist Losartan.
[a] Indicates studies where post hoc analysis show significant risk reduction for CKD progression when proteinuria reduced by greater than 30% at 6 months.

Table 2
Summary of guidelines and position papers for goal BP in people with kidney disease or diabetes from various consensus committees around the world

Group	Goal BP (mm Hg)	Initial Therapy
Am. Society of HTN (2008)	<130/80	ACE inhibitor/ARB[a,b]
Canadian HTN Society (2007)	≤130/80	ACE inhibitor/ARB
Am. Diabetes Assoc. (2005)	<130/80	ACE inhibitor/ARB[a]
Japanese HTN Society (2006)	≤130/80	ARB[a,b]
National Kidney Foundation (2004)	<130/80	ACE inhibitor/ARB[a]
British HTN Society (2004)	≤130/80	ACE inhibitor/ARB
JNC 7 (2003)	<130/80	ACE inhibitor/ARB[a]
ISH/ESC (2003)	<130/80	ACE inhibitor/ARB
Australia-New Zealand (2002)	<130/85	ACE inhibitor
WHO/ISH (1999)	<130/85	ACE inhibitor

Abbreviations: ACE, angiotensin-converting enzyme; ARB, angiotensin-receptor blocker; ESC, European Society of Cardiology; HTN, hypertension; ISH, International Society of Hypertension; JNC 7, Seventh Report of the Joint National Committee on Prevention, Detection, Evaluation, and Treatment of High Blood Pressure; WHO, World Health Organization.
[a] Indicates potential use of initial combination therapy with a thiazide diuretic, if BP is substantially higher than goal.
[b] Calcium antagonists could also be combined.

randomized to the lower target BP of 92 mm Hg, had a slower decline in kidney function, and a lower incidence of renal failure compared with those randomized to a MAP of 107 mm Hg.[34] This difference was apparent within a year after the study ended.

The AASK study adds support to the notion that patients with significant proteinuria benefit from a lower BP target. The primary analysis of AASK demonstrated that patients randomized to a lower BP target of a MAP less than 92 mm Hg derived no additional benefit on CKD slowing over the high BP group. However, a subgroup analysis showed that the lower BP target did preserve kidney function in the small subset of patients with proteinuria less than 1 gm/day, with a trend toward a slower decline in GFR in the cohort of patients with proteinuria greater than 300 mg/day.[35]

Many cite the Ramipril Efficacy in Nephropathy trail (REIN-2) as evidence to contradict lower BP targets in patients with proteinuria.[36] However, this study was grossly underpowered to detect a difference in decline in GFR between the two BP groups, as the median follow-up was only 1.6 years and there was only a 4.8-mm Hg difference in systolic BP difference between treatment groups. All of these trials are limited because the data presented to support the lower BP goal are derived from post hoc analyses.

Perhaps the most supportive evidence to re-evaluate the goal BP in CKD patients comes from the latest 10-year follow-up of the AASK trial. To date, no trial has had an average BP difference of 13/8 mm Hg for a duration of 5 years, and then everyone followed for an additional 5 years with systolic BP levels averaging less than 135 mm Hg in the entire cohort.[37] Even with this level of control, about 65% of the cohort still had progression of CKD, albeit markedly slowed. A potential reason for this was the discovery of masked and nocturnal hypertension that was missed by routine BP measurement.[38] Taken together, these data support the following: (*a*) routine BP measurement are not adequate for determining risk of CKD progression in patients with pre-existing CKD; (*b*) the goal of less than 130/80 mm Hg in CKD cannot be supported by appropriately powered trials in CKD but comes from meta-analyses of these smaller trials and post hoc analyses of larger databases;[15,39] (c) a goal of less than 130/80 mm Hg does have support in the subgroup of patients with MA or proteinuria and CKD. In the long-term follow-up of MDRD and the small subgroup of people (n = 52) in AASK with proteinuria greater than 300 mg/day, there was a slower CKD progression in those randomized to the lower BP goal, which averaged between 127 and 132/77 and 80 mm Hg. This benefit, however, took 5 years to become apparent on average.

Taken together, these data suggest that in patients with baseline GFR values less than 50 mL/min, those with BPs that approach 130/80 mm Hg have slower rates of decline in kidney function among those with advanced proteinuric CKD (**Fig. 2**).

SHOULD PROTEINURIA REDUCTION BE CONSIDERED IN DEVELOPING A BP-LOWERING STRATEGY?

Proteinuria or MA (>300 mg/day) is not an approved surrogate marker for CKD progression by the Food and Drug Administration. The reasons for this were previously mentioned, but proteinuria is felt to be a result of and not a cause of the underlying disease process. Nevertheless, the data are clear that development of proteinuria despite adequate BP control is a clue that CKD is present and progressing. Proteinuria greater than 2.5 g per day is an uncommon consequence of hypertension alone and should prompt consideration of a renal biopsy to determine the etiology of renal disease.

Post hoc analyses of all studies to date, demonstrate that maximal slowing of nephropathy occurs only when proteinuria is reduced in concert with BP.[40] Proteinuria reduction of at least 30% below baseline measurement when treatment started; generally this should occur at 6 months (see **Table 1**). Note, however, that this is not true for patients with CKD and MA, and there is no randomized trial with proteinuria reduction as a primary endpoint linked to nephropathy progression.[16,40] Nevertheless, the totality of the data argues for a strategy that lowers both proteinuria and BP to maximally reduce nephropathy progression.[40,41]

THERAPEUTIC APPROACHES TO HYPERTENSION IN KIDNEY DISEASE

Given the new trial information on CKD progression and information about proteinuria, there have been some proposed changes in management of BP in CKD and they are summarized in this section. The lifestyle approaches to treating BP in those with early CKD have not changed since being published in the 2004 National Kidney Foundation

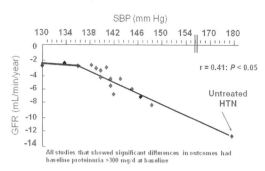

Fig. 2. The relationship between achieved level of BP and rate of decline in renal function in renal outcome trials over the past decade.

(NKF) guidelines.[10,15] The available data, however, suggest that lifestyle modifications alone are inadequate for management of hypertension in patients with CKD.

There are a few aspects of lifestyle management, however, that need emphasis. First, is sodium restriction. High-sodium intake is particularly injurious in African Americans because they excrete a lower sodium load than their White counterparts.[42] This difference of renal-sodium handling is borne out by the results of the dietary approaches to stop hypertension (DASH) diet, where hypertensive Black females had a 6 mm Hg greater reduction in BP compared with hypertensive White females on this low-sodium, high-potassium diet.[43] Care should be given when prescribing the DASH diet to anyone with Stage 4 or higher nephropathy because of risk of hyperkalemia.

Those with CKD are sodium avid, a phenomenon that is amplified in those with diabetes or metabolic syndrome, because the high levels of insulin seen in these conditions affect the tubular reabsorption of sodium.[44–47] Hence, those who are obese or have diabetes are relatively volume expanded.[48] Ingesting large sodium loads also restriction attenuates the antiproteinuric effects of the renin angiotensin aldosterone system blockers (RAAS).[49–51] Therefore, limitation of daily sodium intake to 2 g/day to 4 g/day is a logical initial therapeutic approach with use of a thiazide diuretic in those who do not fully adhere to this recommendation.

Pharmacologic Treatment

The guidelines of both the JNC 7 and the NKF state that management of hypertension in CKD should focus on reducing BP, with the NKF also emphasizing reducing protein excretion. First line agents to achieve these goals are RAAS blockers, ACE inhibitors, or ARBs,[10,15] generally used in concert with either diuretics or calcium antagonists. The American Society of Hypertension has recently updated the existing guidelines summarizing the approach in a position paper. The algorithm summarized in the paper is shown in **Fig. 3**.[10,15,52]

SPECIFIC ANTIHYPERTENSIVE DRUG CLASSES
RAAS Blockers

The RAAS blockers have not been used appropriately by most physicians in the patients who would garner the greatest benefit: that is, those with an eGFR less than 50 mL/min with proteinuria. These are the profiles of people in the outcome studies, yet data from practice databases indicate that these agents are being given with a very low frequency to such patients.

ACE Inhibitors

The mechanism of renal protection from RAAS blockers relates to many factors, including hemodynamic and antifibrotic effects, as well as effects on renal reserve. The nephron responds to a variety of factors, such as increased protein intake, with an elevation in GFR. This is referred to as "renal reserve" because it reflects the ability of the kidney to increase its clearance rate in the presence of higher urea genesis.[53] The increase in GFR is a result of signaling from the macula densa to the afferent glomerular arterioles, resulting in a vasodilator response to various amino acids. ACE inhibitors blunt the rise in GFR that follows a protein load by blocking this afferent arterial dilation.[54] Thus, agents that block the RAAS protect the kidney in a manner similar to the way β-blockers provide cardioprotection.

The first trial to demonstrate a benefit of ACE inhibitors was the Captopril Nephropathy Trial in Type-1 diabetics. This trial demonstrated an almost 75% risk reduction in

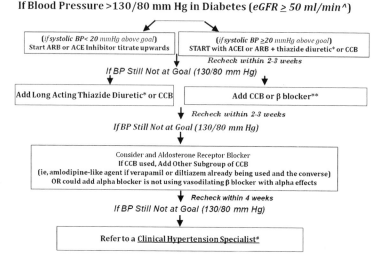

If Blood Pressure >130/80 mm Hg in Diabetes (*eGFR ≥ 50 ml/min^*)

(if systolic BP< 20 mmHg above goal)
Start ARB or ACE Inhibitor titrate upwards

(if systolic BP ≥20 mmHg above goal)
START with ACEI or ARB + thiazide diuretic* or CCB

Recheck within 2-3 weeks

If BP Still Not at Goal (130/80 mm Hg)

Add Long Acting Thiazide Diuretic* or CCB

Add CCB or β blocker**

Recheck within 2-3 weeks

If BP Still Not at Goal (130/80 mm Hg)

Consider and Aldosterone Receptor Blocker
If CCB used, Add Other Subgroup of CCB
(ie, amlodipine-like agent if verapamil or diltiazem already being used and the converse)
OR could add alpha blocker is not using vasodilating β blocker with alpha effects

Recheck within 4 weeks
If BP Still Not at Goal (130/80 mm Hg)

Refer to a Clinical Hypertension Specialist#

Fig. 3. An approach to lower arterial pressure to goal in patients with diabetes or albuminuria. It represents an update of previous guidelines published in 2003/2004 by the JNC 7 and NKF. #, Everyone with diabetes and CKD should be instructed on lifestyle modifications as per the JNC 7. Everyone should also be started on pharmacologic therapy, if blood pressure is greater than 130/80 mm Hg. Note: If BP is less than 20/10 mm Hg above goal (130/80 mm Hg), then ACE inhibitors or ARBs, titrated to maximal doses, alone may be used. *Nondihydropyridine calcium channel blockers (CCBs) (verapamil and diltiazem reduce both CV mortality, proteinuria, and diabetic nephropathy progression independent of ACE inhibitors or ARBs). β-blockers may be substituted for CCBs if the patient has angina, heart failure or arrhythmia, or a high heart rate (ie, >84 beats per minute at rest), necessitating their use. β-blockers with proven efficacy to reduce CV events and the lowest side-effect profile are preferred; of those available, carvedilol and nebivolol meets these criteria. Note that use of a β-blocker with a nondihydropyridine CCB should be avoided in the elderly and those with conduction abnormalities. Otherwise, such combinations are safe and particularly effective for lowering blood pressure. Also note that other agents, such as minoxidil, hydralazine, and clonidine or methyldopa can be used as adjunctive agents to help achieve goal BP. Clonidine should not be used with β-blockers or high-dose verapamil for numerous reasons, not the least of which is a high likelihood of severe bradycardia.

doubling of serum creatinine and in the combined outcome death, dialysis, and kidney transplantation in those treated with captopril when compared with placebo in those whose serum creatinine values were greater than 2 mg/dL. In those with serum creatinine values of less than 1 mg/dL, there was no significant benefit to ACE inhibition when similar BPs were achieved.[55] The REIN trial also demonstrated a 62% reduction in renal disease progression in those with serum creatinine values greater than 2 mg/dL and greater than 3 g/day proteinuria, compared with a 22% reduction in those with MA alone.[56] Similar findings have been noted in meta-analyses of nondiabetic renal disease.[39]

Early clinical trial data suggested that ACE inhibitors may provide additional protection against nephropathy progression, independent of BP, but this has not been borne out in larger clinical trials.[39,57] In a post hoc analysis of the ALLHAT trial, there was no evidence favoring the concept that ACE inhibitors have unique effects, independent of BP control, on preservation of renal function.[57] This difference in renal outcomes among these trials relates to several issues. In earlier studies, all patients had advanced CKD: that is, GFR less than 50 mL/min with more than 500-mg/day protein-uria. The ALLHAT trial was not powered for CKD outcomes and had no proteinuria data, with very few people in advanced Stage 3 and 4 nephropathy. Moreover, early in the ALLHAT, as much 6 mm of mercury difference in systolic BP existed between the ACE-inhibitor group and comparator groups. Consequently, the observed lack of selective benefit of ACE inhibitor treatment is difficult to interpret.

In clinical practice, increases in serum creatinine are commonly seen within a few weeks of starting ACE inhibitors or ARBs, especially in those with advanced nephrop-athy. A rise in serum creatinine limited to 30% to 35% within the first 4 months of start-ing RAAS-blocking therapy, however, correlates with preservation of kidney function over a mean follow-up period of 3 or more years (**Fig. 4**).[15,58] This correlation between a limited early rise in serum creatinine and long-term preservation of kidney function was restricted to patients under the age of 66 years, with baseline serum creatinine values less than or equal to 3.5 mg/dL. If acute increases in serum creatinine of greater than 40% occur in fewer than 4 months of RAAS-blocker therapy, the physician should evaluate the patient for (a) volume depletion (the most common etiology), (b) worsened heart failure, or (c) bilateral renal-artery stenosis.[58] Elevations in serum potassium only become clinically relevant at levels markedly exceeding 6 mEq/L or 5 mEq/L in the presence of digitalis preparations. Data from the recent heart failure trial demonstrated a CV risk reduction in people with CKD with serum potassium levels up to 5.7 mEq/L.[59] Hyperkalemia can be addressed by advising avoidance of high-potassium foods, such as fruits and vegetables, appropriately dosing diuretics, and stopping agents known to increase potassium, such as nonsteroidal anti-inflammatory agents.

ARBs

The RENAAL trial and the IDNT demonstrated that in advanced nephropathy, using an ARB to reduce BP led to a decrease in rate of nephropathy progression greater than that seen with other agents (ie, amlodipine or β-blockers/diuretics).[60,61] The primary composite endpoint for both studies was time to doubling of baseline serum creati-nine, onset of ESRD, or death. In the RENAAL study of 1,513 patients, followed for an average of 3.4 years, and the IDNT of 1,715 patients, followed for an average of

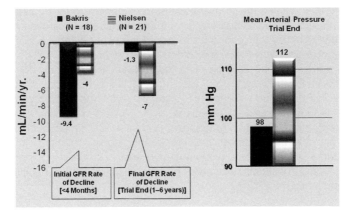

Fig. 4. Initial and long-term change in GFR in patients with Type-2 diabetes initially started on the ACE inhibitor, lisinopril. Note, GFR was measured using ^{99}Tc-diethylenetriamine pentaace-tate. Patient baseline characteristics were similar in both studies.[58] Note as well, with better BP reduction, the GFR dropped more, initially in the study, but the overall rate of decline at 5 years was less in the group with better BP control, in spite of a greater initial fall.

2.7 years, there was a 16% and 37% risk reduction by losartan and irbesartan, respectively, for the primary endpoint. In RENAAL, there was a 28% reduction in time ESRD. It was estimated that losartan could delay the need for dialysis or transplantation for 2 years.[60] Taken together, these trials reinforce the importance of selecting agents that both help achieve BP goal and reduce proteinuria (see **Table 1**).

Data directly comparing renal outcomes of ARBs and ACE inhibitors is limited to one trial that was underpowered and not in a cohort that would yield a meaningful outcome on CKD progression; hence, no difference was noted between the two classes.[62] The COOPERATE trial also compared these classes, but there were major data inconsistencies and hence, the trial is not discussed.[63]

In general, ARBs are generally better tolerated than ACE inhibitors, in that they are associated with a lower incidence of cough (presumably because they do not affect bradykinin), angioedema, taste disturbances, and hyperkalemia.[64]

Direct Renin Inhibitors

Aliskiren is the first and only approved direct renin inhibitor. The mechanism of action of this drug is unique in that it blocks the RAAS by binding to a pocket in renin itself, preventing it from cleaving angiotensinogen to angiotensin I. Aliskiren has a half-life of 24 hours and a side-effect profile similar to that of ARBs.[65] The role for aliskiren in the management of hypertension has yet to be fully determined, but it effectively reduces BP when used alone or in combination with other classes of medications, such as diuretics, ARBs, and CCBs.[66]

Limited data are available describing the use of aliskiren in CKD patients. The Aliskiren in the Evaluation of Proteinuria in Diabetes study compared the effect of aliskiren combined with losartan and losartan combined with placebo on albumin excretion in 599 patients with diabetes. Both groups had similar BPs and the aliskiren group had a 20% reduction in urinary albumin-to-creatinine ratios when compared with the placebo group at 6 months.[67] While these results are promising, we must await the results of the ALTITUDE trial to see if the effects are similar on diabetic nephropathy progression to that of ACE inhibitors and ARBs.

Aldosterone Antagonists

Current recommendations are to use aldosterone antagonists for treating hypertension in patients with advanced heart failure and postmyocardial infarction.[10] However, the role of these medications continues to expand. A post hoc analysis of the Anglo-Scandinavian Cardiac Outcomes Trial-Blood Pressure Lowering Arm demonstrated that adding spironolactone as fourth-line therapy led to a dramatic 21.9/10.5 mm Hg reduction in BP.[68] Others have looked at using aldosterone antagonists as a way to reduce proteinuria. A recent systematic review demonstrated that use of aldosterone antagonist given either alone or in concert with other RAAS agents provided significant reduction in proteinuria as well as BP.[69] It should be noted that patients involved in these studies had reasonable kidney function with estimated GFRs between 57 mL and 67 mL per minute. It is unclear whether aldosterone antagonists can be used in patients with more advanced nephropathy, especially given the risk of hyperkalemia.

DIURETICS

Thiazide diuretics have gained a renewed importance in treating hypertension since the publication of the ALLHAT.[70] Renal outcomes were analyzed post hoc and there was no difference in development of ESRD between the treatment groups.[57]

Although JNC 7 makes no specific recommendation about the particular thiazide diuretic used, strong consideration should be given to using chlorthalidone over hydrochlorothiazide. No trial has ever been designed to directly compare the two medications; however, almost all the major outcome trials supporting diuretics used chlorthalidone.[70,71] Though the two drugs are thought to have similar efficacy, chlorthalidone is likely more potent because of it longer half-life (44 hours for chlorthalidone versus 12 hours for hydrochlorothiazide).[72,73] This difference in duration of action translated into an additional 7-mm Hg reduction in systolic BP when substituted for hydrochlorothiazide.[72]

A potential side effect seen with thiazide diuretics is an increase in blood-glucose levels. The mechanism of this increase is believed to be mediated through hypokalemia, leading to glucose intolerance.[74] However, the increase in glucose at currently used doses is quite small and the risk of new onset diabetes is decreased further when combined with an ACE inhibitor or ARB.[75] Furthermore, no study to date has been able to link thiazide-induced hyperglycemia to worse CV or renal outcomes.

In general, thiazide diuretics are effective in patients that have an estimated GFR greater than 50 mL/min. Loop diuretics should be given to patients with lower levels of renal function. Typically, they should be dosed twice daily unless using the longer-acting torsemide. Diuretic resistance is a commonly encountered problem and relates to either under dosing, severe hypoalbuminemia, or heart failure. Classically, the approach to these patients involves increasing the dose of diuretic to the appropriate level and combining a loop diuretic with a diuretic that acts at the distal tubule. While this approach is reasonable, consideration should be given to using a potassium-sparing diuretic, such as amiloride, with a loop diuretic. The rationale behind this is that the chronic exposure to loop diuretics leads to hypertrophy of the epithelial sodium channel in the cortical collecting duct, the target of amiloride.[76]

CALCIUM CHANNEL BLOCKERS

When used in patients without proteinuric renal disease, both dihydropyridine CCBs (amlodipine, nifedipine) and nondihydropyridine CCBs (verapamil or diltiazem) are effective in lowering BP and both classes have been shown to lower CV events in high-risk populations.[77] These agents appear to have particular efficacy for CV risk reduction when paired with an ACE inhibitor. In the recently published Avoiding Cardiovascular Events through Combination Therapy in Patients Living with Systolic Hypertension (ACCOMPLISH), patients that were high risk for a CV event that were treated with a background of ACE inhibition had a 19% CV event relative-risk reduction when treated with amlodipine, compared with those treated with hydrochlorothiazide.[78] Similarly, verapamil has been shown to be effective in reducing CV outcomes in patients with hypertension and coronary artery disease.[79]

Both preclinical and clinical data demonstrate different renal effects of dihydropyridine CCBs and nondihydropyridine CCBs in patients who have proteinuria, as dihydropyridine CCBs do not reduce albuminuria to the same extent as do nondihydropyridine CCBs.[80,81] The mechanism of this difference relates to differences in glomerular permeability that occur in patients with advanced nephropathy.[82,83] This difference in antiproteinuric effect has translated into worse renal outcomes in advanced nephropathy, with proteinuria treated with dihydropyridine CCBs when compared with those treated with blockers of the RAAS.[83]

CCBs should not be used to decrease protein excretion in those with MA. In the Bergamo Nephrologic Diabetes Complications Trial, which compared nondihydropyridine CCBs with ACE inhibitors, alone or in combination, in patients with hypertension,

Type-2 diabetes mellitus, and normal urinary albumin excretion, no significant effect on reduction of MA was seen by verapamil alone. MA development, the primary endpoint, occurred with similar frequency in the verapamil and placebo group.[84] These results were foreseeable, as neither class of CCBs have anti-inflammatory effects on the vasculature and, as such, are unlikely to have any impact on endothelial damage, the antecedent of MA.[16,85]

In summary, both classes of CCBs should be used aggressively for BP reduction in patients without proteinuric renal disease. In those with advanced proteinuric nephropathy, nondihydropyridine CCBs are preferred, per guidelines, but dihydropyridine CCBs should be used only in combination with an ACE inhibitor or ARB to maximally reduce BP and slow nephropathy progression.[15]

β-ADRENERGIC BLOCKERS

Despite being quite effective at lowering BP, clinicians have been reluctant to use β-blockers because of a significant, adverse metabolic profile. Furthermore, recent data have called into question use of β-blockers for treating hypertension, although the data are focused on atenolol rather than the class.[86] Moreover, recent studies demonstrate that excessive reduction in heart rate may be a problem with this class, although more than 80% of the studies quoted were with atenolol.[87] All advanced nephropathy patients have an increase in sympathetic activity and a high CV event rate. Data clearly indicate a benefit of β-blockers in such patients, yet they are not used, a trend that should change to reduce CV risk.[87]

The emergence of newer β-blockers may expand the role for these agents, especially in diabetes or those with MA. The combined α- and β-blocker, carvedilol, and the β-1 vasodilating agent, nebivolol, have neutral glycemic and lipid parameters. Carvedilol, reduces CV morbidity and mortality and the risk of MA development in those with hypertension and diabetes.[88,89] The mechanism of decreasing MA development likely relates to the antioxidant properties of carvedilol. Thus, vasodilating β-blockers can be used in patients with compelling indications, and are excellent add-on agents to reduce risk and achieve BP targets.

α–ADRENERGIC BLOCKERS

The use of α-adrenergic antagonists, although effective in reducing BP, has not been shown to slow CKD progression or consistently reduce albuminuria in either animal models or patients with Type-2 diabetes.[90] This class of agents also fails to reduce CV events in patients with heart failure, as evidenced by the results of the long-acting α-blocker arm of ALLHAT, which was stopped early because of increased events.[30]

CHALLENGES FOR THE FUTURE

Many physicians fail to use more than one or two medications and then at low doses, hence they fail to achieve BP goal. The average number of agents needed to approach the current guideline goal of less than 130/80 mm Hg for those with CKD in clinical trials is 3.3 agents at maximally tolerated doses (**Fig. 5**). Thus, we must overcome physician inertia and use more fixed-dose combinations if as guidelines state, BP is greater than 20/10 mm Hg above the goal. Data from ACCOMPLISH make a compelling argument for this tenant, and also the use of combinations other than those with a diuretic, as there was an additional 20% CV risk reduction over the diuretic/ACE inhibitor combination.

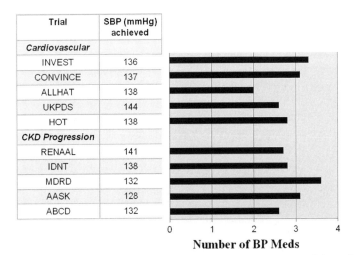

Trial	SBP (mmHg) achieved
Cardiovascular	
INVEST	136
CONVINCE	137
ALLHAT	138
UKPDS	144
HOT	138
CKD Progression	
RENAAL	141
IDNT	138
MDRD	132
AASK	128
ABCD	132

Number of BP Meds

Fig. 5. Number of antihypertensive medications required to achieve BP goals in major clinical trials over the past decade.

There has been concern about the potential risks of aggressive BP lowering, particularly in elderly patients with Type-2 diabetes. Reducing diastolic BP to less than 80 mm Hg has been thought to increase CV risk in this group, but no convincing evidence of this possibility was found in prospective clinical trials.[91,92] Retrospective analyses suggested that there might be a J-shaped relationship between diastolic BP and the rate of CV disease mortality in patients with established symptomatic coronary artery disease or unstable angina. However, a post hoc analyses of two separate renal outcome trials has failed to demonstrate a J curve for BP until levels get to less than 115/55 mm Hg.[93] Thus, the putative J curve should not serve as a deterrent to lowering BP to recommended goals in the absence of any clear evidence of coronary disease or unstable angina.

BP goal should be achieved within 3 to 4 months in most patients, but longer periods may be required in those with previous strokes or autonomic dysfunction. BP should be monitored with patients in both the sitting and the upright position to exclude the possibility of orthostatic hypotension, because autonomic denervation is frequent among patients with Type-2 diabetes who have nephropathy and polyneuropathy.

One of the main reasons for the failure to achieve BP goal is inadequate drug dosing, which is related to emotion-based rather than evidence-based medicine. Physicians recall that there are dose-dependent side-effects of drugs. Although this is true for older antihypertensive agents, it is not true for ACE inhibitors or ARBs. Thus, to optimize CV and renal risk reduction, physicians should set BP, lipid, and glucose goals with their patients and state them on paper, keep a copy in the chart, and give one to the patient. To maximize reduction in CV and renal mortality, the patient and the physician should be aware of treatment goals and discuss progress toward them at each visit.

REFERENCES

1. Schoolwerth AC, Engelgau MM, Hostetter TH, et al. Chronic kidney disease: a public health problem that needs a public health action plan. Prev Chronic Dis 2006;3(2):A57.

2. Coresh J, Selvin E, Stevens LA, et al. Prevalence of chronic kidney disease in the United States. JAMA 2007;298(17):2038–47.

3. Usrd 2007. ADR/reference tables. Available at: http://www.usrds.org-2007.htm. Accessed December 10, 2008.

4. So WY, Kong AP, Ma RC, et al. Glomerular filtration rate, cardiorenal end points, and all-cause mortality in type 2 diabetic patients. Diabetes Care 2006;29(9): 2046–52.

5. Bakris GL. Protecting renal function in the hypertensive patient: clinical guidelines. Am J Hypertens 2005;18(4 Pt 2):112S–9S.

6. Weir MR. The role of combination antihypertensive therapy in the prevention and treatment of chronic kidney disease. Am J Hypertens 2005;18(4 Pt 2):100S–5S.

7. Balu S, Thomas J III. Incremental expenditure of treating hypertension in the United States. Am J Hypertens 2006;19(8):810–6.

8. The cost for Medicare patients with CKD in 2006. Available at: http://www.usrds.org/2008/pdf/V1_05_2008.pdf. Accessed December 10, 2008.

9. Lewington S, Clarke R, Qizilbash N, et al. Age-specific relevance of usual blood pressure to vascular mortality: a meta-analysis of individual data for one million adults in 61 prospective studies. Lancet 2002;360(9349):1903–13.

10. Chobanian AV, Bakris GL, Black HR, et al. The Seventh Report of the Joint National Committee on Prevention, Detection, Evaluation, and Treatment of High Blood Pressure: the JNC 7 report. JAMA 2003;289(19):2560–72.

11. Chua DC, Bakris GL. Is proteinuria a plausible target of therapy? Curr Hypertens Rep 2004;6(3):177–81.

12. Culleton BF, Larson MG, Parfrey PS, et al. Proteinuria as a risk factor for cardiovascular disease and mortality in older people: a prospective study. Am J Med 2000;109(1):1–8.

13. Go AS, Chertow GM, Fan D, et al. Chronic kidney disease and the risks of death, cardiovascular events, and hospitalization. N Engl J Med 2004;351(13): 1296–305.

14. Sarnak MJ, Levey AS, Schoolwerth AC, et al. Kidney disease as a risk factor for development of cardiovascular disease: a statement from the American Heart Association Councils on Kidney in Cardiovascular Disease, High Blood Pressure Research, Clinical Cardiology, and Epidemiology and Prevention. Hypertension 2003;42(5):1050–65.

15. K/DOQI clinical practice guidelines on hypertension and antihypertensive agents in chronic kidney disease. Am J Kidney Dis 2004;43(5 Suppl 1):S1–290.

16. Khosla N, Sarafidis PA, Bakris GL. Microalbuminuria. Clin Lab Med 2006;26(3): 635–53, vi.

17. Bakris GL. Clinical importance of microalbuminuria in diabetes and hypertension. Curr Hypertens Rep 2004;6(5):352–6.

18. Giner V, Tormos C, Chaves FJ, et al. Microalbuminuria and oxidative stress in essential hypertension. J Intern Med 2004;255(5):588–94.

19. Kistorp C, Raymond I, Pedersen F, et al. N-terminal pro-brain natriuretic peptide, C-reactive protein, and urinary albumin levels as predictors of mortality and cardiovascular events in older adults. JAMA 2005;293(13):1609–16.

20. Palaniappan L, Carnethon M, Fortmann SP. Association between microalbuminuria and the metabolic syndrome: NHANES III. Am J Hypertens 2003;16(11 Pt 1): 952–8.

21. Steinke JM, Sinaiko AR, Kramer MS, et al. The early natural history of nephropathy in Type 1 Diabetes: III. Predictors of 5-year urinary albumin excretion rate patterns in initially normoalbuminuric patients. Diabetes 2005;54(7):2164–71.

22. Eknoyan G, Hostetter T, Bakris GL, et al. Proteinuria and other markers of chronic kidney disease: a position statement of the National Kidney Foundation (NKF) and the National Institute of Diabetes and Digestive and Kidney Diseases (NIDDK). Am J Kidney Dis 2003;42(4):617–22.

23. Ibsen H, Olsen MH, Wachtell K, et al. Reduction in albuminuria translates to reduction in cardiovascular events in hypertensive patients: Losartan Intervention for Endpoint Reduction in Hypertension study. Hypertension 2005;45(2): 198–202.

24. Ruggenenti P, Remuzzi G. Time to abandon microalbuminuria? Kidney Int 2006; 70(7):1214–22.

25. Atkins RC, Briganti EM, Lewis JB, et al. Proteinuria reduction and progression to renal failure in patients with type 2 diabetes mellitus and overt nephropathy. Am J Kidney Dis 2005;45(2):281–7.

26. de Zeeuw D, Remuzzi G, Parving HH, et al. Proteinuria, a target for renoprotection in patients with type 2 diabetic nephropathy: lessons from RENAAL. Kidney Int 2004;65(6):2309–20.

27. Lea J, Greene T, Hebert L, et al. The relationship between magnitude of proteinuria reduction and risk of end-stage renal disease: results of the African American Study of Kidney Disease and Hypertension. Arch Intern Med 2005;165(8): 947–53.

28. Gerstein HC. Epidemiologic analyses of risk factors, risk indicators, risk markers, and causal factors. The example of albuminuria and the risk of cardiovascular disease in diabetes. Endocrinol Metab Clin North Am 2002;31(3):537–51.

29. Katz R. Biomarkers and surrogate markers: an FDA perspective. NeuroRx 2004; 1(2):189–95.

30. Diuretic versus alpha-blocker as first-step antihypertensive therapy: final results from the Antihypertensive and Lipid-Lowering Treatment to Prevent Heart Attack Trial (ALLHAT). Hypertension 2003;42(3):239–46.

31. Estacio RO, Jeffers BW, Gifford N, et al. Effect of blood pressure control on diabetic microvascular complications in patients with hypertension and type 2 diabetes. Diabetes Care 2000;23(Suppl 2):B54–64.

32. Bakris GL, Williams M, Dworkin L, et al. Preserving renal function in adults with hypertension and diabetes: a consensus approach. National Kidney Foundation Hypertension and Diabetes Executive Committees Working Group. Am J Kidney Dis 2000;36(3):646–61.

33. Berl T, Hunsicker LG, Lewis JB, et al. Impact of achieved blood pressure on cardiovascular outcomes in the Irbesartan Diabetic Nephropathy Trial. J Am Soc Nephrol 2005;16(7):2170–9.

34. Sarnak MJ, Greene T, Wang X, et al. The effect of a lower target blood pressure on the progression of kidney disease: long-term follow-up of the Modification of Diet in Renal Disease Study. Ann Intern Med 2005;142(5):342–51.

35. Wright JT Jr, Bakris G, Greene T, et al. Effect of blood pressure lowering and antihypertensive drug class on progression of hypertensive kidney disease: results from the AASK trial. JAMA 2002;288(19):2421–31.

36. Ruggenenti P, Perna A, Loriga G, et al. Blood-pressure control for renoprotection in patients with non-diabetic chronic renal disease (REIN-2): multicentre, randomised controlled trial. Lancet 2005;365(9463):939–46.

37. Appel LJ, Wright JT Jr, Greene T, et al. Long-term effects of renin-angiotensin system-blocking therapy and a low blood pressure goal on progression of hypertensive chronic kidney disease in African Americans. Arch Intern Med 2008; 168(8):832–9.

38. Pogue V, Rahman M, Lipkowitz M, et al. Disparate estimates of hypertension control from ambulatory and clinic blood pressure measurements in hypertensive kidney disease. Hypertension 2009;53(1):20–7.

39. Jafar TH, Stark PC, Schmid CH, et al. Progression of chronic kidney disease: the role of blood pressure control, proteinuria, and angiotensin-converting enzyme inhibition: a patient-level meta-analysis. Ann Intern Med 2003;139(4):244–52.

40. Sarafidis PA, Khosla N, Bakris GL. Antihypertensive therapy in the presence of proteinuria. Am J Kidney Dis 2007;49(1):12–26.

41. Toto RD. Proteinuria reduction: mandatory consideration or option when selecting an antihypertensive agent? Curr Hypertens Rep 2005;7(5):374–8.

42. Mishra SI, Jones-Burton C, Fink JC, et al. Does dietary salt increase the risk for progression of kidney disease? Curr Hypertens Rep 2005;7(5):385–91.

43. Sacks FM, Svetkey LP, Vollmer WM, et al. Effects on blood pressure of reduced dietary sodium and the dietary approaches to stop hypertension (DASH) diet. DASH-Sodium Collaborative Research Group. N Engl J Med 2001;344(1):3–10.

44. Nofziger C, Chen L, Shane MA, et al. PPARgamma agonists do not directly enhance basal or insulin-stimulated $Na(+)$ transport via the epithelial $Na(+)$ channel. Pflugers Arch 2005;451(3):445–53.

45. Brands MW, Bell TD, Rodriguez NA, et al. Chronic glucose infusion causes sustained increases in tubular sodium reabsorption and renal blood flow in dogs. Am J Physiol Regul Integr Comp Physiol 2009;296:R265–71.

46. Tiwari S, Sharma N, Gill PS, et al. Impaired sodium excretion and increased blood pressure in mice with targeted deletion of renal epithelial insulin receptor. Proc Natl Acad Sci U S A 2008;105(17):6469–74.

47. Tiwari S, Riazi S, Ecelbarger CA. Insulin's impact on renal sodium transport and blood pressure in health, obesity, and diabetes. Am J Physiol Renal Physiol 2007; 293(4):F974–84.

48. Vedovato M, Lepore G, Coracina A, et al. Effect of sodium intake on blood pressure and albuminuria in Type 2 diabetic patients: the role of insulin resistance. Diabetologia 2004;47(2):300–3.

49. Heeg JE, de Jong PE, van der Hem GK, et al. Efficacy and variability of the antiproteinuric effect of ACE inhibition by lisinopril. Kidney Int 1989;36(2):272–9.

50. Buter H, Hemmelder MH, Navis G, et al. The blunting of the antiproteinuric efficacy of ACE inhibition by high sodium intake can be restored by hydrochlorothiazide. Nephrol Dial Transplant 1998;13(7):1682–5.

51. Vogt L, Waanders F, Boomsma F, et al. Effects of dietary sodium and hydrochlorothiazide on the antiproteinuric efficacy of losartan. J Am Soc Nephrol 2008; 19(5):999–1007.

52. Bakris GL, Sowers JR. ASH position paper: treatment of hypertension in patients with diabetes—an update. J Clin Hypertens (Greenwich) 2008;10(9):707–13.

53. Bosch JP. Renal reserve: a functional view of glomerular filtration rate. Semin Nephrol 1995;15(5):381–5.

54. Tietze IN, Sorensen SS, Ivarsen PR, et al. Impaired renal haemodynamic response to amino acid infusion in essential hypertension during angiotensin converting enzyme inhibitor treatment. J Hypertens 1997;15(5):551–60.

55. Lewis EJ, Hunsicker LG, Bain RP, et al. The effect of angiotensin-converting-enzyme inhibition on diabetic nephropathy. The Collaborative Study Group. N Engl J Med 1993;329(20):1456–62.

56. Ruggenenti P, Perna A, Gherardi G, et al. Renal function and requirement for dialysis in chronic nephropathy patients on long-term ramipril: REIN follow-up trial.

Gruppo Italiano di Studi Epidemiologici in Nefrologia (GISEN). Ramipril efficacy in Nephropathy. Lancet 1998;352(9136):1252–6.

57. Rahman M, Pressel S, Davis BR, et al. Renal outcomes in high-risk hypertensive patients treated with an angiotensin-converting enzyme inhibitor or a calcium channel blocker vs a diuretic: a report from the Antihypertensive and Lipid-Lowering Treatment to Prevent Heart Attack Trial (ALLHAT). Arch Intern Med 2005;165(8):936–46.

58. Bakris GL, Weir MR. Angiotensin-converting enzyme inhibitor-associated elevations in serum creatinine: is this a cause for concern? Arch Intern Med 2000; 160(5):685–93.

59. Pitt B, Bakris G, Ruilope LM, et al. Serum potassium and clinical outcomes in the Eplerenone Post-Acute Myocardial Infarction Heart Failure Efficacy and Survival Study (EPHESUS). Circulation 2008;118(16):1643–50.

60. Brenner BM, Cooper ME, de Zeeuw D, et al. Effects of losartan on renal and cardiovascular outcomes in patients with type 2 diabetes and nephropathy. N Engl J Med 2001;345(12):861–9.

61. Lewis EJ, Hunsicker LG, Clarke WR, et al. Renoprotective effect of the angiotensin-receptor antagonist irbesartan in patients with nephropathy due to type 2 diabetes. N Engl J Med 2001;345(12):851–60.

62. Barnett AH, Bain SC, Bouter P, et al. Angiotensin-receptor blockade versus converting-enzyme inhibition in type 2 diabetes and nephropathy. N Engl J Med 2004;351(19):1952–61.

63. Bidani A. Controversy about COOPERATE ABPM trial data. Am J Nephrol 2006; 26(6):629–32.

64. Mangrum AJ, Bakris GL. Angiotensin-converting enzyme inhibitors and angiotensin receptor blockers in chronic renal disease: safety issues. Semin Nephrol 2004;24(2):168–75.

65. Gradman AH, Schmieder RE, Lins RL, et al. Aliskiren, a novel orally effective renin inhibitor, provides dose-dependent antihypertensive efficacy and placebo-like tolerability in hypertensive patients. Circulation 2005;111(8):1012–8.

66. Musini VM, Fortin PM, Bassett K, et al. Blood pressure lowering efficacy of renin inhibitors for primary hypertension. Cochrane Database Syst Rev 2008;(4): CD007066.

67. Parving HH, Persson F, Lewis JB, et al. Aliskiren combined with losartan in type 2 diabetes and nephropathy. N Engl J Med 2008;358(23):2433–46.

68. Chapman N, Dobson J, Wilson S, et al. Effect of spironolactone on blood pressure in subjects with resistant hypertension. Hypertension 2007;49(4): 839–45.

69. Bomback AS, Kshirsagar AV, Amamoo MA, et al. Change in proteinuria after adding aldosterone blockers to ACE inhibitors or angiotensin receptor blockers in CKD: a systematic review. Am J Kidney Dis 2008;51(2):199–211.

70. Major outcomes in high-risk hypertensive patients randomized to angiotensin-converting enzyme inhibitor or calcium channel blocker vs diuretic: The Antihypertensive and Lipid-Lowering Treatment to Prevent Heart Attack Trial (ALLHAT). JAMA 2002;288(23):2981–97.

71. Wing LM, Reid CM, Ryan P, et al. A comparison of outcomes with angiotensin-converting–enzyme inhibitors and diuretics for hypertension in the elderly. N Engl J Med 2003;348(7):583–92.

72. Khosla N, Chua DY, Elliott WJ, et al. Are chlorthalidone and hydrochlorothiazide equivalent blood-pressure-lowering medications? J Clin Hypertens (Greenwich) 2005;7(6):354–6.

73. Carter BL, Ernst ME, Cohen JD. Hydrochlorothiazide versus chlorthalidone: evidence supporting their interchangeability. Hypertension 2004;43(1):4–9.
74. Zillich AJ, Garg J, Basu S, et al. Thiazide diuretics, potassium, and the development of diabetes: a quantitative review. Hypertension 2006;48(2):219–24.
75. Gress TW, Nieto FJ, Shahar E, et al. Hypertension and antihypertensive therapy as risk factors for type 2 diabetes mellitus. Atherosclerosis Risk in Communities Study. N Engl J Med 2000;342(13):905–12.
76. Kim GH. Long-term adaptation of renal ion transporters to chronic diuretic treatment. Am J Nephrol 2004;24(6):595–605.
77. Turnbull F, Neal B, Ninomiya T, et al. Effects of different regimens to lower blood pressure on major cardiovascular events in older and younger adults: meta-analysis of randomised trials. BMJ 2008;336(7653):1121–3.
78. Jamerson K, Weber MA, Bakris GL, et al. Benazepril plus amlodipine or hydrochlorothiazide for hypertension in high-risk patients. N Engl J Med 2008; 359(23):2417–28.
79. Pepine CJ, Handberg EM, Cooper-DeHoff RM, et al. A calcium antagonist vs a non-calcium antagonist hypertension treatment strategy for patients with coronary artery disease. The International Verapamil-Trandolapril Study (INVEST): a randomized controlled trial. JAMA 2003;290(21):2805–16.
80. Bakris GL, Weir MR, Secic M, et al. Differential effects of calcium antagonist subclasses on markers of nephropathy progression. Kidney Int 2004;65(6): 1991–2002.
81. Toto RD. Management of hypertensive chronic kidney disease: role of calcium channel blockers. J Clin Hypertens (Greenwich) 2005;7(4 Suppl 1):15–20.
82. Boero R, Rollino C, Massara C, et al. Verapamil versus amlodipine in proteinuric non-diabetic nephropathies treated with trandolapril (VVANNTT study): design of a prospective randomized multicenter trial. J Nephrol 2001;14(1):15–8.
83. Nathan S, Pepine CJ, Bakris GL. Calcium antagonists: effects on cardio-renal risk in hypertensive patients. Hypertension 2005;46(4):637–42.
84. Ruggenenti P, Fassi A, Ilieva AP, et al. Preventing microalbuminuria in type 2 diabetes. N Engl J Med 2004;351(19):1941–51.
85. Bakris G. Proteinuria: a link to understanding changes in vascular compliance? Hypertension 2005;46(3):473–4.
86. Lindholm LH, Carlberg B, Samuelsson O. Should beta blockers remain first choice in the treatment of primary hypertension? A meta-analysis. Lancet 2005; 366(9496):1545–53.
87. Kalaitzidis R, Bakris G. Should nephrologists use beta-blockers? A perspective. Nephrol Dial Transplant 2009;24:701–2.
88. Bakris GL, Fonseca V, Katholi RE, et al. Differential effects of beta-blockers on albuminuria in patients with type 2 diabetes. Hypertension 2005;46(6):1309–15.
89. Bakris GL, Fonseca V, Katholi RE, et al. Metabolic effects of carvedilol vs metoprolol in patients with type 2 diabetes mellitus and hypertension: a randomized controlled trial. JAMA 2004;292(18):2227–36.
90. Rachmani R, Levi Z, Slavachevsky I, et al. Effect of an alpha-adrenergic blocker, and ACE inhibitor and hydrochlorothiazide on blood pressure and on renal function in type 2 diabetic patients with hypertension and albuminuria. A randomized cross-over study. Nephron 1998;80(2):175–82.
91. Efficacy of atenolol and captopril in reducing risk of macrovascular and microvascular complications in type 2 diabetes: UKPDS 39. UK Prospective Diabetes Study Group. BMJ 1998;317(7160):713–20.

92. Hansson L, Zanchetti A, Carruthers SG, et al. Effects of intensive blood-pressure lowering and low-dose aspirin in patients with hypertension: principal results of the Hypertension Optimal Treatment (HOT) randomised trial. HOT Study Group. Lancet 1998;351(9118):1755–62.
93. Pohl MA, Blumenthal S, Cordonnier DJ, et al. Independent and additive impact of blood pressure control and angiotensin II receptor blockade on renal outcomes in the Irbesartan Diabetic Nephropathy Trial: clinical implications and limitations. J Am Soc Nephrol 2005;16(10):3027–37.

Current Approaches to Renovascular Hypertension

Stephen C. Textor, MD

KEYWORDS

- Renovascular hypertension • Renal artery stenosis • Stent
- Angioplasty • ACE inhibitor • Angiotensin receptor blocker

Understanding the mechanisms and implications of renovascular disease remains an important challenge for clinicians caring for patients with hypertension. "Renovascular hypertension" is defined as systemic hypertension resulting from renal arterial compromise, often owing to occlusive lesions of the main renal arteries. In classical definitions, the conclusion that hypertension is related directly to an arterial lesion depends on reversal of the hypertension after relief of the obstruction. In practice, obtaining complete "reversal" of hypertension is rarely possible. It is important to recognize that renovascular disease often accelerates preexisting hypertension, can ultimately threaten the viability of the poststenotic kidney, and can impair sodium excretion in subjects with congestive heart failure.

Major advances in vascular imaging allow noninvasive identification of vascular lesions more easily than ever before. At the same time, introduction of effective, well-tolerated antihypertensive drug therapy for renovascular hypertension allows more effective medical management of this disorder than ever before. Although renovascular hypertension appears on lists of "curable" forms of hypertension, outcomes from recent, small prospective trials up to now fail to establish major benefits of revascularization, either performed by endovascular procedures or surgery.[1] These observations leave both patients and physicians uncertain about how best to treat renovascular hypertension, particularly with regard to moving ahead with either endovascular or surgical intervention. In view of this "equipoise" between medical therapy and renal revascularization, the National Institutes of Health in the United States is supporting a major prospective, randomized trial comparing intensive medical therapy alone to intensive therapy plus renal revascularization regarding the Cardiovascular Outcomes for Renal Atherosclerotic Lesions (CORAL). Until these questions are

This work was supported in part by NIH HL 16496 and 1PO1HL085307 from National Heart, Lung and Blood Institute. The content is solely the responsibility of the author and does not necessarily represent the official views of the National Heart, Lung, and Blood Institute or the National Institutes of Health.

Division of Nephrology and Hypertension, West 19, Mayo Clinic, 200 First Street, Rochester, MN 55905, USA

E-mail address: textor.stephen@mayo.edu

more clearly answered, physicians dealing with complex hypertension are understandably uncertain about the value of embarking on expensive, sometimes hazardous, diagnostic workups and vascular intervention.

This article examines the current status regarding prevalence, mechanisms, clinical manifestations and management of renovascular hypertension at this point in time. It should be viewed as a work in progress. As with most complex conditions, clinicians must integrate the results of published literature studies while considering each patient's specific features and comorbid disease risks. Beyond identifying renovascular disease as a cause of secondary hypertension, one must manage renal artery stenosis (RAS) itself as an atherosclerotic vascular complication. This disease warrants follow-up regarding progression and potential for ischemic tissue injury. These elements often determine the role and timing for revascularization. In this respect, atherosclerotic renal artery stenosis is analogous to progressive carotid or aortic aneurysmal disease. Because selection of imaging tools and further diagnostic studies related to management of this condition often depends upon the clinical commitment to act upon those results, the section on imaging and diagnosis is positioned after initial management.

PATHOPHYSIOLOGY

Studies demonstrating that vascular occlusion to the kidneys produces a rise in systemic arterial pressure remain among the seminal observations regarding pathogenic mechanisms for hypertension.[2] Experimental models of renovascular hypertension, including those in which a normal contralateral kidney is exposed to pressure natriuresis (2-kidney-1-clip) and those for which the entire functioning renal mass is beyond a vascular occlusion (1-kidney-1-clip) remain among the most widely studied models of hypertension. For the models with a normal contralateral kidney, hypertension is more predictably angiotensin dependent. These models have been adapted to numerous species including mouse, rat, dog and pig.[3] These are widely accepted as fundamental models of angiotensin-mediated hypertension for studies directed toward vascular remodeling, left-ventricular hypertrophy, small vessel occlusive disease, and renal dysfunction. **Box 1** lists several of the causes of renal artery obstruction recognized as producing this syndrome. Although intrinsic renovascular disorders related to atherosclerotic and fibromuscular disease are most common, it should be recognized that any structural disorder reducing renal perfusion pressure to viable kidney tissue is capable of producing renovascular hypertension.

Activation of the renin-angiotensin system is an essential component of developing renovascular hypertension, at least in the initial stages. Studies in which animals are pretreated with angiotensin-converting enzyme (ACE) inhibition indicate that development of hypertension is delayed so long as ACE inhibition continues. Genetic knockout animals without the angiotensin-1 receptor do not develop renovascular hypertension. Recent transplantation studies indicate that angiotensin receptors in both the systemic vasculature and kidney vasculature participate in this process.[4,5] Measured components of the renin-angiotensin system, eg, plasma renin activity, are elevated only transiently in renovascular hypertension. Observations in both experimental animals and human subjects indicate that renin release is eventually reduced partly related to the rise in systemic, and thereby renal, arterial pressures and/or sodium retention. Recruitment of additional renovascular pressor mechanisms, such as release of endothelin, activation of the sympathetic nervous system, oxidative stress and others also produce sustained rises in arterial pressure that are not directly related to the renin-angiotensin system.

Box 1
Major causes of renovascular hypertension

Atherosclerotic renal artery stenosis

Fibromuscular disease

    Medial fibroplasia

    Perimedial fibroplasia

    Intimal fibroplasia

    Medial hyperplasia

Extrinsic fibrous band

Renal trauma

    Arterial dissection

    Segmental renal infarction

    Page kidney (perirenal fibrosis)

Aortic dissection

Aortic endograft occluding the renal artery

Arterial embolus

Other Medical Disorders:

    Hypercoagulable state with renal infarction

    Takayasu's arteritis

    Radiation-induced fibrosis

    Tumor encircling the renal artery, eg, pheochromocytoma

    Polyarteritis nodosa

How much vascular occlusion is necessary to initiate the "syndrome" of renovascular hypertension? Recent studies confirm the observation that activation of renin release depends on the gradient between the aorta and the poststenotic segments of the renal artery. No renin release can be detected until the gradient is between 10 and 20 mm Hg.[6] Studies with latex casts of arterial segments indicate that reductions in pressure across an occlusive lesion require lumen obstruction in excess of 70% to 75%. Modern imaging studies frequently reveal "incidental" renal arterial occlusive lesions of lesser severity with only minor effects. While the majority of clinical cases of renovascular hypertension are produced by main renal artery lesions from atherosclerosis or forms of fibromuscular dysplasia, it should be recognized that any lesion that reduces kidney perfusion pressures can lead to similar results. Less common cases include renal artery occlusion related to trauma (with or without arterial dissection), extrinsic compression such as a perivascular tumor, intrinsic obstruction such as produced by an aortic endograft that partially occludes the renal arteries, aortic dissection, and so forth (**Box 1** and **Fig. 1**).

EPIDEMIOLOGY AND CLINICAL CHARACTERISTICS OF RENOVASCULAR HYPERTENSION

The hallmarks of renovascular hypertension include the onset and progression of blood pressure elevation outside the ranges typical of essential hypertension. Hence, hypertension appearing in younger individuals, eg, children or young adults, or the recent onset of hypertension in previously normotensive older individuals older than 55 raises

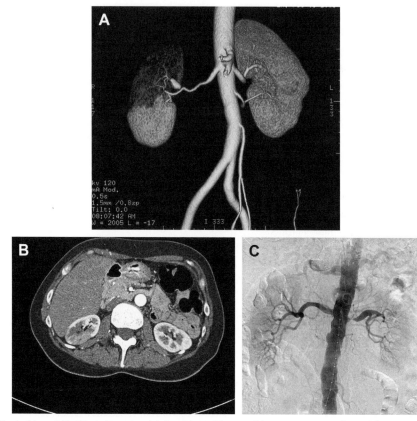

Fig. 1. (*A* and *B*) CT angiogram obtained in a 45-year-old woman presenting with new-onset renovascular hypertension. Aneurysmal dilation and vascular occlusion beyond a fibromuscular lesion is present in the right kidney associated with loss of perfusion to the entire upper pole of the kidney. Antihypertensive therapy in this instance can be achieved using agents that block the renin-angiotensin system. Although such cases are unusual, they underscore the broad range of lesions that can produce the syndrome of renovascular hypertension. (*C*) Aortogram demonstrating high-grade stenosis affecting the left renal artery. Quantitative measurements indicated more than 86% lumen obstruction. This individual was randomized to medical therapy in the CORAL trial (see text).

this diagnostic concern. Congenital anomalies and/or segmental infarction have been observed commonly in infants and children with hypertension. With the rise in childhood obesity, blood pressure elevations are now observed in more children than ever before. Hence, renovascular disease is not the single most likely cause of hypertension at any age. Prospective studies from a hypertension unit in the United Kingdom targeting 96 younger individuals identified secondary hypertension in 18.1%, most of which were renovascular hypertension (75%).[7] Actual cure rate was only 2 of 13 subjects (15% of renovascular cases), which represented only 3.2% of the screened population. Whether extensive diagnostic studies and renovascular intervention is always warranted in such cases remains controversial as discussed later in this article.

Fibromuscular disease (FMD) affecting the renal arteries occurs in 3% to 5% of normotensive individuals presenting as potential kidney donors.[8,9] It appears as a cause of hypertension most commonly in younger females, sometimes during pregnancy. Smoking is thought to lead to progression and worsening arterial pressures in this group. Rarely, FMD leads to complete or segmental occlusion **(Fig. 1**A and B), but most individuals have normal kidney function and it rarely leads to loss of glomerular filtration rate.

The most common and problematic cause is atherosclerotic renovascular disease. Recent interventional series indicate that atherosclerosis constitutes 84% of patients identified with renal artery stenosis **(Fig. 1**C).[10] Epidemiologic observations suggest that atherosclerotic lesions exceeding 60% occlusion (by Doppler ultrasound) affect the kidney in 6.8% of a community-based sample of subjects older than 65.[11] When the renal arteries are studied as part of clinical angiography for other disorders, occlusive lesions are found in nearly 20% of patients with coronary disease and more than 35% in patients with clinically significant aortic or peripheral vascular disease.[12] In this regard, the extent of renal arterial disease appears to reflect the overall disease burden related to atherosclerotic disease elsewhere. High-grade atherosclerotic renal artery disease predicts long-term survival based on several cohort studies, regardless of whether or not revascularization is undertaken.[13]

Hypertensive specialists recognize that atherosclerotic renovascular disease is associated with accelerated and more severe target organ injury than essential hypertension. Careful studies of office and ambulatory blood pressure levels indicate that circadian pressure rhythms are commonly disturbed in subjects with RAS. Such individuals often lack a nocturnal fall in arterial pressure (therefore are classified as "non-dippers") and may have paradoxically elevated nocturnal pressures.[14] The severity of left ventricular hypertrophy, impairment of kidney function, and other manifestations of vascular disease are increased for such patients. Increased adrenergic activity as measured by efferent sympathetic nerve traffic is common in this disorder and is associated with wider variability in blood pressure as compared with essential hypertension. Sometimes this appears as paroxysmal hypertension, easily confused with pheochromocytoma. Endothelial dysfunction with impaired vascular relaxation develops in patients with renovascular hypertension.[15] In experimental models, disturbances in endothelial function are magnified by cholesterol feeding as a manifestation of early atherosclerosis. All of these characteristics can improve after revascularization, and in some cases with statin therapy.[16] Whether similar outcomes can be achieved using medical therapy that blocks the neurohormonal pathways activated with renovascular disease is not yet clear and is one of the major objectives of randomized controlled studies including CORAL.

Studies of Medicare claims indicate that individuals with newly identified renovascular disease develop other cardiovascular events at a higher rate than those without renovascular disease over a 2-year period.[17] It should be emphasized that clinical events are most commonly related to new cardiovascular disease including coronary events, myocardial infarction, and heart failure. These are more common by far than reduction in kidney function in absolute terms **(Fig. 2)**.

The role of renovascular disease limiting sodium excretion warrants special consideration. Structural occlusion of the renal artery sufficient to reduce renal perfusion pressure itself enhances sodium retention by slowing blood flow and filtration and enhancing peritubular forces leading to solute reabsorption. Activation of the renin-angiotensin-aldosterone system tends to retain sodium further. Angiotensin II directly increases sodium transport, an effect magnified by the reduction in blood flow related to its vascular effects. Aldosterone activates distal sodium retention by activating sodium-potassium ATPase. These combined forces have long been recognized as reducing sodium excretion in the poststenotic kidney. In subjects with an intact contralateral kidney sodium excretion may be

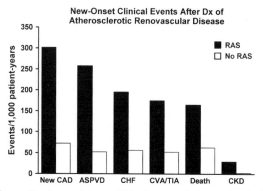

Fig. 2. Incidence of new Medicare claims within 2 years of diagnosis of atherosclerotic renal artery stenosis. Patients with renal artery disease are more likely to have new coronary, stroke, congestive heart failure, and chronic kidney disease (CKD) than those without renal arterial disease. Adverse cardiovascular outcomes are far more likely than those related specifically to kidney disease. (*Data from* Kalra PA, Guo H, Kausz AT, et al. Atherosclerotic renovascular disease in United States patients aged 67 years or older: risk factors, revascularization and prognosis. Kidney Int 2005;68:293–301.)

increased as a result of "pressure natriuresis" induced by systemic hypertension.[18] Early studies using bilateral ureteral cannulation to examine individual kidney function confirmed that demonstration of lateralization of sodium excretion could predict improvement in renovascular hypertension after surgery.[19] As the contralateral kidney becomes subject to intrinsic parenchymal injury or the effects of circulating sodium-retaining hormones, it may lose the ability to excrete sodium effectively. This form of functional sodium retention has been invoked to explain why the rise in plasma renin activity may be transient and why lateralization of renin secretion can be demonstrated only after sodium-depleting maneuvers. Hence, many of the early studies of renal vein lateralization depend on administration of potent diuretics such as furosemide to identify the pressor role of the stenotic kidney. Perhaps even more importantly, bilateral renal artery disease (or stenosis to a solitary functioning kidney) limits kidney function and sodium excretion. This is sometimes manifest as transient episodes of severe hypertension and circulatory congestion that magnify left ventricular dysfunction and congestive heart failure, so-called "flash" pulmonary edema.[20] The combination of reduced cardiac pump function and renovascular disease can be difficult to manage. Although no controlled, prospective trials have been performed for such patients, several series suggest that recurrent hospitalizations for circulatory congestion can be reduced after renal revascularization.[21] Thus, renovascular hypertension can present a broad range of neurohormonal pressor systems and impaired sodium and volume control.

Perhaps the most common presentation of renovascular hypertension is "resistant hypertension." Recent consensus statements define this condition as failure to achieve goal blood pressures (usually considered <140/90 mm Hg or lower for high-risk conditions), despite optimal doses of three or more antihypertensive agents, including a diuretic. Common features to such patients include older age, systolic hypertension, obesity, obstructive sleep apnea, and other manifestations of renal dysfunction.[22] The fact that most such patients have multiple comorbidities makes it more difficult to assign a causative role for any specific condition, including renovascular disease.

MANAGEMENT OF RENOVASCULAR HYPERTENSION

Optimizing antihypertensive therapy and overall cardiovascular risk is an essential initial step in managing renovascular hypertension (**Box 2**). Much of the impetus for embarking on further diagnostic and therapeutic maneuvers depends on whether blood pressure control and renal function can be maintained readily. Because actual "cure" of hypertension is rarely achieved (defined as normal blood pressure without requiring antihypertensive therapy), it may be argued that if blood pressure and renal function are managed easily, little is to be gained by elaborate diagnostic procedures. Conversely, failure to achieve acceptable levels of arterial pressure adds strength to the potential benefit of even partial improvement achievable with successful renal revascularization. Hence, the response to therapy is an important element in deciding on the benefits of renal revascularization when high-grade arterial lesions are present.

THE ROLE OF ANGIOTENSIN BLOCKADE

Blockade of the renin-angiotensin system is now established as an important element in the treatment of renovascular hypertension. Before agents such as angiotensin-converting enzyme (ACE) inhibitors were available, renovascular hypertension commonly presented as "untreatable" hypertension. Series of emergency room

---

Box 2
Management of renovascular hypertension

Antihypertensive Drug Therapy

Blockade of the renin-angiotensin system:

    Angiotensin-converting enzyme inhibitors (ACE)

    Angiotensin receptor blockers (ARB's)

    Direct renin inhibitors? (Aliskiren)

Calcium channel blocking agents

Diuretics

Mineralocorticoid receptor blockade

Additional classes: Beta-blockade, alpha-receptor blockade, sympatholytic agents, vasodilators

Cardiovascular Risk Reduction:

Removal of tobacco use

Treatment of dyslipidemia: statins, fibrates, others

Treatment of obesity: obstructive sleep apnea

Management of glucose intolerance/diabetes

Renal Revascularization: Selected Cases

Endovascular revascularization

    PTRA: primarily fibromuscular dysplasia

    PTRA with stenting: atherosclerotic disease

Surgical: renal artery bypass/endarterectomy (now usually reserved for complex aorto-renal disease, aneurysmal disease, failed endovascular stent procedures, and so forth

Nephrectomy: open or laparoscopic removal of pressor kidney, usually nonfunctional

patients with hypertensive emergencies routinely appeared with accelerated phase hypertension, later identified as renovascular in origin.[23] A few small series of patients with episodic, malignant-phase hypertension were identified that were subjected to bilateral nephrectomy as a life-saving measure.[24] With the introduction of agents now capable of interrupting this system, such measures are rarely necessary. Based on the potential adverse effects of angiotensin to magnify vascular injury, myocardial damage and remodeling and increase the risk of adverse cardiovascular outcomes, many argue that administration of ACE inhibitors should be part of managing nearly all patients with significant cardiovascular risk, based on data from the HOPE trial and others.[25] These observations have been extended to angiotensin-receptor blocking agents (ARBs) based on results from studies directly comparing ACE inhibition with angiotensin receptor blockade.[26] Whether neurohormonal disturbances resulting directly from renovascular disease are a major factor in the cardiovascular risk intervention in these patients remains an important question. As a result, blockade of the renin-angiotensin system is a core element in determining the effects of renal revascularization. All patients participating in the CORAL trial are provided an angiotensin receptor blocker as a cornerstone of therapy. Whether direct renin-inhibition with agents such as aliskiren will have the same effect is logical, but as yet unproven. Blockade of the renin-angiotensin system is therefore important, but often not sufficient, to control hypertension in patients with renovascular hypertension. Therapy with additional antihypertensive agents, particularly diuretics, is essential.

It must be emphasized that removal of the renin-angiotensin system is not without drawbacks. Initial consensus regarding application of ACE inhibitors was difficult to achieve, in part because of the well-recognized potential of these agents to lower glomerular filtration rate as a result of loss of angiotensin II effects at the efferent arteriole. As noted above, renin release can be observed when sufficient lumen obstruction to produce a pressure gradient between the pre- and poststenotic segment of 10% to 20%. This can occur with only a minor disruption of blood flow to the kidney that requires less than 10% of its blood flow for metabolic demands. Early studies in the dog demonstrated that as renal blood flow becomes reduced with a progressive occlusion, sustaining transcapillary filtration pressures depend on maintaining efferent arteriolar constriction. This constriction is modulated largely by the vascular effects of angiotensin II. Blockade of angiotensin II production (with the use of an ACE inhibitor) or its receptor (with an angiotensin receptor blocking drug) reduces efferent arteriolar tone and allows blood flow past the capillary surface with insufficient pressure to form urine. As a result, the poststenotic kidney may develop "functional acute renal insufficiency," despite having adequate blood flow for metabolic demands.

When arterial obstruction is extreme, simply reducing perfusion pressure sometimes can reduce poststenotic blood flow beyond that required for metabolic demands in the kidney. This can develop with any form of antihypertensive therapy and is not limited to agents that block the renin-angiotensin system.[27] Early experimental studies in rats emphasized the potential for irreversible damage to the kidney to develop beyond a renal artery clip in animals treated with ACE inhibitors, leading some to refer to such therapy as "medical nephrectomy."[28] These experiences highlight the potential for renovascular disease to both activate pressor mechanisms and to ultimately threaten the poststenotic kidney with insufficient blood supply. Surveys of pharmacy records related to administration of agents that block the renin-angiotensin system indicate that although these drugs allow effective blood pressure control and reduced clinical events such as stroke, death, congestive heart failure, and initiation of permanent dialysis, they are associated nonetheless with a definite incidence of acute renal failure, sometimes leading to drug withdrawal.[29] Postmarketing surveys indicate that risk factors for adverse events include older age groups, preexisting renal dysfunction, and episodes of acute illness leading to volume depletion (such as diarrhea or reduced intake during diuretic administration).[30]

MANAGEMENT OF ATHEROSCLEROTIC DISEASE RISK

As a practical matter, much renovascular hypertension develops in the setting of preexisting cardiovascular risk, including essential hypertension, dyslipidemia, diabetes, and smoking. Because the major causes of morbidity and mortality remain related to cardiovascular outcomes including stroke and coronary events, management includes intensive efforts to reduce these risks. These include discontinuation of smoking, initiation of statin therapy, low-dose aspirin, and weight and diabetes control as appropriate. It must be recognized that identification of involvement of the renal vessels with atherosclerosis itself predicts higher mortality and intensifies the importance of risk management. The CORAL trial specifically seeks to address the additive effects of renal artery revascularization regarding cardiovascular events after ensuring adequate and intensive management of these risk factors. For that reason, drug therapy to block angiotensin and statins to lower cholesterol is provided and each treatment site is provided "report cards" related to adequacy of risk factor control.

THE ROLE OF RENAL REVASCULARIZATION

In the past, renovascular hypertension was often viewed as a secondary cause of hypertension that warranted diagnosis specifically with the goal of restoring blood flow to the kidney to "cure" hypertension. Although logical, this argument has not been supported by studies of clinical outcomes. Clinicians caring for patients with hypertension must balance the pros and cons of vascular intervention carefully, as summarized by a recent American Heart Association symposium (**Box 3**). These sometimes relate directly to the expertise available locally for either endovascular or surgical intervention within a specific institution or region. Previous studies emphasize that rates of peripheral arterial intervention differ by up to 14 fold within different regions of the country.[31] Few prospective trial data are available to define either the populations most likely to benefit or the true risk/benefit profiles for these procedures.

The reasons for this ambiguity are complex. Rapid expansion of both imaging and interventional expertise has led to more common diagnoses of renal arterial lesions and a greater enthusiasm for endovascular procedures than ever before. Medicare claims data indicate a rise of more than fourfold between 1996 and 2005 as we have reviewed.[32] These developments led the Centers for Medicare and Medicaid Services (CMS) to commission a review of the data to support these procedures published in 2006. It concluded "available evidence was neither adequate nor sufficiently applicable to current practice to clearly support one treatment approach over another...."[1]

FIBROMUSCULAR DYSPLASIAS

Most clinicians favor considering endovascular intervention in the form of PTRA for fibromuscular disease affecting the main renal arteries. This disorder often produces hypertension in younger individuals, most often women. A recent series of 69 subjects indicated that PTRA achieved patency over 90% initially and 87% during follow-up over 6 years, although repeat procedures are needed in up to 25% of patients.[33] The potential for relief of hypertension (although rarely complete cure) is substantial and this approach may reduce long-term antihypertensive therapy requirements. It

---

Box 3

Clinical Factors favoring Medical Therapy with or without revascularization for Renovascular Disease

1. *Favoring Medical therapy with Revascularization:*

   a. Progressive decline in GFR during treatment of hypertension

   b. Failure to achieve adequate blood pressure control despite optimal medical therapy

   c. Rapid or recurrent decline in GFR associated with reduced systemic blood pressure

   d. Decline in GFR associated with ACE inhibition/ARB therapy

   e. Recurrent congestive heart failure out of proportion to left ventricular dysfunction

2. *Favoring Medical Therapy and Surveillance without revascularization*

   a. Controlled blood pressure with stable renal function

   b. Stable renal arterial disease without evident progression

   c. Advanced age and/or limited life expectancy

   d. Extensive comorbidity

   e. High risk or previous atheroembolic disease

   f. Other concomitant parenchymal renal disease likely to explain renal dysfunction, eg, diabetic nephropathy

GFR, glomerular filtration rate. *Data from* American Heart Association Atherosclerotic Peripheral Vascular Disease Symposium recommendations {8267}. Circulation 2008;118:2873–8.

---

must be emphasized that FMD can extend into smaller branch vessels and may not be amenable to intervention for technical reasons. Similarly, these lesions have a predilection for developing aneurysms that should not be stressed mechanically. In some cases, embolization of the aneurysm or surgical resection should be considered.[34] Normally, stents are not suitable for FMD unless needed to repair a vessel dissection. Recent surgical series for complex anatomy or failed PTRA intervention indicate 27% with effective "cure" and improved in 67%.[34] Most recent series suggest that up to 74% will have improved blood pressure levels following PTRA. Kidney function is most often normal in subjects with FMD and does not materially change after PTRA.

Atherosclerotic disease of the renal arteries presents a more complex picture. With the widespread application of endovascular stenting, most (95% to 98%) lesions can be successfully dilated to restore blood flow. Atherosclerosis commonly involves both the aorta and orificial components of the renal arteries. Dilation of these plaques commonly releases atheroembolic debris of varying sizes. Ex vivo studies suggest that many steps of an interventional procedure, including initial placement of guidewires, are capable of releasing microembolic material.[35] The results of restoring renal artery patency in these cases are not completely predictable. Previous studies with both surgical and endovascular procedures indicate that blood pressure control may be more easily achieved, sometimes with fewer medications. Current goal levels for blood pressure nearly always require further antihypertensive drug therapy, so complete cure without residual treatment is rare. In some patients with reduced glomerular filtration rate, kidney function may improve substantially with restoration of main vessel patency. This occurs in 25% to 28% of cases depending on the definition for "improvement." Most patients have no discernible change in kidney function. Most series report a smaller group of patients, ranging between 12% and 20%, that experience a loss of kidney function after renal artery revascularization, most often attributed to atheroemboli.[36] In such cases, loss of renal function can progress rapidly and may progress to end-stage renal disease (ESRD) requiring dialysis. As a result, the appropriate application of endovascular stenting procedures for atherosclerotic renal artery disease remains controversial.

The Agency for Healthcare Research and Quality (AHRQ) review of published literature commissioned by CMS concluded that data were insufficient to consider the role of revascularization of proven benefit. At least four prospective, randomized trials of endovascular stenting for renal artery stenosis have been undertaken in the past several years. Preliminary results of the largest of these (the Angioplasty and Stenting in Renal Atherosclerotic Lesions [ASTRAL]) conducted in the United Kingdom have been presented in abstract form. This trial was intended to evaluate changes in renal function. Subjects were eligible if the clinicians were "uncertain" about optimal therapy. The mean serum creatinine was more than 2.0 mg/dL at entry and the average degree of stenosis was estimated to be 76% lumen occlusion. Remarkably, no differences among 806 patients assigned to medical therapy with or without stenting could be detected regarding blood pressure control, renal function, hospitalization for congestive heart failure, or mortality[37] during a median follow-up period exceeding 2 years. More than 600 subjects with more stringent entry criteria have been enrolled in CORAL with a target date to finish enrollment of more than 1000 subjects by the final quarter of 2009.

How should clinicians interpret these results in the interim? As noted above, some patients develop functional acute renal insufficiency during antihypertensive drug therapy that can improve after successful revascularization. The AHRQ summaries acknowledged that occasional removal of antihypertensive drug therapy and recovery of kidney function were reported only in patients subjected to renal revascularization.[1] It is inescapable that some patients derive major benefits from successfully restoring renal blood flow. What must be acknowledged is that these benefits are not universal (or even common) and do entail both risk and considerable expense. In this respect, we view them as important interventions similar to other vascular procedures such as those applied to aortic or carotid disease. Revascularization should be considered mainly for individuals with vascular disease likely to progress and likely to benefit from the procedure at acceptable levels of risk. How best to identify patients likely to benefit remains an elusive goal. To a great extent, this is defined by failure of medical therapy alone, as summarized in **Boxes 2** and **3**.

DIAGNOSTIC EVALUATION OF RENOVASCULAR HYPERTENSION

The hallmark of identifying renovascular hypertension is the demonstration of structural and functional occlusion of the renal vessels. How to achieve this optimally remains an elusive goal. We have argued that selection of imaging studies should reflect precisely the questions to be answered, because not all of these can be equally addressed with certainty.[38] As a result, many patients undergo multiple noninvasive studies before reaching a diagnostic and/or therapeutic angiogram. Our own approach is to emphasize—in advance—the precise goals of the diagnostic study and the commitment to act upon the findings if positive.

Major advances in vascular imaging over the past decade allow positive identification of renovascular disease more easily than ever before. Although a detailed discussion of each technique is beyond the scope of this discussion, several points may be worth mentioning.

Renal Artery Duplex (Doppler) Ultrasound

Renal artery duplex (Doppler) ultrasound remains among the most widely available and least costly studies to identify hemodynamically significant vascular lesions.

Ultrasound examination is a proven technology for evaluating the kidney and reliably detects obstructive uropathy, asymmetry in size, cortical thickness, location, and many parenchymal abnormalities. As such it remains among the first studies considered by nephrologists evaluating patients with reduced glomerular filtration. When used to evaluate renovascular disease, results remain operator and center dependent. The results are most useful when "positive," ie, when major flow accelerations are detected and verified in a major renal artery. Although moderate increases in velocity (above 180 to 200 cm/sec) generally correlate with stenosis above 60%, these are approximate. Recent modifications to allow entry into CORAL require velocities above 300 cm/sec (**Fig. 3**), when confirmed by a central laboratory. Because the location and course of renal arteries can be complex, a negative study is less reassuring that no lesion is present. Previous claims that resistive index, a measure of relative systolic and diastolic flow patterns, predict the clinical outcomes of renal revascularization have not been universally confirmed.[39] Detection of a low resistive index, however, does suggest relatively preserved parenchymal blood flow.

Captopril Renography

Captopril renography remains widely available as an imaging technique. This method does not image the vasculature directly, but provides functional assessment of overall perfusion and function. Early studies indicated that entirely normal studies reliably excluded renovascular disease.[40] Recent inclusion of renography in prospective trials failed to predict clinical outcomes.[41,42] When renal function is abnormal, asymmetries in renal flow and function can develop for many reasons unrelated to renovascular disease. When considering nephrectomy or evaluating the relative contribution of a given kidney to overall glomerular filtration rate, renography can assess each kidney's level of function separately.

MR Angiography

Although relatively expensive, MR imaging has become a major imaging tool to reliably evaluate size, structure, and vascular anatomy. Gadolinium-enhanced imaging is now less commonly used because of concerns about nephrogenic systemic fibrosis.

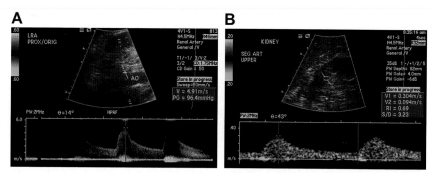

Fig. 3. (*A*) Doppler ultrasound velocity at the origin of the vessel was measured at 4.91 m/s (or 491 cm/s) consistent with vascular occlusion exceeding 85%. (*B*) Segmental artery Doppler waveforms demonstrate a delayed upstroke in the distal vessels (defined as "tardus parvus), but excellent diastolic blood flow with a calculated "resistive index" of 0.69. Demonstration of a low resistive index has been proposed as a measure of the viability of the poststenotic kidney and likely benefit from revascularization regarding kidney function and blood pressure (see text).

Newer technologies promise to allow high-resolution imaging of the major renal vessels without contrast, however, and allow definition of vascular patterns without radiation exposure. Both MR and CT angiography (see the next section) can reliably define "normal" major vessels, thereby assuring the patient that bilateral disease is not present. This fact can be critically important in planning long-term medical therapy.

CT Angiography

Application of multi-detector CT and rapid image acquisition now allow excellent vascular and parenchymal imaging with moderate radiation and contrast exposure (see **Fig. 1**A and B). Although expensive, CT angiography can provide detailed estimation of function, blood flow, anatomic variation and approachability.

Intra-Arterial Angiography

Intra-arterial angiography remains the "gold standard" by which renovascular lesions are identified and subjected to quantitative assessment (see **Fig. 1**C). It is usually reserved for the time of planned endovascular intervention, although some centers include aortic imaging as part of coronary angiography. The additional contrast usually is minor and several studies indicate little incremental risk to imaging the renal arteries, so long as selective instrumentation is avoided.

When should an identified renovascular lesion be subjected to instrumentation and dilation, with or without stenting? This remains a troubling question. Prediction of a positive blood pressure response remains elusive—and less pressing in the era of effective antihypertensive drug therapy than it was 2 decades ago. We have proposed a series of criteria that may be addressed by both clinicians and patients that may facilitate this decision (**Box 3**).

A variety of biomarkers have been proposed to identify patients likely to have clinical improvement in blood pressure after renal revascularization. These include measurement of renal vein renin levels, brain natriuretic peptide (BNP),[43] captopril-stimulated renin values, and changes in glomerular filtration after ACE inhibition. Although useful when strongly positive, these strategies often fail to add critical information when applied to unselected populations. The strongest predictor of clinical benefit until now remains the short duration of hypertension.

SUMMARY OF CURRENT THINKING ON RENOVASCULAR HYPERTENSION

Taken together, it should be apparent that advances in medical therapy, vascular imaging and endovascular procedures have changed the landscape of renovascular hypertension. Many cases presenting simply as new-onset hypertension with normal kidney function can be treated simply with existing antihypertensive drug therapy, usually including agents that block the renin-angiotensin system. Renovascular disease remains an important predictor of cardiovascular risk and warrants intensive therapy to reduce this risk including aspirin, statins, tobacco withdrawal, and diabetes and weight control, in addition to attention to blood pressure. For patients with complex disease, changing levels of kidney function, or failure to respond to antihypertensive therapy, further diagnostic studies with a commitment to restoring renal perfusion may be entirely appropriate. The magnitude of the risks and benefits remain controversial. They depend greatly on the comorbid conditions of the individual subject. Further studies directed toward how best to estimate recovery potential for renal function and the long-term outcomes for specific patient groups will be essential for optimal application of newer interventional procedures.

REFERENCES

1. Balk E, Raman G, Chung M, et al. Effectiveness of management strategies for renal artery stenosis: a systematic review. Ann Intern Med 2006;145:901–12.
2. Garovic V, Textor SC. Renovascular hypertension and ischemic nephropathy. Circulation 2005;112:1362–74.
3. Lerman LO, Schwartz RS, Grande JP, et al. Noninvasive evaluation of a novel swine model of renal artery stenosis. J Am Soc Nephrol 1999;10:1455–65.
4. Cervenka L, Horacek V, Vaneckova I, et al. Essential role of AT1-A receptor in the development of 2K1C hypertension. Hypertension 2002;40:735–41.
5. Crowley SD, Gurley SB, Oliverio MI, et al. Distinct roles for the kidney and systemic tissues in blood pressure regulation by the renin-angiotensin system. J Clin Invest 2005;115(4):1092–9.
6. De Bruyne B, Manoharan G, Pijls NHJ, et al. Assessment of renal artery stenosis severity by pressure gradient measurements. J Am Coll Cardiol 2006;48:1851–5.
7. Little MA, O'Brien E, Owens P, et al. A longitudinal study of the yield and clinical utility of a specifically designed secondary hypertension investigation protocol. Ren Fail 2003;25:709–17.
8. Neymark E, LaBerge JM, Hirose R, et al. Arteriographic detection of renovascular disease in potential renal donors: incidence and effect on donor surgery. Radiology 2000;214:755–60.
9. Cragg AH, Smith TP, Thompson BH, et al. Incidental fibromuscular dysplasia in potential renal donors: long-term clinical follow-up. Radiology 1989;172:145–7.
10. Krijnen P, van Jaarsveld BC, Steyerberg EW, et al. A clinical prediction rule for renal artery stenosis. Ann Intern Med 1998;129:705–11.
11. Hansen KJ, Edwards MS, Craven TE, et al. Prevalence of renovascular disease in the elderly: a population based study. J Vasc Surg 2002;36:443–51.
12. Fisher JEE, Olin JW. Renal artery stenosis: clinical evaluation. In: Creager MA, Loscalzo J, editors. Vascular medicine: a companion to Braunwald's heart disease. Philadelphia: Saunders/Elsevier; 2006. p. 335–47.
13. Conlon PJ, Athirakul K, Kovalik E, et al. Survival in renal vascular disease. J Am Soc Nephrol 1998;9:252–6.
14. Iantorno M, Pola R, Schinzari F, et al. Association between altered circadian blood pressure profile and cardiac end-organ damage in patients with renovascular hypertension. Cardiology 2003;100:114–9.
15. Mounier-Vehier C, Cocheteux B, Haulon S, et al. Changes in renal blood flow reserve after angioplasty of renal artery stenosis in hypertensive patients. Kidney Int 2004;65:245–50.
16. Chade AR, Rodriguez-Porcel M, Grande JP, et al. Mechanisms of renal structural alterations in combined hypercholesterolemia and renal artery stenosis. Ateriroscler Thromb Vasc Biol 2003;23:1295–301.
17. Kalra PA, Guo H, Kausz AT, et al. Atherosclerotic renovascular disease in United States patients aged 67 years or older: risk factors, revascularization and prognosis. Kidney Int 2005;68:293–301.
18. Textor SC, Lerman LO. Renal artery disease: pathophysiology. In: Creager MA, Dzau VJ, Loscalzo J, editors. Vascular medicine: a companion to Braunwald's heart disease. Philadelphia: Saunders-Elsevier; 2006. p. 323–34.
19. Stamey TA, Nudelman JJ, Good PH, et al. Functional characteristics of renovascular hypertension. Medicine 1961;40:347–94.
20. Missouris CG, Belli AM, MacGregor Ga. "Apparent" heart failure: a syndrome caused by renal artery stenoses. Heart 2000;83:152–5.

21. Gray BH, Olin JW, Childs MB, et al. Clinical benefit of renal artery angioplasty with stenting for the control of recurrent and refractory congestive heart failure. Vasc Med 2002;7:275–9.
22. Taler SJ, Textor SC, Augustine JE. Resistant hypertension: comparing hemodynamic management to specialist care. Hypertension 2002;39:982–8.
23. Davis BA, Crook JE, Vestal RE, et al. Prevalence of renovascular hypertension in patients with grade III or IV hypertensive retinopathy. N Engl J Med 1979;301: 1273–6.
24. Lazarus JM, Hampers CL, Bennett AH, et al. Urgent bilateral nephrectomy for severe hypertension. Ann Intern Med 1972;76:733–9.
25. Hackam DG, Spence JD, Garg AX, et al. The role of renin-angiotensin system blockade in atherosclerotic renal artery stenosis and renovascular hypertension. Hypertension 2007;50:998–1003.
26. Yusuf S, Teo KK, Pogue J, et al. Telmisartan, ramipril, or both in patients at high risk for vascular events. N Engl J Med 2008;358:1547–59.
27. Textor SC, Novick AC, Steinmuller DR, et al. Renal failure limiting antihypertensive therapy as an indication for renal revascularization. Arch Intern Med 1983;143: 2208–11.
28. Jackson B, Franze L, Sumithran E, et al. Pharmacologic nephrectomy with chronic angiotensin converting enzyme inhibitor treatment in renovascular hypertension in the rat. J Lab Clin Med 1990;115:21–7.
29. Hackam DG, Duong-Hua ML, Mamdani M, et al. Angiotensin inhibition in renovascular disease: a population-based cohort study. Am Heart J 2008;156: 549–55.
30. Speirs CJ, Dollery CT, Inman WHW, et al. Postmarketing surveillance of enalapril II: investigation of the potential role of enalapril in deaths with renal failure. Br Med J 1988;297:830–2.
31. Axelrod DA, Fendrick AM, Birkmeyer JD, et al. Cardiologists performing peripheral angioplasties: impact on utilization. Eff Clin Pract 2001;4:191–8.
32. Textor SC. Renovascular hypertension in 2007: where are we now? Curr Cardiol Rep 2007;9:453–61.
33. Alhadad A, Mattiasson I, Ivancev K, et al. Revascularisation of renal artery stenosis caused by fibromuscular dysplasia: effects on blood pressure during 7-year follow-up are influenced by duration of hypertension and branch artery stenosis. J Hum Hypertens 2005;19:761–7.
34. Carmo M, Bower TC, Mozes G, et al. Surgical management of renal fibromuscular dysplasia: challenges in the endovascular era. Ann Vasc Surg 2005;19:208–17.
35. Hiramoto J, Hansen KJ, Pan XM, et al. Atheroemboli during renal artery angioplasty: an ex-vivo study. J Vasc surg 2005;41:1026–30.
36. Scolari F, Ravani P, Pola A, et al. Predictors of renal and patient outcomes in atherembolic renal disease: a prospective study. J Am Soc Nephrol 2003;14:1584–90.
37. Wheatley K, Kalra PA, Moss J, et al. Lack of benefit of renal artery revascularization in atheroslerotic renovascular disease (ARVD): results of the ASTRAL Trial. J Am Soc Nephrol 2008;19:47A.
38. Textor SC. Pitfalls in imaging for renal artery stenosis. Ann Intern Med 2004;141: 730–1.
39. Krumme B, Hollenbeck M. Doppler sonography in renal artery stenosis—does the Resistive Index predict the success of intervention? Nephrol Dial Transplant 2007;22:692–6.
40. Elliot WJ, Martin WB, Murphy MB. Comparison of two non-invasive screening tests for renovascular hypertension. Arch Intern Med 1993;153:755–64.

41. Postma CT, van Oijen AH, Barentsz JO, et al. The value of tests predicting reno-vascular hypertension in patients with renal artery stenosis treated by angio-plasty. Arch Intern Med 1991;151:1531–5.

42. Soulez G, Therasse E, Qanadli SD, et al. Prediction of clinical response after renal angioplasty: respective value of renal Doppler sonography and scintigraphy. Am J Roentgenol 2004;181:1029–35.

43. Silva JA, Chan AW, White CJ, et al. Elevated brain natriuretic peptide predicts blood pressure response after stent revascularization in patients with renal artery stenosis. Circulation 2005;111:328–33.

Obesity and Hypertension: Mechanisms, Cardio-Renal Consequences, and Therapeutic Approaches

Efrain Reisin, MD*, Avanelle V. Jack, MD

KEYWORDS

- Obesity • Hypertension • Renal and cardiovascular disease
- Nonpharmacological and pharmacological therapies

Obesity and its relationship to hypertension is growing worldwide and is considered today to be a pandemic.[1]

In the United States the prevalence of overweight (body mass index [BMI] >25) in the adult population is 66.6% according to the report of the National Health and Nutrition Examination Survey (NHAANES 2003-2004).[2] The prevalence of obesity (BMI $\geq$ 31) has more than doubled to 32.9% since 1980,[2] and the prevalence of hypertension in the obese population in the United States has been shown to be 40.8%.[3] Other studies have shown that when compared with normal-weight adults, individuals with a BMI higher than 40 have greater than seven times the likelihood of being hypertensive.[4]

This increasing trend in the prevalence of obesity and obesity hypertension has not only been described in the western industrialized hemisphere but also in China and other populous countries in Asia.[5] In a recent study by the Obesity in Asia Collaboration Group, the authors conclude that the strength of the association between obesity and blood pressure was greater among Asians than among whites and Pacific Islanders.[6]

Obesity is characterized by multiple metabolic-endocrine alterations extensively described previously in the article that discusses hypertension and the metabolic

Section of Nephrology and Hypertension, Department of Medicine, Louisiana State University Health Sciences Center, 2020 Gravier Street, 7th Floor, Suite D, Room 734, New Orleans, LA 70112, USA
* Corresponding author.
E-mail address: docneph@aol.com (E. Reisin).

Med Clin N Am 93 (2009) 733–751
doi:10.1016/j.mcna.2009.02.010
0025-7125/09/$ – see front matter © 2009 Elsevier Inc. All rights reserved.

syndrome. This article focuses on the impact of obesity hypertension on the cardio-vascular and renal systems. It also summarizes the nonpharmacological and pharma-cological approaches used to control hypertension in the obese population.

THE IMPACT OF OBESITY ON THE HEART

The hemodynamic changes in obesity hypertension are characterized by an increased systemic blood volume, a redistribution of this volume to the cardiopulmonary area of the circulation, and a consequential increase in cardiac output.[7] The normal compen-satory response to an elevated cardiac output, which should be a drop in peripheral vascular resistance in response to elevated blood volume, is blunted in the obese hypertensive, revealing an inappropriately normal total peripheral resistance.[8,9] As a consequence, both the increased blood volume with resulting increased cardiac output, and the relatively higher than expected vascular peripheral resistance contribute to the hemodynamic changes that define obesity hypertension (**Fig. 1**).

VASCULAR ADAPTATIONS

In healthy, nonobese subjects, insulin may inhibit voltage-gated Ca2+ influx and stim-ulate glucose transport and phosphorylation of glucose to glucose-6-phosphate, which further activates Ca2+ efflux.[10] The decrease in net intracellular calcium will originate a decrease in peripheral resistance. This pattern is abolished in obese individuals as a consequence of insulin resistance, leading to a vascular resistance that we have considered to be inappropriately normal.[11]

Insulin resistance, a metabolic disarray that characterizes obesity, is also associ-ated with an increased secretion of cytokines by the adipocyte.[12] These changes,

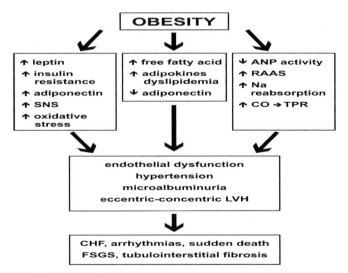

Fig. 1. Mechanisms of cardiac and kidney injury in obesity hypertension. ANP, atrial natri-uretic peptide; CHF, congestive heart failure; CO, cardiac output; FSGS, focal segmental glo-merulosclerosis; LVH, left ventricular hypertrophy; RAAS, rennin angiotensin-aldosterone system; SNS, sympathetic nervous system; TPR, total peripheral resistance. (*Modified from* Morse S, Zhang R, Thakur V, et al. Hypertension and the metabolic syndrome. Am J Med Sci 2005;330(6):303–10; with permission.)

together with oxidative stress and certain neurohumoral factors, are the possible inter-mediary mechanisms that may lead to vascular endothelial dysfunction, dyslipidemia, and vascular inflammation.[13] All these metabolic changes, together with hypertension, contribute to the development of atherosclerotic cardiovascular disease.[14]

CARDIAC ADAPTATIONS

In animal studies, leptin, a hormone produced by the adipose tissue that may be impli-cated in the development of hypertension in obese patients, has direct effects on rat neonatal ventricular myocytes.[15] The stimulation of endothelin ET1 production and the generation of reactive oxygen species (ROS) induce hypertrophy of the myocyte.[16] The effects of leptin on hypertension, however, are still controversial,[17] and more inves-tigation in humans is needed to clarify the obesity-leptin hypertension relationship.

In patients with hypertension, the pressure overload results in myocyte thickening and concentric hypertrophy.[18] Eccentric hypertrophy is the result of volume overload, wall thickening, and cavity dilatation[18] that will cause fiber elongation.[19] Obesity hypertension cause concentric-eccentric left ventricular hypertrophy, changes that were confirmed by autopsy[20] and prospective clinical studies.[21] The combined hemo-dynamic burden, according to some investigators increases the risk for congestive heart failure and may also increase the risk for the development of cardiac arrhythmias.[22]

The electrocardiographic changes are characterized by mild, leftward shifts in P, QRS, and T waves with a low QRS voltage, T wave flattering, left atrial abnormalities, and the prolongation of QT intervals.[23] These electrophysiological changes may be responsible for the increase in sudden death previously described in the obese pop-ulation who participated in the Framingham Study.[21]

In summary, obesity can cause systemic hemodynamic changes with structural vascular and cardiac adaptations. The coexistence of obesity hypertension triggers a double burden on the heart,[9] resulting in concentric-eccentric left ventricular hyper-trophy and electrophysiological changes, which increase the risk for congestive heart failure (CHF) and sudden cardiac death as a result of arrhythmias.[9] However, the rela-tionship between obesity hypertension and CHF is still controversial, as some new studies propose that elevated BMI paradoxically seems to have a favorable impact on survival after the onset of heart failure.[24]

THE IMPACT OF OBESITY ON THE KIDNEY

Several clinical and animal researchers have linked chronic kidney disease and micro-albuminuria with metabolic syndrome and obesity.[25,26] According to Framingham data, each unit increase in BMI after a mean follow-up of 18.5 years was associated with a 1.2-fold increase in the risk for kidney disease.[27] Autopsy studies from obese patients have shown a high incidence of glomerulomegaly and focal segmental glo-merulosclerosis (FSGS) an incidence that increases over a 10-year period.[28,29] The pattern of progression of the obesity-related focal segmental glomerulosclerosis, however, has shown a more indolent evolution to end-stage renal disease than in patients with idiopathic focal segmental glomerulosclerosis.[29]

HEMODYNAMIC AND MECHANICAL EFFECTS

Earlier studies in dogs with diet-induced obesity have shown an increase in sodium retention at the level of the loop of Henle that may be caused by a decreased natri-uresis (a consequence of an increase in the clearance of atrial natriuretic peptide by the adipose cells), insulin resistance, hyperinsulinemia, increased sympathetic activity, and activation of the renin angiotensin-aldosterone system (RAAS).[30] Microscopic examination of the animal kidneys revealed an increase in the interstitial cells and expression of the extracellular matrix between tubules in the renal medulla, changes that may cause a higher fluid hydrostatic pressure.[30] All these metabolic-hemodynamic-hormonal changes at the kidney level explain the shift of pressure natriuresis toward a higher blood pressure.[30]

In humans, Reisin and colleagues[31] proved that obesity is associated with increased renal blood flow. Other investigators[32] found a decreased renal vascular resistance and increase in the glomerular filtration rate (GFR) with an increased filtration per nephron and a consequential hyperperfusion and hyperfiltration. Chagnac and colleagues[33] conclude that in obese normotensive subjects, the higher hydrostatic pressure is responsible for hyperfiltration because the GFR increases more than renal plasma flow, resulting in an elevated filtration fraction (FF).

Consequently, in humans, like in animals, higher FF raises the post glomerular aortic pressure in peritubular arterioles with an increase in sodium chloride reabsorption and a decrease in NaCl delivery to the macula densa, changes that originate the activation of tubular-glomerular feedback and hyperfiltration.

Together with the previously described renal hemodynamic changes that harm the kidney in obese subjects, the occurrence of metabolic-hormonal changes in these individuals also plays a very important role in kidney injury. High-circulating free fatty acid (FFA) and the elevated cellular uptake of fatty acid (FA) inhibit the secretion of adiponectin, a protective protein expressed by the adipocyte.[34,35] As a consequence of these changes, the reactive compounds originated by the excess of FA in the cells, including the fatty acyl Co A, diacylglycerol, and ceramide, cause kidney injury through reactive oxygen scavering, cytotoxicity, and cell apoptosis.[36] A damage of the proximal tubular cells contributes to tubular-interstitial inflammation and fibrosis.[37] This evolution of events closes the linkage between high FFA–abdominal obesity–microalbuminuria and renal injury.[36–38]

Moreover, leptin can stimulate tumor growth factor α (TGF-α) synthesis and type 4 collagen production and can cause cellular proliferation in the glomerular endothelial cells.[39–41] Leptin also up-regulates TGF-β type 2 receptor, stimulates type 1 collagen production, and may induce proteinuria and FSGS.[40] The visceral adipocyte has been also associated with an increase expression of angiotensinogen tumor necrosis factor alpha, resistin, leptin, and PAI-1.[39–41] Together leptin and all the cytokines are responsible for endothelial injury kidney damage.[40–42]

In summary, obesity, through increased activity of the sympathetic activity and RAAS, decreases natriuresis that, together with insulin and leptin resistance, leads to renal sodium retention, hyperperfusion, and hyperfiltration. All these hemodynamic changes, together with high-circulating FFA, lower secretion of adiponectin. The damage caused by the reactive compounds originated by the excess of FA in the cells contributes to the development of the glomerulomegaly, FSGS, tubulointerstitial inflammation, and fibrosis that characterize the renal damage in obese hypertensive individuals.

TREATMENT OF HYPERTENSION IN OBESE PATIENTS
Lifestyle Modifications

Weight loss
The major goal of management of both overweight and obesity is to reduce the age-related rate of weight gain. This challenging task will require a complex combination of

healthy behaviors, including a decrease in sedentary activities, an increase in physical activity, and a reduction in calorie and alcohol intake (**Table 1**).[43–45] The emphasis for weight management should be on avoidance of excess total energy intake with the addition of an increased regular pattern of physical activity.[43–45] Reducing food portion sizes and limiting fat intake can assist in reducing overall calorie intake. Specific nutrient intakes for individuals should be based on lipoprotein levels and the presence of coexisting heart disease, diabetes, and other risk factors.[45]

In an earlier study, Reisin and colleagues[46] showed that in 75% of obese hypertensive patients consuming a low-calorie diet in which salt intake was not reduced, an average weight loss of 22 pounds was followed by controlled blood pressure. Some of these patients who maintained their weight loss, showed a persistent pressure reduction 12 to 18 months later.[47]

Adoption of the well-studied low-sodium Dietary Approaches to Stop Hypertension diet (DASH) eating plan provides healthy foods that can be used to promote weight loss, reduce blood pressure in both hypertensive and prehypertensive individuals, and reduce low-density lipoprotein cholesterol.[48] The DASH study has also shown that a reduction of NaCl intake under 100 mEq a day increases the effect of this diet on blood pressure reduction.[48] This augmented effect may cause an extratherapeutic benefit to the obese hypertensive individuals considered to be salt-sensitive patients.[44]

Table 1 Recommended lifestyle modifications for obesity hypertension		
Modification	Recommendations	Approximate SBP Reduction, Range[a]
Weight reduction	Maintain normal body weight (body mass index, 18.5–24.9 kg/m^2)	5–20 mm Hg/10 kg weight loss
Adopt DASH eating plan	Consume a diet rich in fruits, vegetables, and low-fat dairy products with a reduced content of saturated and total fat.	8–14 mm Hg
Dietary sodium reduction	Reduce dietary sodium intake to no more than 100 mEq/L per day (2.4 g sodium or 6 g sodium chloride)	2–8 mm Hg
Physical activity	Engage in regular aerobic physical activity such as brisk walking (at least 30 min per day, most days of the week).	4–9 mm Hg
Moderation of alcohol consumption	Limit consumption to no more than 2 drinks per day (1 oz or 30 mL ethanol [eg, 24 oz beer, 10 oz wine, or 3 oz 80-proof whiskey]) in most men, and to no more than 1 drink per day in women and lighter-weight persons.	2–4 mm Hg

Abbreviations: DASH, Dietary Approaches to Stop Hypertension; SBP, systolic blood pressure.
[a] The effects of implementing these modifications are dose and time dependent and could be greater for some individuals.
Reproduced from Chobanian AV, Bakris G, Black HR, et al. The Seventh Report of the Joint National Committee on Prevention, Detection, Evaluation, and Treatment of High Blood Pressure. The JNC 7 Report. JAMA 2003;289(19):2564; with permission.

The Framingham Heart Study showed that weight loss of 5 pounds or greater was associated with reductions in cardiovascular risk of about 40% and that a 10% reduction in body weight can reduce disease risk factors.[49]

In the Dietary Intervention Study in Hypertension (DISH),[50] hypertensive patients were separated into three groups: weight reduction, dietary sodium restriction, or no intervention as controls. The average weight loss in the weight reduction group was 4.5 kg after 1 year, and 60% of them remained normotensive without antihypertensive medication. When daily sodium intake was reduced to 40 mEq, 46% of them remained normotensive without antihypertensive medication. Only 30% of the control group remained normotensive without medication. The beneficial effects of weight reduction occurred in both sexes and also in both white and African-American subjects. The authors concluded that weight loss was the best nonpharmacological intervention for obese hypertensive patients.

The Trial of Nonpharmacological Interventions in the Elderly (TONE) has shown that elderly hypertensive subjects (defined as having systolic [SBP] and diastolic [DBP] blood pressure lower than 145/85 mm Hg when treated with antihypertensive medications) benefit from weight reduction, after the withdrawal of the antihypertensive medications, and have fewer cardiovascular events compared with subjects treated with the usual care.[51] The Trial of Hypertension Prevention (TOHP) included a weight reduction intervention arm and concluded that an average 2 kg of weight loss was associated with a 3.7/2.7 mm Hg drop in systolic and diastolic blood pressure (SBP and DBP).[52] The TOHP II study showed that patients with a larger decrease in weight, averaging 4.4 kg, had a reduction of 5 and 7 mm Hg in SBP and DBP, respectively.[53] In the same study, subjects who have maintained their weight reduction for more than 3 years have shown a persistent blood pressure reduction.[53] These last two studies have enrolled normotensive subjects with DBP in the range of 80–89 mm Hg, and SBP/ DBP lower than 140 mm Hg/80–89 mm Hg, respectively.[51,53] Neter and colleagues,[54] in a meta-analysis of 25 studies on the effect of weight loss on hypertension, concluded that each kg loss of body weight was followed by 1 mm Hg of blood pressure reduction.

The lack of large data on long-term maintenance of weight loss leaves some authors unconvinced that weight loss is effective in treating hypertension;[55] however, Befort and colleagues[56] proved that although some weight regain is expected, if the methods used to lose the initial weight are continued, the weight loss maintenance can be achieved.

We agree with Harsha and Bray[57] that weight loss is not only effective in reducing blood pressure and improving other metabolic abnormalities, but it is also the most effective approach in the spectrum of lifestyle modifications. We believe that weight loss can frequently obviate the need for antihypertensive drugs, and for those patients requiring antihypertensive medications, weight loss can also help to decrease the number and dosage of drugs, thereby decreasing both the side effects and treatment cost.

Sodium restriction

Earlier studies have shown a direct relationship between sodium consumption and the prevalence of hypertension. These studies have also shown a low incidence of hypertension in populations with low salt intake.[58] More recent research, however, has proven that the relationship between salt and hypertension is positively correlated in subjects considered to be sodium-sensitive, but not in those subjects considered to be sodium resistant. Sodium sensitivity is deemed to be a deficiency that may have a genetic basis,[59] and is explained by different mechanisms including the ability of the kidneys to regulate fluid volume, increased sympathetic activity, blunted renin-aldosterone and norepinephrine response to sodium intake or volume depletion, suppressed kalikreen-kinin system, or excess activation of the arginine vasopressin pressor systems.[60]

We have previously discussed the results of large studies like DASH[48] and DISH,[50] in which the addition of a low salt diet to caloric restriction caused an extratherapeutic effect in obese hypertensive patients.

In a recent publication,[61] caloric restriction was combined with regular aerobic exercise and metformin therapy to compare the decrease in blood pressure in obese salt-sensitive individuals with obese salt-resistant hypertensive individuals. Weight loss and the correction of metabolic abnormalities lowers blood pressure only in salt-sensitive but not in salt-resistant subjects. The authors conclude that correcting adiposity in salt-sensitive patients lowers blood pressure by making the blood pressure insensitive to dietary salt. Moreover, it is possible that some sodium-resistant phenotype subjects are protected from obesity-induced increases in blood pressure.

In summary, we believe that salt restriction may improve blood pressure in the obese hypertensive individual because most of these subjects appear to be affected by a sodium-sensitive phenotype.

Exercise

Physical activity is a key feature of the treatment of hypertension in obese patients. Increased physical activity, when combined with a reduction in calories, is essential to weight loss success.[44,62] Available studies have also shown that adequate dynamic endurance training may decrease the SBP and DBP in hypertensive patients by 11 and 6 mm Hg, respectively.[63] Based on the available evidence, the recommendation is to engage in regular physical activity for at least 30 minutes per day most days of the week.[45,64] In addition, physical activity is critical to the maintenance of weight loss and is important for overall reduction in cardiovascular risk.[64]

Exercise programs appear to be beneficial at any age and are associated with overall reductions in cardiovascular disease outcomes by about 50%.[45] The cardiovascular disease benefits of slow walking appear to be comparable with those of walking faster, suggesting that the most important predictor of benefit was walking time, not speed.[65]

Reduction in Alcohol Intake

Earlier cross-sectional studies have shown that systolic and diastolic hypertension are significantly related to alcohol intake and to drinking patterns. Blood pressure levels were higher in subjects who consumed up to three drinks a day than in those who drank heavily only on weekends,[66,67] and the prevalence of hypertension was not related to the type of alcoholic beverage imbibed.[68]

Klatsky and colleagues[66] have shown a J-shaped curve with higher blood pressures in subjects who reported having less than one drink a day compared with those who drank up to three drinks a day. Other investigators have also proved that alcohol restrictions reduce blood pressure.[69,70]

The mechanistic evidences to explain the increase in blood pressure related to alcohol include the effects of alcohol on intracellular sodium, baroreflexes, cellular calcium transfer, magnesium depletion, and impaired insulin sensitivity.[71] Current recommendations from the European Society of Hypertension and Cardiology advise limiting the alcohol consumption in hypertensive subjects who drink alcohol to no more than 20 to 30 g of ethanol per day for men and no more than 10 to 20 g for women.[72] In obese hypertensive subjects, low levels of drinking will help to reduce the daily caloric intake, which, like exercise, will facilitate weight loss success.

The Benefits of Lifetime Modifications on the Cardiovascular and Renal Abnormalities

Among all of the lifetime modifications recommended for the improvement in blood pressure for obese hypertensive patients, weight loss, in some studies, together with an increase in exercise activity or with a sodium restriction, have shown the most significant impact on the cardio-renal abnormalities described in obese hypertensive patients. This benefit works by a positive effect on some of the deleterious metabolic, endocrinic, and hemodynamic alterations that occur in obesity hypertension. Weight reduction, in addition to the control of blood pressure, may induce reduction in insulin and leptin resistance; decrease the sympathetic, rennin, and aldosterone activities; and in addition cause an increased natriuresis.[73,74]

In an earlier study,[75] we showed that a weight loss of only 20 pounds results in lower total circulating and cardio pulmonary blood volumes, without changing total peripheral resistance. These improvements were related to a decrease venous return, cardiac output, heart rate, and stroke volume.

In recent research investigating the effect of weight loss after bariatric surgery, the authors have shown that weight reduction normalizes aortic function studied by two-dimensional echocardiographic techniques. Weight loss also reduces left ventricular hypertrophy and improves left ventricular diastolic function over a follow-up of 3 years.[76] Other investigators[77] have shown that weight loss improved significantly the endothelial dysfunction measured by flow-mediated dilatation in the forearm. They conclude that this change was triggered by an increase in endothelial nitric oxide production that occurs after weight loss.

In a bench research with obese Zucker rats, a model that shares many common characteristics with human obesity and Type 2 diabetes mellitus, we showed that the group of animals treated with a low-caloric diet had a decrease in proteinuria with a reduction in the immunohistochemical α-smooth muscle actin staining in cortical and medullary interstitium, a marker of interstitial fibrosis.[78]

In other studies from our laboratory, Obese Zucker rats treated with a low-caloric normal protein intake, have shown a lower weight than the control group at the end of the treatment, and a reduction in proteinuria, glomerular damage index, and mesangial expansion.[79]

A clinical study in obese adults treated with a hypocaloric diet without a protein restriction, have shown that after losing weight, proteinuria significantly decreases.[80] Other investigators have shown that in patients with proteinuria induced by a different type of proteinuric kidney disease, weight loss significantly correlates with decreased proteinuria.[81] Chagnac and colleagues[82] performed serial direct GFR measurements in normotensive morbidly obese subjects who underwent gastric bypass surgery; the study showed that weight loss decreased renal plasma flow and GFR.

In conclusion, in an animal model of obesity hypertension, weight reduction leads to a decrease in proteinuria and improvement in the glomerulosclerosis and interstitial fibrosis. At the same time, clinical studies suggest that weight loss decreases proteinuria and improves glomerular filtration.

Pharmacologic Intervention

Most obese patients find that weight reduction is difficult to maintain, and previous studies have reported a high dropout rate in the first 1 to 2 years of a weight loss program.[44] When obese patients are unable to tolerate or unwilling to comply with weight reduction, or when weight reduction alone cannot control HTN, then antihypertensive drug therapy should be used (**Table 2**).

Table 2
Mechanisms, benefits, and disadvantages of antihypertensive drug therapy in obesity

Agent	Mechanisms – Benefits	Disadvantage
ACE I, ARBs	↑ natriuresis, ↓RAAS, ↓TPR, ↑ IS, ↓SA, ↓LR, ↓ proteinuria Neutral Metabolic Effect	Large studies are lacking
Direct renin inhibitors	May have the same positive effects as ACE I, ARBs	Large studies are lacking
Thiazide diuretics	↑ natriuresis, ↓ CO, ↓ TPR	In large dosage: ↑ TG, ↑
LDL, ↑ UA,	May be effective in small dosage associated with other agents	↓ IS
Ca-channel blockers	↑ natriuresis, ↓TPR, ↓LR Dihydropiridone ↑ proteinuria Neutral metabolic effect Non dihydropiridone may ↓ proteinuria	—
Beta blockers	↓ RA, ↓ SA ↓ CO May improve CV morbidity-mortality New β blockers with alpha blocking effects may ↓ TPR and have neutral metabolic effects	↑ TPR, ↑ TG, ↓IS, Difficult weight loss —
Central-acting alpha 2 agonist	↓ natriuresis, ↓TPR, ↓ S. efferent activity	Many side effects
Alpha 1 adrenergic blockers	↓ TPR, ↓ SA, ↓ IS, ↓ leptin, ↓ TC	More CHF in ALLHAT

Abbreviations: ↓, decrease; ↑, increase; ACEI, angiotensin-converting enzyme inhibitor; CO, cardiac output; IS, insulin sensitivity; IR, insulin resistance; LDL, low density lipoprotein; LR, leptin resistance; LVH, left ventricular hypertrophy; RAAS, renin-angiotensin-aldosterone system; SA, sympathetic activity; TPR, total peripheral resistance; TG, triglycerides; TC, total cholesterol; UA, uric acid.
Modified from Richards RJ, Thakur V, Reisin E, et al. Obesity-related hypertension: its physiological basis and pharmacological approaches to its treatment. J Hum Hypertens 1996;10(Suppl 3):S59–64; with permission.

The ideal medications to treat HTN in obese patients would be those that specifically target the pathogenic factors, protect the renal and cardiovascular end organs, and do not enhance the existing metabolic abnormalities. However, there are currently only a few prospective studies examining the efficacy and safety of antihypertensive agents in obese patients,[83] and clinical studies have never been performed to evaluate the specific cardiovascular and renal benefits in obese hypertensive subjects. Consequently, in the following review, we discuss the working mechanisms of each antihypertensive compound with an emphasis on the specific metabolic, endocrinic, and cardiovascular-renal advantage that each drug may offer to the obese hypertensive subject.

Angiotensin-Converting Enzyme Inhibitors, Angiotensin 2 Type 1 Receptor Blockers, and Renin Inhibitors

Angiotensin-converting enzyme inhibitors (ACEI) and angiotensin 2 type 1 receptor blockers (ARBs) block the renin angiotensin system, facilitate natriuresis and diuresis, control glomerular hyperfiltration, decrease proteinuria, protect kidney function, and reduce left ventricular hypertrophy. ACEI and ARBs also improve insulin sensitivity and reduce plasma levels of insulin, norepinephrine, and leptin in obese hypertensive subjects.[44]

Earlier studies demonstrate renin angiotensin-aldosterone system expression in adipose tissues.[83] These local systems may have different regulatory mechanisms in lean compared with obese hypertensive subjects.[43] ACEI and ARBs appear to be the most appropriate drugs for treating obesity HTN.[84] Many studies confirm the neutral or positive metabolic properties of ACEI and ARBs; these compounds are not associated with weight gain or adverse effect on lipids or glycemic control.[43]

We have previously published the first large, prospective, multicenter, double-blind trial (TROPHY)[85] performed in obese hypertensive patients, comparing the therapeutic effect of the ACEI lisinopril with hydrochlorothiazide (HCTZ). At the end of 3 months, follow-up with both antihypertensives effectively lowered systolic and diastolic blood pressure. Lisinopril was more effective than HCTZ in white and younger subjects, whereas HCTZ was more effective in African-American patients. More than half of the patients controlled with lisinopril only needed 10 mg/day treatment, whereas 46% of those treated with HCTZ required a high dose (50 mg/day) to control blood pressure. The TROPHY trial also evaluated ambulatory blood pressure response and showed that both antihypertensive medications significantly lowered systolic and diastolic blood pressure.[86] Insulin and lipid profile were similar in both groups of obese patients, but the plasma glucose was increased in the HCTZ group.[70] We concluded that the use of ACEI in obese subjects may generate a more rapid rate of response of blood pressure control with fewer side effects.[85,86]

A more recent trial in obese patients showed that the combination of the ACEI, trandolapril, and the nondihydropyridine calcium channel blocker, verapamil, reduced the risk of new-onset diabetes in obese subjects as compared with the combination of the ARB losartan and HCTZ.[87] Some studies in experimental models have shown that some ARBs, like telmisartan[88] and irbesartan,[89] may induce a partial peroxisome proliferator activated receptor (PPAR) gamma agonism that may increase insulin sensitivity.

The direct renin inhibitor, aliskiren, was added in a clinical study to obese uncontrolled patients treated with HCTZ monotherapy. The antihypertensive effects and side effects were compared with those of other groups of patients who received antihypertensive additional therapy with a calcium channel blocker, ARBs, or a placebo. The authors concluded that all the arms have similar reduction in blood pressure but that the association of a direct renin inhibitor and HCTZ were better tolerated.[90]

We believe that ACI or ARBs should be the initial pharmacologic approach in patient with obesity-related hypertension.

Diuretics

The hypotensive effect of thiazides is attributed initially to a reduction of intravascular and extracellular fluid volumes. Over time, this action on volume becomes less important, and the more chronic action of thiazides results chiefly from a reduction in peripheral vascular resistance.[91]

Most studies have used HCTZ in obesity HTN for only short terms (several months), and most patients require a high dose of thiazide for good pressure control.[85,86] The prolonged use of such a high dose of thiazide will likely exacerbate some preexisting metabolic abnormalities in obese patients, such as hyperlipidemia and other diabetogenic effects.[92,93]

We agree that the impact of the antihypertensive drugs on some of the important mechanisms that characterize obesity-related hypertension should be taken into consideration when treating hypertension; however, obese hypertensive subjects are considered to be salt-sensitive and resistant to the antihypertensive medications.

Consequently, a low dose of thiazide diuretics might be used as a second- or third-step therapy to increase the antihypertensive efficacy.[94]

Calcium Channel Blockers

Calcium channel blockers (CCBs) inhibit the slow inward calcium channels, which cause relaxation of smooth-muscle arterial walls and myocardial cells. CCBs also induce a mild natriuresis and diuresis and are considered to be neutral in their effects on glucose and insulin resistance.[95] An earlier study showed that a long-acting CCB effectively control blood pressure in 76% of extremely obese and 72% of moderately obese patients. The responsive rate was similar in obese and nonobese hypertensive patients.[96]

Dihydropyridine CCBs may increase glomerular hyperfiltration by inducing dilatation of the preglomerular afferent arteriole, a hemodynamic change that may increase proteinuria.[97] Studies with nondihydropyridone CCBs, however, have shown them to decrease the proteinuria in hypertensive patients.[97] More long-term clinical studies are needed to elucidate the value and safety of the CCBs in the treatment of obesity hypertension.

Alpha-1 Adrenergic Blockers

Alpha adrenergic blockers have neutral or favorable effects on insulin resistance and dyslipidemia.[43] In one small study, a combined alpha and beta blockade using doxazosin and atenolol reduced blood pressure significantly more in obese hypertensive patients than in lean hypertensive patients.[98] However, following the high rate of heart failure caused by the doxazosin arm in the Antihypertensive Lipid-Lowering Treatment to Prevent Heart Attack Trial (ALLHAT), the alpha adrenergic blockers are no longer recommended as first-line treatment for hypertension.[99]

Centrally Acting Alpha-2 Agonists

The centrally acting antihypertensive agents (eg, clonidine) induce inhibition of the release of norepinephrine to postganglionic adrenergic nerve stimulation and reduce the sympathetic afferent activity.[100] In an earlier, small, prospective study of obese hypertensive African-American women,[101] we found that the diuretic clorthalidone controls blood pressure more effectively than clonidine. In another study[102] performed in very obese hypertensive patients, clonidine was found to lower blood pressure and plasma norepinephrine concentration more significantly than a placebo. The many adverse effects reported in patients treated with clonidine, such as drowsiness, sedation, and dry mouth, limit its use.[43]

Beta Blockers

The hemodynamic and hormonal characteristic of obesity-related hypertension such as increased cardiac output, stroke volume, cardiac work, norepinephrine levels, and increased sympathetic nervous system tone may be improved with beta blocker compounds that may also improve cardiovascular morbidity and mortality.[103] In obese patients, however, beta blockers may exacerbate the dyslipidemia, decrease insulin resistance, and make weight loss difficult to accomplish by inhibiting the catecholamine activity on fatty acid metabolism and reducing the satiety signal to the appetite center. All these metabolic changes may ultimately cause more weight gain.[104]

The antihypertensive efficacy of beta blockers in obese patients remains controversial. Small studies have shown that metoprolol was not effective in controlling blood pressure,[105] whereas atenolol showed a beneficial effect.[106] Consequently, the classic beta blockers are not recommended in obese patients for the control of blood pressure.

The new vasodilating beta blockers, carvedilol and nebivolol, may not share the previously described metabolic side effects; on the contrary, they have a neutral effect on glucose metabolism and a favorable effect on lipid profile.[107] Studies on the use of these drugs in obese patients are still not available.

OTHER THERAPEUTIC APPROACHES
Obstructive Sleep Apnea

Obstructive sleep apnea (OSA) is associated with obesity. The association between sleep apnea and hypertension in obese subjects is seen in all gender, ethnic, and age groups.[108] Therefore, understanding the pathophysiology of OSA may lead to noninvasive treatment modalities that may control blood pressure.[43] Treatment of OSA with continuous positive airway pressure has been shown to decrease daytime and nocturnal blood pressures in obese hypertensive subjects and also may reduce cardiovascular events and improve quality of life.[43,93]

Antiobesity Agents

The National Heart, Lung, and Blood Institute (NHLBI) guidelines recommended that overweight individuals with a BMI greater than 27 and concomitant obesity-related risk factors or disease, as well as those with a BMI greater than 30 and no concomitant disease will be considered candidates for weight loss and intervention strategies, including pharmacologic treatments, if they fail to lose weight after a 6-month trial of lifestyle modifications.[62] Sibutramine, a serotonin, dopamine, and norepinephrine reuptake inhibitor is associated with a substantial dose-dependent increase in blood pressure and heart rate in some patients.[109] NHLBI guidelines recommend against using sibutramine in hypertensive obese patients.[110] However, the Hypertension Obesity Sibutramine (HOS) study recently published[109] evaluates the interaction between sibutramine and a combination antihypertensive treatment that included three arms: felodipine and ramipril, verapamil and trandolapril, metoprolol and HCTZ. The authors analyzed the effect of each one of those regimens on sibutramine weight loss. The HOS study demonstrated that in obese hypertensive patients, the combination treatment with ACEI and the dihydropyridine and nondihydropyridine CCBs were better than a beta blocker and diuretic combination treatment in supporting the weight reduction and metabolic improvements induced by sibutramine. The antihypertensive action was similar in the three groups of patients.[109]

The other antiobesity drug, orlistat, an inhibitor of pancreatic lipase that decreases fat absorption, has a limited use owing to gastrointestinal adverse effects.[110]

Reliance on antiobesity pharmacotherapy as a main therapeutic approach is premature; no long-term data are yet available in obese hypertensive patients.

SUMMARY

The increasing prevalence of obesity in the industrialized world is causing an alarming epidemic. Almost 70% of American adults are overweight or obese. The link between increasing body weight and hypertension is well established. Obesity hypertension through metabolic, endocrinic, and systemic hemodynamic alteration causes structural vascular and cardiac adaptations that trigger concentric, eccentric left ventricular hypertrophy and electrophysiological changes, which may increase the risk for congestive heart failure and sudden cardiac death as a result of arrhythmias.

The increased renal blood flow in conjunction with a decreased renal vascular resistance causes renal hyperperfusion and hyperfiltration. Such changes lead to glomerulomegaly, focal segmental glomerulosclerosis, tubulointerstitial inflammation, and fibrosis that characterize the renal damage in obese hypertensive subjects.

We propose that weight reduction, with the addition of other nonpharmacological approaches that included exercise and reduction in alcohol intake, should be the first choice to treat obesity hypertension. Salt restriction may be helpful only in salt-sensitive patients.

The benefits of diet in obese patients include improvement of insulin sensitivity, reduction in sympathetic nervous and renin angiotensin system activities, and restoration of leptin sensitivity. As a consequence of these and other metabolic changes, the previously described systemic and renal hemodynamic alterations improved and the cardiovascular and renal morphological changes induced by obesity were lessened.

After reviewing the medications available, we believe that owing to the cardiovascular and renal morbidity and mortality that characterized obesity hypertension, the ACEI or ARBs offer the best cardio-renal protection and should be the pharmacologic treatment of choice. If these alone do not control BP adequately, then a low-dose diuretic should be added as a second approach.

Although we strongly believe in our proposal, more multicenter long-term clinical pharmacological trials are needed to evaluate the efficacy and safety of the antihypertensive approaches in the treatment of obesity hypertension.

ACKNOWLEDGMENTS

Special thanks to Michelle Holt for her editorial review and to Kim Adams for her secretarial assistance. Efrain Reisin, MD, is a consultant for Forest Research Institute.

REFERENCES

1. Francischetti EA, Genelhu VA. Obesity-hypertension: an ongoing pandemic. Int J Clin Pract 2007;61(2):269–80.
2. Ogden CL, Carroll MD, Curtin LR, et al. Prevalence of overweight and obesity in the United States, 1999–2004. JAMA 2006;295(13):1549–55.
3. Ong KL, Cheung BM, Man YB, et al. Prevalence, awareness, treatment, and control of hypertension among United States adults 1999–2004. Hypertension 2007;49(1):69–75.
4. Romero R, Bonet J, de la Sierra A, et al. Esopoh Study Investigators. Undiagnosed obesity in hypertension: clinical and therapeutic implications. Blood Press 2007;16(6):347–53.
5. Asia Pacific Cohort Studies Collaboration. The burden of overweight and obesity in the Asia-Pacific region. Obes Rev 2007;8(3):191–6.
6. Obesity in Asia Collaboration. Is central obesity a better discriminator of the risk of hypertension than body mass index in ethnically diverse populations? J Hypertens 2008;26(2):169–77.
7. Frohlich ED, Susic D. Mechanisms underlying obesity associated with systemic and renal hemodynamics in essential hypertension. Curr Hypertens Rep 2008; 10(2):151–5.
8. Messerli FH, Christie, DeCarvallho JG, et al. Obesity and essential hypertension: hemodynamics, intravascular volume, sodium excretion and plasma renin activity. Arch Intern Med 1981;141(1):81–5.

9. Reisin E, Frohlich ED. Hemodynamics in obesity. In: Zanchetti A, Tarazi RC, editors. Handbook of hypertension: pathophysiology of hypertension. cardiovascular aspects, vol. 7. Amsterdam: Elsevier Science Publishers; 1987. p. 280–97.

10. Zemel MB. Nutritional and endocrine modulation of intracellular calcium: implications in obesity, insulin resistance and hypertension. Mol Cell Biochem 1998;188(1–2):129–36.

11. Baron AD. Hemodynamic actions of insulin. Am J Physiol Endocrinol Metab 1994;267:E187–202.

12. Licata G, Scaglione R, Capuana G, et al. Hypertension in obese subjects: distinct hypertensive subgroup. J Hum Hypertens 1990;4(1):37–41.

13. Romero JC, Reckelhoff JF. State-of-the-art lecture: role of angiotensin and oxidative stress in essential hypertension. Hypertension 1999;34(4 Pt 2):943–9.

14. DeFronzo RA, Ferrannini E. Insulin resistance: a multifaceted syndrome responsible for NIDDM, obesity, hypertension, dyslipidemia, and atherosclerotic cardiovascular disease. Diabetes Care 1991;14(3):173–94.

15. Rajapurohitam V, Gan XT, Kirshenbaum LA, et al. The obesity-associated peptide leptin induces hypertrophy in neonatal rat ventricular myocytes. Circ Res 2003;93(4):277–9.

16. Karmazyn M, Purdham DM, Rajapurohitam V, et al. Leptin as a cardiac hypertrophic factor: a potential target for therapeutics. Trends Cardiovasc Med 2007;17(6):206–11.

17. Patel SB, Reams GP, Spear RM, et al. Leptin: linking obesity, the metabolic syndrome, and cardiovascular disease. Curr Hypertens Rep 2008;10(2):131–7.

18. Frohlich ED. The heart in hypertension: a 1991 overview. Hypertension 1991; 18(5 Suppl):62–8.

19. Messerli FH, Sundgaard-Riise K, Reisin ED, et al. Dimorphic cardiac adaptation to obesity and arterial hypertension. Ann Intern Med 1983;99(6):757–61.

20. Smith HL, Willius FA. Adiposity of the heart: a clinical pathologic study of 136 obese patients. Arch Intern Med 1933;52:910–31.

21. Kannel WB, Cobb J. Left ventricular hypertrophy and mortality—results from the Framingham Study. Cardiology 1992;81(4–5):291–8.

22. Dunn FG, McLenachan J, Isles CG, et al. Left ventricular hypertrophy and mortality in hypertension: an analysis of data from the Glasgow Blood Pressure Clinic. J Hypertens 1990;8(8):775–82.

23. Anand RG, Peters RW, Donahue TP. Obesity and dysrhythmias. J Cardiometab Syndr 2008;3(3):149–54.

24. Artham SM, Lavie CJ, Patel HM, et al. Impact of obesity on the risk of heart failure and its prognosis. J Cardiometab Syndr 2008;3(3):155–61.

25. Chen J, Muntner P, Hamm LL, et al. The metabolic syndrome and chronic kidney disease in US adults. Ann Intern Med 2004;140:167–74.

26. Palaniappan L, Carnethon M, Fortmann SP. Association between microalbuminuria and the metabolic syndrome: NHANES III. Am J Hypertens 2003; 16(11 Pt 1):952–8.

27. Fox CS, Larson MG, Leip EP, et al. Predictors of new-onset kidney disease in a community-based population. JAMA 2004;291(7):844–50.

28. Verani RR. Obesity-associated focal segmental glomerulosclerosis: pathological features of the lesion and relationship with cardiomegaly and hyperlipidemia. Am J Kidney Dis 1992;20(6):629–34.

29. Kambham N, Markowitz GS, Valeri AM, et al. Obesity-related glomerulopathy: an emerging epidemic. Kidney Int 2001;59(4):1498–509.

30. Hall JE. Mechanisms of abnormal renal sodium handling in obesity hypertension. Am J Hypertens 1997;10(5 Pt 2):49S–55S.

31. Reisin E, Messerli FG, Ventura HO, et al. Renal haemodynamic studies in obesity hypertension. J Hypertens 1987;5(4):397–400.
32. Ribstein J, du Cailar G, Mimran A. Combined renal effects of overweight and hypertension. Hypertension 1995;26(4):610–5.
33. Chagnac A, Weinstein T, Korzets A, et al. Glomerular hemodynamics in severe obesity. Am J Physiol Renal Physiol 2000;278(5):F817–22.
34. Morse SA, Zhang R, Thakur V, et al. Hypertension and the metabolic syndrome. Am J Med Sci 2005;330(6):303–10.
35. Thakur V, Morse S, Reisin E. Functional and structural renal changes in the early stages of obesity. Contrib Nephrol 2006;151:135–50.
36. Bagby SP. Obesity-initiated metabolic syndrome and the kidney: a recipe for chronic kidney disease? J Am Soc Nephrol 2004;15(11):2775–91.
37. Kamijo A, Kimura K, Sugaya T, et al. Urinary free fatty acids bound to albumin aggravate tubulointerstitial damage. Kidney Int 2002;62(5):1628–37.
38. Unger RH. Minireview: weapons of lean body mass destruction: the role of ectopic lipids in the metabolic syndrome. Endocrinology 2003;144(12):5159–65.
39. Wisse BE. The inflammatory syndrome: the role of adipose tissue cytokines in metabolic disorders linked to obesity. J Am Soc Nephrol 2004;15(11):2792–800.
40. Wolf G, Chen S, Han DC, et al. Leptin and renal disease. Am J Kidney Dis 2002; 39:1–11.
41. Wolf G, Ziyadeh FN. Leptin and renal fibrosis. Contrib Nephrol 2006;151:175–83.
42. Zhang R, Reisin E. Obesity-hypertension: the effects on cardiovascular and renal systems. Am J Hypertens 2000;13:1308–14.
43. Wofford MR, Smith G, Minor DS. The treatment of hypertension in obese patients. Curr Hypertens Rep 2008;10(2):143–50.
44. Reisin E, Hutchinson HG. Obesity-hypertension: effects on the cardiovascular and renal system—the therapeutic approach. In: Oparil S, Weber MA, editors. Hypertension. Philadelphia: W.B. Saunders; 1999. p. 206–10.
45. Chobanian AV, Bakris GL, Black HR, et al. The seventh report of the Joint National Committee on prevention, detection, evaluation, and treatment of high blood pressure: the JNC 7 report. JAMA 2003;289(19):2560–72.
46. Reisin E, Abel R, Modan M, et al. Effect of weight loss without salt restriction on the reduction of blood pressure in overweight hypertensive patients. N Engl J Med 1978;298(1):1–6.
47. Reisin E, Frohlich ED. Effects of weight reduction on arterial pressure. J Chronic Dis 1982;35(12):887–91.
48. Appel LJ, Moore TJ, Obarzanek E, et al. A clinical trial of the effects of dietary patterns on blood pressure. DASH Collaborative Research Group. N Engl J Med 1997;336(16):1117–24.
49. Kannel WB, Brand N, Skinner JJ Jr, et al. The relation of adiposity to blood pressure and development of hypertension. The Framingham study. Ann Intern Med 1967;67(1):48–59.
50. Gillum RF, Prineas RJ, Jeffery RW, et al. Nonpharmacologic therapy of hypertension: the independent effects of weight reduction and sodium restriction in overweight borderline hypertensive patients. Am Heart J 1983;105(1):128–33.
51. Whelton PK, Appel LJ, Espeland MA, et al. Sodium reduction and weight loss in the treatment of hypertension in older persons: a randomized controlled trial of nonpharmacologic interventions in the elderly (TONE). TONE Collaborative Research Group. JAMA 1998;279(11):839–46.
52. The Trials of Hypertension Prevention Collaborative Research Group. The effects of nonpharmacological interventions on blood pressure of persons with high

normal levels. Results of the trial of hypertension prevention. Phase I. JAMA 1992;267:1213–20.

53. Stevens VJ, Obarzanek E, Cook NR, et al. Long-term weight loss and changes in blood pressure: results of the trials of hypertension prevention, phase II. Ann Intern Med 2001;134(1):1–11.

54. Neter JE, Stam BE, Kok FJ, et al. Influence of weight reduction on blood pressure: a meta-analysis of randomized controlled trials. Hypertension 2003; 42(5):878–84.

55. Mark AL. Dietary therapy for obesity: an emperor with no clothes. Hypertension 2008;51(6):1426–34.

56. Befort CA, Stewart EE, Smith BK, et al. Weight maintenance, behaviors and barriers among previous participants of a university-based weight control program. Int J Obes (Lond) 2008;32(3):519–26.

57. Harsha DW, Bray GA. Weight loss and blood pressure control (Pro). Hypertension 2008;51(6):1420–5.

58. Kawasaki T, Delea CS, Bartter FC, et al. The effect of high-sodium and low-sodium intakes on blood pressure and other related variables in human subjects with idiopathic hypertension. Am J Med 1978;64(2):193–8.

59. Weinberger MH. Salt sensitivity of blood pressure in humans. Hypertension 1996;27(3 Pt 2):481–90.

60. Elijovich F, Laffer CL. Salt sensitivity. In: Izzo JL, Sica DA, Black HR, editors. Hypertension primer. The essentials of high blood pressure. Basic science, population science, and clinical management. 4th edition. Dallas (TX): American Heart Association; 2008. p. 156–9.

61. Hoffmann IS, Alfieri AB, Cubeddu LX. Salt-resistant and salt-sensitive phenotypes determine the sensitivity of blood pressure to weight loss in overweight/obese patients. J Clin Hypertens 2008;10(5):355–61.

62. National Institutes of Health. National Heart, Lung, and Blood Institutes. Clinical guidelines on the identification, evaluation, and treatment of overweight and obesity in adults—the evidence report. Obes Res 1998;6(Suppl 2): 51S–209S.

63. Fagard R, Bielen E, Hespel P, et al. Physical exercise in hypertension. In: LaraLaragh JH, Renner BM, editors. Hypertension pathophysiology, diagnosis and management. New York: Raven Press Ltd; 1990. p. 1985–8.

64. American Heart Association Nutrition Committee, Lichtenstein AH, Appel LJ, et al. Diet and lifestyle recommendations revision 2006: a scientific statement from the American Heart Association Nutrition Committee. Circulation 2006; 114(1):82–96.

65. Trapp EG, Chisholm DJ, Freund J, et al. The effects of high-intensity intermittent exercise training on fat loss and fasting insulin levels of young women. Int J Obes (Lond) 2008;32(4):684–91.

66. Klatsky AL, Friedman GD, Siegelaub AB, et al. Alcohol consumption and blood pressure Kaiser-Permanente Multiphasic Health Examination data. N Engl J Med 1977;296(21):1194–200.

67. Gordon T, Kannel WB. Drinking and its relation to smoking, BP, blood lipids, and uric acid. The Framingham study. Arch Intern Med 1983;143(7):1366–74.

68. Fuchs FD. Vascular effects of alcoholic beverages: is it only alcohol that matters? Hypertension 2005;45(5):851–2.

69. Puddey IB, Parker M, Beilin LJ, et al. Effects of alcohol and caloric restrictions on blood pressure and serum lipids in overweight men. Hypertension 1992;20(4): 533–41.

70. Parker M, Puddey IB, Beilin LJ, et al. Two-way factorial study of alcohol and salt restriction in treated hypertensive men. Hypertension 1990;16(4):398–406.
71. Klatsky AL, Gunderson E. Alcohol and hypertension: a review. J Agric Saf Health 2008;2(50):307–17.
72. Mancia G, De Backer G, Dominiczak A, et al. Guidelines for the management of arterial hypertension: the Task Force for the Management of Arterial Hypertension of the European Society of Hypertension (ESH) and of the European Society of Cardiology (ESC). J Hypertens 2007;25(6):1105–87.
73. Poirier P, Giles TD, Bray GA, et al. Obesity and cardiovascular disease: pathophysiology, evaluation, and effect of weight loss. Arterioscler Thromb Vasc Biol 2006;26(5):968–76.
74. Reisin E. Obesity-hypertension: non pharmacologic and pharmacologic therapeutic modalities. In: Laragh JH, Brenner BM, editors. Hypertension, pathophysiology, diagnosis and management. 2nd edition. New York: Raven Press; 1955. p. 2683–91.
75. Reisin E, Frohlich ED, Messerli FH, et al. Cardiovascular changes after weight reduction in obesity hypertension. Ann Intern Med 1983;98(3):315–9.
76. Ikonomidis I, Mazarakis A, Papadopoulos C, et al. Weight loss after bariatric surgery improves aortic elastic properties and left ventricular function in individuals with morbid obesity: a 3-year follow-up study. J Hypertens 2007;25(2): 439–47.
77. Pierce GL, Beske SD, Lawson BR, et al. Weight loss alone improves conduit and resistance artery endothelial function in young and older overweight/obese adults. Hypertension 2008;52(1):72–9.
78. Richards RJ, Porter JR, Inserra F, et al. Effects of dehydroepiandrosterone and quinapril on nephropathy in obese Zucker rats. Kidney Int 2001;59(1):37–43.
79. Liao J, Richards R, Zhang R, et al. Effects of a modified low calorie diet in metabolic changes and kidney histology in young obese Zucker rats. J Am Soc Nephrol 2007;18:823 A.
80. Praga M, Hernández E, Andrés A, et al. Effects of body-weight loss and captopril treatment on proteinuria associated with obesity. Nephron 1995;70(1):35–41.
81. Morales E, Valero MA, León M, et al. Beneficial effects of weight loss in overweight patients with chronic proteinuric nephropathies. Am J Kidney Dis 2003; 41(2):319–27.
82. Chagnac A, Weinstein T, Herman M, et al. The effects of weight loss on renal function in patients with severe obesity. J Am Soc Nephrol 2003;14(6):1480–6.
83. Reisin E, Tuck ML. Obesity-associated hypertension: hypothesized link between etiology and selection of therapy. Blood Press Monit 1999;4(Suppl 1):S23–6.
84. Kershaw EE, Flier JS. Adipose tissue as an endocrine organ. J Clin Endocrinol Metab 2004;89(6):2548–56.
85. Reisin E, Weir MR, Falkner B, et al. Lisinopril versus hydrochlorothiazide in obese hypertensive patients: a multicenter placebo-controlled trial. Treatment in Obese Patients With Hypertension (TROPHY) Study Group. Hypertension 1997;30(1 Pt 1):140–5.
86. Weir MR, Reisin E, Falkner B, et al. Nocturnal reduction of blood pressure and the antihypertensive response to a diuretic or angiotensin converting enzyme inhibitor in obese hypertensive patients. TROPHY Study Group. Am J Hypertens 1998;11(8 Pt 1):914–20.
87. Bakris G, Molitch M, Hewkin A, et al. Differences in glucose tolerance between fixed-dose antihypertensive drug combinations in people with metabolic syndrome. Diabetes Care 2006;29(12):2592–7.

88. Benson SC, Pershadsingh HA, Ho CI, et al. Identification of telmisartan as a unique angiotensin II receptor antagonist with selective PPAR gamma-modulating activity. Hypertension 2004;43(5):993–1002.

89. Di Filippo C, Lampa E, Tufariello E, et al. Effects of irbesartan on the growth and differentiation of adipocytes in obese Zucker rats. Obes Res 2005;13(11): 1909–14.

90. Jordan J, Engeli S, Boye SW, et al. Direct renin inhibition with aliskiren in obese patients with arterial hypertension. Hypertension 2007;49(5):1047–55.

91. Wilson IM, Freis ED. Relationship between plasma and extracellular fluid volume depletion and the antihypertensive effect of chlorothiazide. Circulation 1959;20: 1028–36.

92. Johnson BF, Saunders R, Hickler R, et al. The effects of thiazide diuretics upon plasma lipoproteins. J Hypertens 1986;4(2):235–9.

93. Pollare T, Lithell H, Berne C. A comparison of the effects of hydrochlorothiazide and captopril on glucose and lipid metabolism in patients with hypertension. N Engl J Med 1989;321(13):868–73.

94. Redon J, Cifkova R, Laurent S, et al. The metabolic syndrome in hypertension: European Society of Hypertension position statement. J Hypertens 2008; 26(10):1891–900.

95. Richards RJ, Thakur V, Reisin E. Obesity-related hypertension: its physiological basis and pharmacological approaches to its treatment. J Hum Hypertens 1996; 10(Suppl 3):S59–64.

96. Tuck ML, Bravo EL, Krakoff LR, et al. Endocrine and renal effects of nifedipine gastrointestinal therapeutic system in patients with essential hypertension. Results of a multicenter trial. The Modern Approach to the Treatment of Hypertension Study Group. Am J Hypertens 1990;3(12 Pt 2):333S–41S.

97. Bakris GL, Weir MR, Secic M, et al. Differential effects of calcium antagonist subclasses on markers of nephropathy progression. Kidney Int 2004;65(6): 1991–2002.

98. Wofford MR, Anderson DC Jr, Brown CA, et al. Antihypertensive effect of alpha- and beta-adrenergic blockade in obese and lean hypertensive subjects. Am J Hypertens 2001;14(7 Pt 1):694–8.

99. ALLHAT Collaborative Research Group. Major cardiovascular events in hypertensive patients randomized to doxazosin vs chlorthalidone: the antihypertensive and lipid-lowering treatment to prevent heart attack trial (ALLHAT). JAMA 2000;283(15):1967–75.

100. Jarrott B, Conway EL, Maccarrone C, et al. Clonidine: understanding its disposition, sites and mechanism of action. Clin Exp Pharmacol Physiol 1987;14(5):471–9.

101. Reisin E, Weed SG. The treatment of obese hypertensive black women: a comparative study of chlorthalidone versus clonidine. J Hypertens 1992; 10(5):489–93.

102. Tuck ML. Obesity, the sympathetic nervous system, and essential hypertension. Hypertension 1992;19(1 Suppl):I67–77.

103. Lithell H. Hypertension and hyperlipidemia. A review. Am J Hypertens 1993; 6(11 Pt 2):303S–8S.

104. Gress TW, Nieto FJ, Shahar E, et al. Hypertension and antihypertensive therapy as risk factors for type 2 diabetes mellitus. Atherosclerosis Risk in Communities Study. N Engl J Med 2000;342(13):905–12.

105. MacMahon SW, Macdonald GJ, Bernstein L, et al. Comparison of weight reduction with metoprolol in treatment of hypertension in young overweight patients. Lancet 1985;1(8440):1233–6.

106. Fagerberg B, Berglund A, Andersson OK, et al. Cardiovascular effects of weight reduction versus antihypertensive drug treatment: a comparative, randomized, 1-year study of obese men with mild hypertension. J Hypertens 1991;9(5): 431–9.
107. Sarafidis PA, Bakris GL. Do the metabolic effects of beta blockers make them leading or supporting antihypertensive agents in the treatment of hypertension? J Clin Hypertens (Greenwich) 2006;8(5):351–6.
108. Weiss JW, Remsburg S, Garpestad E, et al. Hemodynamic consequences of obstructive sleep apnea. Sleep 1996;19(5):388–97.
109. Scholze J, Grimm E, Herrmann D, et al. Optimal treatment of obesity-related hypertension: the Hypertension-Obesity-Sibutramine (HOS) study. Circulation 2007;115(15):1991–8.
110. Snow V, Barry P, Fitterman N, et al. Clinical Efficacy Assessment Subcommittee of the American College of Physicians. Pharmacologic and surgical management of obesity in primary care: a clinical practice guideline from the American College of Physicians. Ann Intern Med 2005;142(7):525–31.

Barriers to and Determinants of Medication Adherence in Hypertension Management: Perspective of the Cohort Study of Medication Adherence Among Older Adults

Marie A. Krousel-Wood, MD, MSPH[a,b,c,]*, Paul Muntner, PhD[d],
Tareq Islam, MPH[b], Donald E. Morisky, ScD, MSPH[e], Larry S. Webber, PhD[f]

KEYWORDS

- Medication adherence • Hypertension • Morisky scale
- Cohort • Older adults • Blood pressure control
- Pharmacy fill adherence • Barriers

The project described was supported by Grant Number R01 AG022536 from the National Institute on Aging. The content is solely the responsibility of the authors and does not necessarily represent the official views of the National Institute on Aging or the National Institutes of Health.

[a] Center for Health Research, Ochsner Clinic Foundation, 1514 Jefferson Highway, New Orleans, LA 70121, USA

[b] Department of Epidemiology, Tulane University School of Public Health and Tropical Medicine, 1430 Tulane Avenue, Suite 2041, New Orleans, LA 70112, USA

[c] Department of Family and Community Medicine, Tulane University School of Medicine, 1430 Tulane Avenue TB3, New Orleans, LA 70112, USA

[d] Department of Community and Preventive Medicine, Mount Sinai School of Medicine, 1 Gustave Levy Place, Box 1057, New York, NY 10029, USA

[e] Department of Community Health Sciences, UCLA School of Public Health, 650 Charles E. Young Drive South, Los Angeles, CA 90095, USA

[f] Department of Biostatistics, Suite 2001, Tulane University School of Public Health and Tropical Medicine, 1430 Tulane Avenue, New Orleans, LA 70112, USA

* Corresponding author. Center for Health Research, Ochsner Clinic Foundation, 1514 Jefferson Highway, New Orleans, LA 70121.

E-mail address: mawood@ochsner.org (M.A. Krousel-Wood).

Although there has been recent progress in the prevention, detection and treatment of hypertension, it persists as a major public health challenge, affecting approximately one billion persons worldwide and about 70 million people in the United States.[1–3] Hypertension is a significant and often asymptomatic chronic disease, which requires persistent adherence to prescribed medication to reduce the risks of stroke, cardiovascular disease, and renal disease.[4] Effective medical therapy and evidence-based treatment guidelines for hypertension are readily available; yet, hypertension management at the population level is not optimal.[5] For example, over 36% of United States adults treated for hypertension have uncontrolled blood pressure.[3] Low patient adherence to antihypertensive medication is the most significant modifiable patient-related barrier to achieving controlled blood pressure.[6]

Barriers to medication adherence are multifactorial and include complex medication regimens, convenience factors (eg, dosing frequency), behavioral factors, and issues with treatment of asymptomatic diseases (eg, treatment side effects).[7] There is a lack of understanding of which patient groups are at greatest risk of low adherence, how barriers to medication-taking behavior influence low adherence, and what interventions are most effective in overcoming barriers and improving adherence rates in different patient populations.

The Cohort Study of Medication Adherence in Older Adults (CoSMO), a prospective study among older adults with essential hypertension who are enrolled in a single managed care organization, is designed to investigate barriers to, and determinants of, antihypertensive medication adherence and lay the groundwork for interventions to improve adherence and clinical outcomes. The specific aims of CosMO are (a) to assess the effect of psychosocial, behavioral, quality of life, and clinical factors on changes in medication adherence over 2 years of follow-up; (b) to assess health care system barriers, uses of prescribed and over-the-counter medications, complementary/alternative therapies, and lifestyle modification on medication adherence and change in adherence; and (c) to determine the relationship of medication adherence with future medical and psychosocial outcomes, including blood pressure control, cardiovascular disease incidence, all-cause mortality, quality of life, and health care use.

The purpose of this article is to describe the design and methods of CoSMO and to present baseline demographic characteristics, as well as levels of medication adherence and blood pressure control for the overall study population and for demographic subgroups. The associations of self-reported medication adherence to pharmacy fill adherence and blood pressure control in older insured adults, which have not been well documented previously, are presented. A framework for understanding the barriers for adherence to antihypertensive medications is reviewed.

COLLECTION OF DATA TO UNDERSTAND BARRIERS TO ANTIHYPERTENSIVE MEDICATION ADHERENCE

A sample size of 2,000 participants was selected to provide adequate statistical power to detect clinically important and meaningful differences between persons with and without low adherence to their antihypertensive medication. CoSMO has 80% power to detect prevalence ratios of low medication adherence, as low as 1.2 for cross-sectional analyses, and as low as 1.4 for longitudinal analyses of reductions in medication adherence, depending on the prevalence of low medication adherence, the percent of the population reducing adherence, and the prevalence of the exposure or barrier being studied.

The catchment area for CoSMO reflects a demographically diverse group of individuals in urban and suburban areas. Recruitment was conducted from August 21, 2006 to September 30, 2007. Participants, 65 years and older with essential hypertension, were randomly selected from the roster of a large managed-care organization in southeastern Louisiana. An introductory letter with a reply card including an opt-out option was mailed to potentially eligible participants, based on the review of administrative criteria from the managed care organization (MCO) database ($n = 7,020$). Administrative criteria from the MCO's database used to initially assess eligibility included:

Men and women aged 65 years of age or older enrolled in the Medicare Risk product;

At least one encounter in calendar year 2005 with a primary or secondary diagnosis of essential hypertension (ICD-9 code 401) in the outpatient administrative database;

At least one antihypertensive medication prescription filled in calendar year 2005;

Continuously enrolled in the MCO for at least 2 years at the time of the baseline survey;

No ICD-9 diagnosis (ICD-9 codes 290, 291–294, 317–319, 331) of cognitive impairment;

No ICD-9 diagnosis of malignancy or human immunodeficiency virus (ICD-9 codes 140–172.9, 174–195.8, 200–208.99, 042–044.9).

For those not opting out and with valid contact information, eligibility was confirmed using a brief telephone questionnaire. Eligibility criteria confirmed with each participant included:

English speaking
Community dwelling
Current diagnosis of and prescribed medication for hypertension
Current enrollment in the MCO
No cognitive impairment via a cognitive function screener[8]

There were 1,373 individuals deemed ineligible for the study and 2,279 individuals refused to participate (**Fig. 1**). We were unable to reach 1,174 individuals because of invalid contact information, likely resulting from displacement following Hurricane Katrina. A total of 2,194 participants enrolled in the study. Those who refused compared with those who participated in the survey were more likely to be male (50.4% versus 41.5%, respectively; $P<.001$), white (84.5% versus 68.8%, respectively; $P<.001$), and older (76.3 years versus 74.5 years, respectively; $P<.001$). Those who we were unable to reach compared with their counterparts who participated in the study were more likely to be male (45.1% versus 41.5%, respectively; $P = .043$), white (77.5% versus 68.8%, respectively; $P<.001$), and older (75.2 years versus 74.5 years, respectively; $P = .001$).

All participants provided verbal informed consent, and CoSMO was approved by the Ochsner Clinic Foundation Institutional Review Board and the privacy committee of the MCO. Participants completed a survey at baseline and will be followed longitudinally and resurveyed both 1 and 2 years following their baseline interview to assess changes in adherence, barriers, risk factors and outcomes.

Study measures were collected through participant surveys, clinic and hospital electronic medical records (EMR), and the MCO's administrative databases. The baseline survey was administered by telephone using trained interviewers and lasted

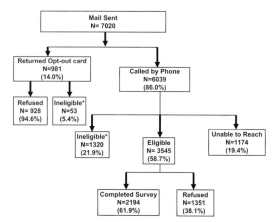

Fig. 1. Recruitment flowchart for CoSMO. *Reasons for ineligibility were as follows: no confirmed diagnosis of hypertension (22.9%), hard of hearing (16.4%), too ill to complete survey (12.6%), deceased (11.5%), cognitive screen failure (11.1%), not currently prescribed antihypertensive medication (8.4%), no longer using the managed care organization's insurance (6.9%), non-English speaker (5.8%), confined to a nursing home (1.9%), moved out of state (1.1%), current treatment for cancer (1%), or miscellaneous reason (<1%).

30 to 45 minutes. A complete outline of the study measurements is provided in **Table 1**. Of relevance to the current analyses, the participant survey included assessment of socio-demographic factors, medication adherence, and clinical variables. In addition, information regarding comorbid conditions and medication complexity was downloaded from the administrative databases of the MCO. Blood pressure data were abstracted from the outpatient EMR. These domains are described in detail below.

Socio-Demographics

Participant age, gender, race, level of education, marital status, and number of dependents were obtained through the telephone survey. If self-reported race was missing ($n = 37$), it was determined using data in the participant's medical records.[9] The socio-demographic factors were categorized as follows: age, less than 75 years of age and greater than or equal to 75 years of age; race, white and black; education, high-school graduate and not a high-school graduate; marital status, married and not married; and dependents, one or more and none.

Medication Adherence

Self-reported medication adherence was measured with the eight-item Morisky Medication Adherence Scale (MMAS).[10] This adherence measure was designed to facilitate the identification of barriers to and behaviors associated with adequate adherence to chronic medications. In a previous study, the scale has been determined to be reliable ($\alpha = 0.83$) and significantly associated with blood-pressure control ($P<.05$) in low income, mostly minority, and under-served individuals with hypertension (ie, low adherence levels were associated with lower rates of blood-pressure control).[10] Also, the MMAS has been shown to have high concordance with antihypertensive medication pharmacy fill rates in a managed-care population similar to the current study population.[11] MMAS scores can range from 0 to 8, with low adherence defined as MMAS scores less than 6; medium adherence as scores of 6 to less than 8, and high-adherence scores as a score of 8.[10]

Pharmacy fill data were extracted for the year before completion of the baseline survey and included a listing of all antihypertensive prescriptions filled, date filled, drug class, and number of pills dispensed. Medication possession ratio (MPR) is the sum of the days' supply obtained between the first pharmacy fill and the last fill, with the supply obtained in the last fill excluded, divided by the total number of days in this time period.[11] Provided each participant had at least three pharmacy fills in a drug class in the time period, MPR was calculated for each antihypertensive medication class and averaged across all classes to assign a single MPR to each participant. Pharmacy fill nonpersistency was defined as an MPR less than 0.8.[11–15] There were 2,087 participants who had at least three pharmacy fills used to calculate MPR.

Other Risk Factors

Duration of hypertension was assessed through self-report. Cholesterol tests and values were obtained from the EMR. Using ICD-9 codes recorded in the MCO's administrative database in the year before each survey, a weighted comorbidity score was generated using the Charlson comorbidity index.[16,17] Body mass index (BMI) was calculated from self-reported height and weight. The number and classes of antihypertensive medications were downloaded from the managed-care pharmacy database.

Blood Pressure

Using standard data collection forms and trained record abstractors, blood-pressure levels (including systolic and diastolic values, patient position, and date of blood pressure measurement) were abstracted from the primary care clinics' EMR for the year preceding the survey. The mean blood pressure was calculated for the seated measurements on two different dates closest to the survey date. Using established guidelines,[1] uncontrolled blood pressure was defined as systolic blood pressure greater than or equal to 140 mm Hg or diastolic blood pressure greater than or equal to 90 mm Hg. Blood-pressure data were available for 1,908 participants.

Staff Training and Quality Control

All study staff successfully completed a training program in human subjects' protection, data collection strategies, and on the study protocol. Additional training sessions for the telephone surveyors provided instructions on computer-assisted administration and data entry of the study questionnaire. Baseline surveys were recorded using *Versadial* technology (VS Logger, version 3.0 release, 2008, Irvine, California), and data were entered into a Microsoft Access database. A 10% random sample of recorded surveys was selected for audit and quality check; any discrepancies or illogical values identified were reviewed by the investigative team.

Statistical Analyses

Characteristics of the study population were calculated, overall and by age group (<75 and ≥75 years of age), gender, and race. Data analyses were limited to black and white participants; 14 participants reporting another race were excluded from the current analyses. Significance in the differences in demographics, clinical factors, uncontrolled blood pressure, and low adherence across age group, gender, and race were determined using *t*-tests and chi-square tests. Log binomial regression models that included adjustment for age, gender, and race were used to determine the prevalence ratio of antihypertensive medication nonpersistency by MPR and uncontrolled blood pressure associated with low and medium adherence by MMAS,

Table 1
Study measurements for CoSMO

Variable Domain	Study Measurements	Source
Risk factors		
Socio-demographics	Age, gender, race, education, marital status, dependents, social support,[56] knowledge of hypertension[57]	Survey
Clinical	Duration of hypertension, body mass index; Severity of hypertension-JNC 7,[1] cholesterol; Comorbidities[16,17]	Survey Medical record Administrative data
Behavioral	Smoking status, alcohol use, sexual function,[58] depression,[59-62] coping,[63] stress[64]	Survey
Medication complexity, source and self-efficacy	Antihypertensive medication, dose, frequency, and drug class; hypertensive medication change over prior year; Medication source, pill-splitting practices, medication-taking self efficacy[20]	Pharmacy data Survey
Self-management	Provider blood pressure checks, lifestyle modifications –NHANES,[65] complementary/alternative therapy use,[66] home blood pressure monitoring	Survey
Health care system issues	Perception of primary care provider, satisfaction with access to care and communication;[67-70] Number of visits to health care provider in past year, co-payment, pharmacy benefit package	Survey Survey and administrative data

Life events	Life experiences in the last 12 months-Holmes-Rahe scale[71]	Survey
Hurricane Katrina	Damage to residence,[72] hurricane coping self-efficacy,[73] posttraumatic stress disorder,[74,75] primary cause of stress before and after the disaster, distance from and visits with family and friends[76]	Survey
Adherence		
Medication adherence	Self-report adherence[10] Pharmacy fill[11]	Survey Pharmacy data
Outcomes		
Blood pressure control	Systolic blood pressure (mm Hg); diastolic blood pressure (mm Hg)	Medical record
Quality of life	Quality of life scales: physical, social, role-physical, role-mental, mental health, energy and fatigue, pain, general health, physical summary, and mental summary[77-80]	Survey
Cardiovascular events	Heart failure, myocardial infarction, end-stage renal disease, stroke, transient ischemic attack, atrial fibrillation, peripheral vascular disease	Administrative data, medical record, and survey
Mortality	All-cause and disease-specific mortality	National Death Index
Health care use	Emergency department, in-patient, out-patient, home health, rehabilitation, pharmacy and laboratory encounters	Administrative data

Abbreviations: JNC 7, Joint National Committee on Prevention, Detection, Evaluation and Treatment of High Blood Pressure–7th report; NHANES, National Health and Nutrition Examination Survey.

using those with high adherence as the reference group. Analyses were performed using SAS 9.1 (Cary, North Carolina).

NEW FINDINGS REGARDING ANTIHYPERTENSIVE MEDICATION ADHERENCE IN OLDER ADULTS

Baseline characteristics of the CoSMO participants are presented in **Table 2**. Those younger than 75 years, compared with those 75 years and older, were more likely to be black, a high-school graduate, married, have at least one dependent, a lower co-morbidity score, and a higher BMI. Women enrolled in the study, compared with men, were significantly older, less likely to be married, less likely to have hypertension for more than 10 years, and have higher cholesterol levels, higher BMI, and a lower co-morbidity score. Blacks, compared with whites, were significantly younger, less likely to be a high-school graduate and married, more likely to have a hypertension diagnosis longer than 10 years, have filled two or more antihypertensive medications in the prior year, and have a higher comorbidity score, higher cholesterol levels, and a higher BMI.

Overall, using MMAS, 14.1% of study participants had low adherence and 34.2% and 51.7% had medium and high adherence, respectively. Low medication adherence was more common among participants who were younger than 75 years of age, were black, and had a higher BMI (BMI data not shown in **Table 2**; $P<.01$). Nonpersistent MPR was more common among black participants. Those older than 75 years, women, and blacks had a higher mean systolic blood pressure; those younger than 75 years and blacks had a higher mean diastolic blood pressure. Overall, 33.7% of the participants had uncontrolled blood pressure. Blacks had a significantly higher prevalence of uncontrolled blood pressure ($P<.05$). Marginally significant associations for gender ($P = .08$) and duration of hypertension (data not shown in **Table 2**; $P = .09$) were also identified: women and participants with duration of hypertension greater than 10 years were more likely to have uncontrolled blood pressure.

Prevalence ratios (PR) of nonpersistent MPR and uncontrolled blood pressure by category of medication adherence are presented in **Table 3**. After adjustment for age, race, and gender, and compared with participants with high adherence by MMAS, participants with low adherence by MMAS were 2.71 (95% CI: 2.31–3.18) times more likely to have nonpersistent MPR (P-trend <0.001). Also after age, race, and gender adjustment, participants with low-medication adherence by MMAS were 1.20 (95% CI 1.00–1.43) times more likely to have uncontrolled blood pressure when compared with those participants with high-medication adherence by MMAS. Results were markedly similar after additional adjustment for duration of hypertension and BMI (data not presented). In addition, the association between adherence as measured by MPR and uncontrolled blood pressure was similar: participants with nonpersistent MPR were 1.17 (95% CI 1.02–1.34) more likely to have uncontrolled blood pressure (data not presented in tables).

DISCUSSION

Relatively little is known about the relationship of demographics to medication adherence in older adults, and few studies have examined the validity of self-report adherence measures in the elderly.[18] In the CoSMO study of older adults with hypertension, a substantial portion had low adherence to their antihypertensive medications and uncontrolled blood pressure. Black participants and individuals less than 75 years old had lower adherence levels compared with whites and individuals 75 years or older. Black participants had a significantly higher prevalence of uncontrolled blood pressure compared with their white counterparts. The current study of 2,180 participants confirms a strong association between self-report adherence using the eight-item MMAS and pharmacy fill adherence using MPR, which was previously described in a small sample of hypertensive adults.[11] Additionally, this study reports a significant association between self-reported low adherence by MMAS and uncontrolled blood pressure determined by clinic blood pressure readings, an association which has not been well-documented in an insured older population.

The baseline results of CoSMO support earlier findings that demographic and other risk-factor differences in medication adherence and blood-pressure control are present even in insured groups. Some work has been done to assess barriers to medication adherence in selected populations,[19–21] yet there is a paucity of information about which barriers affect different people. Understanding differences in barriers to medication adherence within demographic subgroups may help target interventions to overcome patient-specific barriers to adherence and to improve clinical outcomes.[22–24] Several studies have found demographic disparities in medication adherence with lower adherence reported among younger individuals,[25,26] men,[25,27] and blacks.[26,28,29] Numerous barriers to medication adherence have been identified, including the asymptomatic nature of hypertension,[21] depression,[30] other noncardiovascular comorbidities,[31] lack of knowledge regarding hypertension and its treatment,[32] beliefs about hypertension and its treatment,[21] complexity and cost of medication regime,[33–35] use of complementary and alternative medicine,[34,36] health care system perceptions by the patient,[37] sexual dysfunction,[38] side effects of medication,[39,40] forgetfulness,[10,41] poor quality of life,[2] inadequate social support,[19,42] caring for dependents,[28] and more recently, disaster-related barriers.[43,44] For example, preliminary analyses in the CoSMO population have identified clinically relevant associations between the presence of depressive symptoms and low antihypertensive medication adherence. CoSMO will explore these barriers and their direct and indirect influence on medication adherence, blood-pressure control, and outcomes, overall and in demographic subgroups. Barriers to medication adherence may be categorized into patient-specific (eg, forgetfulness, beliefs), medication-specific (eg, complexity of medication), logistic (eg, frequency of clinic visits and pharmacy fills), and disease-specific (eg, absence of symptoms for hypertension) barriers, which may provide a framework to facilitate communication with patients about medication adherence in clinical settings and may assist in developing multicomponent behavioral interventions for further investigation.[21]

Multiple strategies to improve medication adherence with the ultimate goal of improving rates of blood-pressure control have been investigated; yet, no single intervention has emerged as superior.[45–50] Interventions aimed at overcoming barriers to adherence have been classified into several broad groups: patient educational interventions (eg, didactic teaching), patient behavioral interventions (eg, patient motivation, support, reminders, drug packaging, simplification of dosing), provider interventions, and complex or combined patient interventions (eg, educational coupled with behavioral interventions).[24] Although there is heterogeneity in the individual trials conducted to date, systematic reviews of the trials have revealed patient behavioral interventions,[47,48,50] provider education interventions,[46,47,51] and combination patient interventions[45,49] resulted in substantial improvements in adherence behaviors and, in some studies, blood-pressure control. The benefits of patient educational interventions alone on medication adherence have been inconclusive.[18,45,46,48] Given that several barriers may influence medication adherence and no single intervention has been identified as the gold standard for improving antihypertensive medication adherence, a patient-centered approach that tailors interventions to overcome patient-specific barriers to medication adherence is warranted.[22–24,48,49]

Table 2
Socio-demographics, other risk factors, medication adherence, and blood pressure levels for CoSMO

	Overall (n = 2,180)[a]	Age		Gender		Race	
		<75 yrs (n = 1,111)	≥75 yrs (n = 1,069)	Men (n = 905)	Women (n = 1,275)	White (n = 1,510)	Black (n = 670)
Socio-demographics							
Age, years; mean standard deviation (SD)	75.0 (5.6)	70.6 (2.6)	79.7 (3.7)[d]	74.7 (5.4)	75.3 (5.6)[c]	75.4 (5.7)	74.3 (5.2)[d]
Female gender, %	58.5	57.0	60.1	0	100	53.0	70.9[d]
Black race, %	30.7	34.4	26.9[d]	21.6	37.3[d]	0	100
High-school graduate, %	79.3	82.7	75.7[d]	81.0	78.0	86.6	62.8[d]
Married, %	56.7	66.1	47.1[d]	77.1	42.3[d]	61.4	46.3[d]
At least one or more dependents, %	40.5	45.8	34.9[d]	53.0	31.5[d]	42.0	36.9[c]
Other risk factors							
Cigarette smoking, %	5.6	7.0	4.0[d]	6.2	5.1	5.4	5.8
Hypertension duration >10 years, %	62.8	62.4	63.3	65.3	61.0[c]	60.9	67.0[d]
Comorbid index score ≥2%	49.6	45.8	53.6[d]	56.3	44.8[d]	48.1	52.9[c]
BMI, kg/m², mean (SD)	29.0 (5.7)	30.2 (6.0)	27.8 (5.0)[d]	28.7 (5.0)	29.2 (6.1)[c]	28.4 (5.4)	30.4 (6.0)[d]
Total cholesterol, mg/dl; mean (SD)	178 (36)	178 (36)	178 (36)	164 (34)	188 (35)[d]	176 (37)	183 (33)[d]

Two or more classes of anti-hypertensive medication used in the prior year, %	83.6	82.4	84.8	82.2	84.5	82.5	86.0[c]
Adherence							
Low medication adherence, %	14.1	16.4	11.8[d]	13.0	14.9	12.3	18.4[d]
Nonpersistent MPR (<0.8), %	27.0	27.1	27.0	26.4	27.5	21.9	38.5[d]
Blood pressure[b]							
Blood pressure							
Systolic blood pressure; mean (SD)	135 (14)	134 (13)	135 (14)[c]	133 (13)	136 (14)[d]	134 (13)	137 (14)[d]
Diastolic blood pressure; mean (SD)	75 (9)	76 (8)	74 (9)[c]	75 (9)	75 (9)	74 (9)	77 (8)[d]
Uncontrolled blood pressure, %	33.7	32.0	35.4	31.4	35.3	31.9	37.7[c]

n = 1,908 for blood pressure; n = 2,087 for medication possession ratio.

[a] Excludes persons with race other than white or black (n = 14).

[b] Blood pressure (BP) included all participants with at least two BP recordings on different days and used the two BP readings closest to the participant survey date to determine uncontrolled BP, n = 1,908; Uncontrolled BP was defined as mean systolic BP and diastolic BP $\geq$ 140/90 mm Hg.

[c] $P < 0.05$.

[d] $P < 0.01$.

Table 3
Associations of MMAS scores with medication possession ratio and uncontrolled blood pressure in CoSMO

	Morisky Medication Adherence Scale (MMAS) score category			
	Low (<6)	Medium (6 to <8)	High (8)	P-Value
n	291	709	1,087	N/A
Nonpersistent MPR (<0.8)[a]				
Prevalence, %	55%	28%	19%	<0.001
Prevalence ratio (95% CI)[c]	2.71 (2.31–3.18)	1.42 (1.20–1.69)	1.00 (ref)	<0.001
n	266	644	998	N/A
Uncontrolled blood pressure[b]				
Prevalence, %	38	35	32	0.13
PR (95% CI)[c]	1.20 (1.00–1.43)	1.07 (0.93–1.23)	1.00 (ref)	<0.04

Uncontrolled BP was defined as mean systolic BP and diastolic BP $\geq$ 140/90 mm Hg.
Abbreviation: CI, confidence interval.
[a] Included all participants with pharmacy fill data available for calculation of MPR, $n = 2,087$.
[b] Included all participants with at least two BP recordings on different days and used the two BP readings closest to the participant survey date to determine uncontrolled BP, $n = 1,908$.
[c] Adjusted for age, gender and race.

It is important for physicians and other health care providers to consider low medication adherence as a factor contributing to poor blood pressure control, to communicate the importance of medication adherence in light of patient-specific barriers (ie, tailored approach) with their patients, to consider strategies a priori that might lessen the effect of barriers on medication adherence and to actively engage patients in the selection of strategies to improve adherence.[24] However, clinicians often do not ask about medication adherence.[52] Important limiting factors for providers considering adherence in their clinical decision-making are lack of time, doubt that low adherence is a cause of uncontrolled blood pressure, and uncertainty about how to accurately determine adherence and use this information in clinical practice.[11,53] Determining patient adherence to antihypertensive medications in outpatient settings is an important first step for clinicians in understanding the effectiveness of the treatments they prescribe, identifying barriers to treatment, and improving blood-pressure control. Validated and short self-report measures, such as MMAS, which provides information on factors affecting adherence such as forgetfulness and medication side effects, may be useful in clinical settings.[23] The baseline results of CoSMO reveal that the new eight-item self-report MMAS performed well with respect to its association with pharmacy fill adherence and blood-pressure control in older insured adults, thus supporting its use in clinical settings to identify low adherers to antihypertensive medications.

The study results should be interpreted with the following limitations in mind. While, in the future, longitudinal data will be available from CoSMO, the analyses presented here were cross-sectional, as data on change in medication adherence are not yet available. The current study was limited to English-speaking older adults with health insurance who were able to complete the baseline telephone survey. The association of MMAS with pharmacy fill was not perfect and may be a result of short-comings of self-report measures (eg, recall and social desirability bias) and inability of pharmacy fill data to capture nuances of medication-taking behavior (eg, pill-splitting, taking medications on alternate days, stopping a medication because of side effects, and hospitalization).[11,53] The association of MMAS with uncontrolled blood pressure is conservative and the true association between low adherence and poor blood-pressure control is likely larger than we report. Blood-pressure measurements were abstracted from the EMR of primary care visits. Challenges of accurate blood-pressure measurements in clinical settings have been documented, and missing data and misclassification are possible.[54] The possible concern regarding missing data in the medical records is minimized because of the mandatory use of the EMR for all outpatient encounters at the primary institution providing care for the managed-care participants.[55] Nevertheless, our findings of associations between low adherence and poor blood-pressure control are consistent with previous studies on middle-aged and disadvantaged patients, which captured blood pressure as part of a standardized study protocol.[10] Our study extends these findings to a population of older insured adults with diverse racial background.

The design of CoSMO has several strengths. The study population includes a large number of black and white patients and is diverse with respect to other socio-demographics and the presence of cardiovascular risk factors. The prospective cohort design, large sample size, and breadth of the data being collected for this study provide the infrastructure for addressing many important questions. An added advantage of the current study is the ability to analyze these relationships across age, race, and gender subgroups to distinguish whether groups of older patients are at greater risk of low adherence. The restriction of our sample to older adults in the managed-care organization minimizes the confounding effects of health insurance, access to medical care, and employment status among older adults. Because hypertension is a prevalent disease, the results of this study may be useful in the evaluation and management of a substantial segment of the population.

SUMMARY AND FUTURE DIRECTIONS

Low adherence to antihypertensive medication is common and contributes to poor blood-pressure control and adverse outcomes. There is lack of understanding of how patient-specific barriers influence low medication adherence and how effective interventions can be targeted to overcome barriers and improve adherence behavior in adults with hypertension. The CoSMO study is designed to provide data on the factors influencing medication adherence and lay the groundwork for interventions to improve antihypertensive medication adherence and clinical outcomes. Important next steps to move the field of antihypertensive medication adherence forward include understanding longitudinal changes in adherence, impact of low adherence on physiologic measures, and development of tailored interventions that overcome patient-specific barriers.

ACKNOWLEDGMENTS

The authors gratefully acknowledge the contributions of the CoSMO Advisory Panel members, including Edward Frohlich MD (Ochsner Clinic Foundation, New Orleans, Louisiana), Jiang He MD, PhD (Tulane School of Public Health and Tropical Medicine, New Orleans, Louisiana), Richard Re MD (Ochsner Clinic Foundation, New Orleans, Louisiana), Paul K Whelton MD (Loyola University Medical Center, Chicago, Illinois).

REFERENCES

1. Chobanian AV, Bakris GL, Black HR, et al. The seventh report of the Joint National Committee on Prevention, Detection, Evaluation, and Treatment of High Blood Pressure. JAMA 2003;289:2560–72.

2. Krousel-Wood M, Thomas S, Muntner P, et al. Medication adherence: a key factor in achieving blood pressure control and good clinical outcomes in hypertensive patients. Curr Opin Cardiol 2004;19:357–62.
3. Ong KL, Cheung BM, Man YB, et al. Prevalence, awareness, treatment, and control of hypertension among United States adults 1999–2004. Hypertension 2007;49:69–75.
4. Hamilton GA. Measuring adherence in a hypertension clinic trial. Eur J Cardiovasc Nurs 2003;2:219–28.
5. Dusing R. Overcoming barriers to effective blood pressure control in patients with hypertension. Curr Med Res Opin 2006;22(8):1545–53.
6. Borzecki AM, Oliveria SA, Berlowitz DR. Barriers to hypertension control. Am Heart J 2005;149:785–94.
7. Osterberg L, Blaschke T. Adherence to medication. N Engl J Med 2005;353:487–97.
8. Callahan CM, Unverzaqt FW, Hui SL, et al. Six-item screener to identify cognitive impairment among potential subjects for clinical research. Med Care 2002;40:771–81.
9. Stanley E, Wood RF, Kergosien L, et al. A comparison of self reported versus administrative race data [abstract]. J Investig Med 2008;56:485.
10. Morisky DE, Ang A, Krousel-Wood MA, et al. Predictive validity of a medication adherence measure in an outpatient setting. J Clin Hypertens 2008;10:348–54.
11. Krousel-Wood MA, Islam T, Webber LS, et al. New medication adherence scale versus pharmacy fill rates in hypertensive seniors. Am J Managed Care 2009;15:59–66.
12. Kopjar B, Sales AEB, Pineros SL, et al. Adherence with statin therapy in secondary prevention of coronary heart disease in veterans administration male population. Am J Cardiol 2003;92:1106–8.
13. Rizzo JA, Simons WR. Variations in compliance among hypertensive patients by drug class: implications for health care costs. Clin Ther 1997;19:1446–57.
14. Sikka R, Xia F, Aubert RE. Estimating medication persistency using administrative claims data. Am J Manag Care 2005;11:449–57.
15. Simpson E, Beck C, Richard H, et al. Drug prescriptions after acute myocardial infarction: dosage, compliance, and persistence. Am Heart J 2003;145:438–44.
16. Charlson ME, Pompei P, Ales KL, et al. A new method of classifying prognostic comorbidity in longitudinal studies: development and validation. J Chronic Dis 1987;40:373–83.
17. Deyo RA, Cherkin DC, Ciol MA. Adapting a clinical comorbidity index for use with ICD-9-CM administrative databases. J Clin Epidemiol 1992;45:613–9.
18. Russell C, Conn V, Jantarakupt P. Older adult medication compliance: integrated review of randomized controlled trials. Am J Health Behav 2006;30:636–50.
19. Fongwa MN, Evangelista LS, Hays RD, et al. Adherence treatment factors in hypertensive African American women. Vasc Health Risk Manag 2008;4(1):157–66.
20. Ogedegbe G, Mancuso CA, Allegrante JP, et al. Development and evaluation of a medication adherence self-efficacy scale in hypertensive African-American patients. J Clin Epidemiol 2003;56:520–9.
21. Ogedegbe G, Harrison M, Robbins L, et al. Barriers and facilitators of medication adherence in hypertensive African Americans: a qualitative study. Ethn Dis 2004;14:3–12.
22. Harmon G, Lefante J, Krousel-Wood MA. The role of providers in improving patient adherence to antihypertensive medications. Curr Opin Cardiol 2006;21:310–5.

23. Hawkshead J, Krousel-Wood MA. Techniques for measuring medication adherence in hypertensive patients in outpatient settings: advantages and limitations. Dis Manage Health Outcomes 2007;15:109–18.
24. Krousel-Wood M, Hyre A, Muntner P, et al. Methods to improve medication adherence in hypertensive patients: current status and future directions. Curr Opin Cardiol 2005;20:296–300.
25. Marentette MA, Gerth WC, Billings DK, et al. Antihypertensive persistence and drug class. Can J Cardiol 2002;18:649–56.
26. Monane M, Bohn RL, Gurwitz JH, et al. The effects of initial drug choice and comorbidity on antihypertensive therapy compliance: results from a population-based study in the elderly. Am J Hypertens 1997;10:697–704.
27. Caro JJ, Salas M, Speckman JL, et al. Persistence with treatment for hypertension in actual practice. CMAJ 1999;160:31–7.
28. Hyre A, Krousel-Wood MA, Muntner P, et al. Prevalence and predictors of poor antihypertensive medication adherence in an urban health clinic setting. J Clin Hypertens 2007;9:179–86.
29. Sharkness CM, Snow DA. The patient's view of hypertension and compliance. Am J Prev Med 1992;8:141–6.
30. Wang PS, Bohn RL, Knight E, et al. Noncompliance with antihypertensive medications: the impact of depressive symptoms and psychosocial factors. J Gen Intern Med 2002;17:504–11.
31. Wang PS, Avorn J, Brookhart MA, et al. Effects of noncardiovascular comorbidites on antihypertensive use in elderly hypertensives. Hypertension 2005;46:273–9.
32. Egan BH, Lackland DT, Cutler NE. Awareness, knowledge and attitudes of older Americans about high blood pressure: implications for health care policy, education, and research. Arch Intern Med 2003;163:681–7.
33. Iskedjian M, Einarson TR, MacKeigan LD, et al. Relationship between daily dose frequency and adherence to antihypertensive pharmacotherapy: evidence from meta-analysis. Clin Ther 2002;24:302–16.
34. Brown CM, Segal R. The effects of health and treatment perceptions on the use of prescribed medication and home remedies among African American and white American hypertensives. Soc Sci Med 1996;43:903–17.
35. Steinman MA, Sands LP, Covinsky KE. Self-retriction of medications due to cost in seniors without prescription coverage: a national survey. J Gen Intern Med 2001;16:793–9.
36. Gohar F, Greenfield SM, Beevers DG, et al. Self-care and adherence to medication: a survey in the hypertension outpatient clinic. BMC Complement Altern Med 2008;8:4.
37. World Health Organization. Hypertension in adherence to long-term therapies evidence for action. Geneva Switzerland: World Health Organization; 2003. p. 107–14.
38. Grimm RH, Grandits GA, Prineas RJ, et al. Long-term effects on sexual function of five antihypertensive drugs and nutritional hygenic treatment in hypertensive men and women. Treatment of Mild Hypertension Study. Hypertension 1997;29:8–14.
39. Wassertheil-Smoller S, Blaufox MD, Oberman A, et al. Effects of antihypertensives on sexual function and quality of life: the TAIM study. Ann Intern Med 1991;114:613–20.
40. Gregoire JP, Moisan J, Guibert R, et al. Tolerability of antihypertensive drugs in a community-based setting. Clin Ther 2001;23:715–26.
41. Morisky DE, Green W, Levine DM, et al. Concurrent and predictive validity of a self-reported measure of medication adherence. Med Care 1986;24:67–74.

42. Schroeder K, Fahey T, Hollinghurst S, et al. Nurse-led adherence support in hypertension: a randomized controlled trial. Fam Pract 2005;22:144–51.
43. Islam T, Muntner P, Webber LS, et al. Cohort study of medication adherence in older adults: extended effects of Hurricane Katrina on medication adherence among older adults. Am J Med Sci 2008;336(2):105–10.
44. Krousel-Wood M, Islam T, Muntner P, et al. Medication adherence in older patients with hypertension after Hurricane Katrina: implications for clinical practice and disaster management. Am J Med Sci 2008;336:99–104.
45. McDonald HP, Garg AX, Haynes RB. Interventions to enhance patient adherence to medication prescriptions: scientific review. JAMA 2002;288(22):2868–79.
46. Morrison A, Wertheimer A, Berger M. Interventions to improve antihypertensive drug adherence: a quantitative review of trials. Formulary 2000;35:234–55.
47. Roter DL, Hall JA, Merisca R, et al. Effectiveness of interventions to improve patient compliance: a meta-analysis. Med Care 1998;36(8):1138–61.
48. Schroeder K, Fahey T, Ebrahim S. How can we improve adherence to blood pressure-lowering medication in ambulatory care? Systematic review of randomized controlled trials. Arch Intern Med 2004;164(7):722–32.
49. Takiya LN, Peterson AM, Finley RS. Meta-analysis of interventions for medication adherence to antihypertensives. Ann Pharmacother 2004;38(10):1617–24.
50. Wetzels GE, Nelemans P, Schouten JS, et al. Facts and fiction of poor compliance as a cause of inadequate blood pressure control: a systematic review. J Hypertens 2004;22(10):1849–55.
51. Inui TS, Yourtee EL, Williamson JW. Improved outcomes in hypertension after physician tutorials: a controlled trial. Ann Intern Med 1976;84:646–51.
52. Bokhour BG, Belowitz DR, Long JA, et al. How do providers assess antihypertensive medication adherence in medical encounters? J Gen Intern Med 2006;21:577–83.
53. Grymonpre R, Cheang M, Fraser M, et al. Validity of a prescription claims database to estimate medication adherence in older persons. Med Care 2006;44:471–7.
54. Jones DW, Appel LJ, Sheps SG, et al. Measuring blood pressure accurately. New and persistent challenges. JAMA 2003;289:1027–30.
55. Elder NC, Hickner J. Missing clinical information. The system is down. JAMA 2005;293:617–9.
56. Sherbourne CD, Stewart AL. The MOS social support survey. Soc Sci Med 1991;32:705–14.
57. Williams MV, Baker DW, Parker RM, et al. Relationship of functional health literacy to patients' knowledge of their chronic disease: a study of patients with hypertension and diabetes. Arch Intern Med 1998;158:166–72.
58. Labbate LA, Lare SB. Sexual dysfunction in male psychiatric outpatients: validity of the Massachusetts General Hospital Sexual Functioning Questionnaire. Psychother Psychosom 2001;70:221–5.
59. Kim MT, Han HR, Hill MN, et al. Depression, substance use, adherence behaviors, and blood pressure in urban hypertensive black men. Ann Behav Med 2003;26:24–31.
60. Knight RG, Williams S, McGee R, et al. Psychometric properties of the Center for Epidemiologic Studies Depression Scale (CES-D) in a sample of women in middle life. Behav Res Ther 1997;35:373–80.
61. Radloff LS. The CES-D scale: a self-report depression scale for research in the general population. Applied Psychological Measurement 1977;1:385–401.

62. Roberts RE, Vernon SW, Rhoades HM. Effests of language and ethnic status on reliability and validity of the CES-D with psychiatric patients. J Nerv Ment Dis 1989;177:581–92.

63. Fernander A, Duran R, Saab P, et al. Assessing the reliability and validity of the John Henry Scale in an urban sample of African-Americans and white-Americans. Ethn Health 2003;8:147–61.

64. Cohen S, Kamarck T, Mermelstein R. A global measure of perceived stress. J Health Soc Behav 1983;24:385–96.

65. 2003–04 Blood Pressure Questionnaire-BPQ_C. Available at: http://www.cdc.gov/nchs/data/nhanes/nhanes_03_04/sp_bpq_c.pdf. Accessed February 15, 2008.

66. Lengacher C, Bennett MP, Kipp KE, et al. Design and testing of the use of a complementary and alternative therapies survey in women with breast cancer. Oncol Nurs Forum 2003;30:811–21.

67. Davies AR, Ware JE. GHAA's Consumer Satisfaction Survey and User's Manual. 2nd edition. Washington, DC: Group Health Association of America, Inc.; 1991. p. 1–48

68. Jatulis DE, Bundek NI, Legorreta AP. Identifying predictors of satisfaction with access to medical care and quality of care. Am J Med Qual 1997;12:11–8.

69. Krousel-Wood MA, Re R, Abdoh A, et al. Patient and physician satisfaction in a clinical study of telemedicine in a hypertensive patient population. J Telemed Telecare 2001;7:206–11.

70. Meng YY, Jatulis DE, McDonald JP, et al. Satisfaction with access to and quality of health care among Medicare enrollees in a health maintenance organization. West J Med 1997;166:242–7.

71. Holmes TH, Rahe RH. The social readjustment rating scale. J Psychosom Res 1967;11:213–8.

72. Inui A, Kitaoka H, Majima M, et al. Effects of the Kobe Earthquake on stress and glycemic control in patients with diabetes mellitus. Arch Intern Med 1998;158:274–8.

73. Benight C, Ironson G, Durham R. Psychometric properties of a hurricane coping self-efficacy measure. J Trauma Stress 1999;12:379–86.

74. Ruggiero KJ, Del Ben K, Scotti JR, et al. Psychometric properties of the PTSD checklist—civilian version. J Trauma Stress 2003;16:495–502.

75. Weathers FW, Huska JA, Keane TM. PCL-C for DSM-IV Boston: National Center for PTSD-Behavioral Division; 1991.

76. Bland SH, Parinaro E, Krogh V, et al. Long term relations between earthquake experiences and coronary heart disease risk factors. Am J Epidemiol 2000; 151:1086–90.

77. Krousel-Wood MA, Re RN. Health status assessment in a hypertension section of an internal medicine clinic. Am J Med Sci 1994;308:211–7.

78. McHorney CA, Ware JE, Rogers W, et al. The validity and relative precision of MOS short-and long-form health scales and Dartmouth COOP chart. Results from the Medical Outcomes Study. Med Care 1992;30:MS253–65.

79. Ware JE, Sherbourne CD. The MOS 36-item short-form health survey (SF-36): I. Conceptual framework and item selection. Med Care 1992;30:473–83.

80. Ware JE, Snow KK, Kosinski M, et al. SF-36 Health survey-manual and interpretation guide. Boston: New England Medical Center; 1993.

Index

Note: Page numbers of article titles are in **boldface** type.

A

Adherence, medication. *See* Medication adherence.
Adhesion molecules, in arterial wall stiffness, 610
Adiponectin deficiency, atherosclerosis in, 683–684
Adipose tissue. *See also* Obesity.
   angiotensinogen in, 571
African American Study of Kidney Disease (AASK), 699–701
Aging
   arterial. *See* Arteries, aging of.
   diastolic dysfunction in, 647–664
   heart failure prevention in, 671
   hypertension prevalence in, 650
Alcohol intake, blood pressure and, 739
Aldosterone
   action of, 571, 574
   antagonists of, for hypertension, 706
Aliskiren, for hypertension, 561
   in chronic kidney disease, 706
   in obesity, 742
Alkoxy radicals, structure of, 621
Alpha-1 adrenergic blockers, for hypertension, in obesity, 741, 743
Alpha-2 agonists, centrally acting, for hypertension, in obesity, 741, 743
Alpha blockers, for hypertension, in chronic kidney disease, 708
Amlodipine, for hypertension, 689
   in cardiovascular disease prevention, 615
   in chronic kidney disease, 700, 707
   in diastolic dysfunction, 656, 658–659
   metabolic effects of, 577
Angiography, in renovascular hypertension, 728–729
Angioplasty and Stenting in Renal Atherosclerotic Lesions trial, 727
Angiotensin (1-7), action of, 562
Angiotensin II. *See also* Renin-angiotensin-aldosterone system.
   in arterial aging, 592–597
   intracellular, 563
   reactive oxygen species and, 573, 627–628
   receptors for, 561–562
   vascular disease due to, 559–563
Angiotensin II-receptor blockers
   action of, 560–561
   for cardiometabolic syndrome, 575–576
   for diastolic dysfunction, 657

Med Clin N Am 93 (2009) 771–786
doi:10.1016/S0025-7125(09)00050-9
0025-7125/09/$ – see front matter © 2009 Elsevier Inc. All rights reserved.

medical.theclinics.com

Angiotensin (*continued*)
    for hypertension
        in chronic kidney disease, 701, 705–706
        in heart failure prevention, 671
        in obesity, 741–742
        renovascular, 724
Angiotensin type 1 receptor. *See* AT-1 receptor.
Angiotensin-converting enzyme, ACE2 homolog of, 562
Angiotensin-converting enzyme inhibitors, for hypertension, 689–690
    for cardiovascular disease prevention, 615
    in chronic kidney disease, 701, 703–705
    in diastolic dysfunction, 656–657
    in heart failure prevention, 671
    in obesity, 741–742
    renovascular, 723–724
    with cardiometabolic syndrome, 575–576
Anglo-Scandinavian Cardiac Outcomes Trial, 615, 706
Annexin, in left ventricular hypertrophy, 643
Antihypertensive and Lipid-Lowering Treatment to Prevent Heart Attack Trial (ALLHAT), 576, 658, 671, 699, 704–705, 743
Antihypertensive drugs. *See* Hypertension, treatment of.
Antiobesity agents, 744
Antioxidants, 623
Aorta
    aging of
        angiotensin II signaling in, 592–597
        macroscopic structure of, 584, 586
        microscopic structure of, 584–585, 587–588
    hemodynamics of, alterations for risk reduction, 614–615
    hypertension effects on, 530
    pulse pressure in
        cardiovascular disease risk and, 611–615
        diffusion, 609–611
        factors affecting, 606–609
    systolic blood pressure in, 606–609
    weakness of, in Marfan syndrome, 562–563
Apoptosis, of cardiomyocytes, 639–641, 667
Appropriate Blood Pressure Control in Diabetes (ABCD) trial, 699
Arrhythmias, 545–546, 658
Arteries
    aging of, **583–604**
        angiotensin II signaling in, 592–597
        aorta, 584–588, 592–596
        arterial blood pressure determinants in, 597–598
        calpain-1 in, 594
        compliance in, 591
        endothelial function and, 589–590, 598–599
        exaggerated, 598–600
        hypertension and, 598–600
        macroscopic structure in, 584, 586
        vmatrix metalloproteinases in, 595

mechanisms of, 609–611
microscopic structure in, 584–588, 592
monocyte chemotactic protein-1 in, 596
pulse wave reflections in, 607–608
reflected pulse wave evaluation of, 591–592
stiffness in, 591–592, 599, 653, 656
transforming growth factor-beta 1 in, 595–596
ventricular coupling with, 599–600
large. *See* Aorta; Large arteries.
remodeling of, 608–609
wall of, pulse pressure and, 609–611
Arterioles, high resistance, 607
AT-1 receptor, 561–563
angiotensin II interactions with, 571
in arterial aging, 592–593
AT-1 receptor antagonists, for hypertensive heart disease, 643
Atenolol, for hypertension
in cardiovascular disease prevention, 615
in chronic kidney disease, 708
in obesity, 743
Atherosclerosis
coronary, myocardial ischemia in, 683–684
formation of
angiotensin II in, 559–563
oxidized low-density lipoprotein in, 562
prevention of, 555
renovascular hypertension in, 718, 721, 725–727
risk for, 547–549
T lymphocytes in, 629–630
Atrial natriuretic peptide, in obesity, 548
Atrium
enlargement of, in hypertension, 652
volume of, measurement of, 656
Autophagy, of cardiomyocytes, 639–641
Avoiding Cardiovascular Events through Combination Therapy in Patients Living with Systolic Hypertension (ACCOMPLISH), 577, 656–657, 707

B

Baroreflex, reactive oxygen species effects on, 628
Benazepril, for hypertension, 577, 656
Benidipine, for hypertension, 689
Bergamo Nephrologic Diabetes Complications Trial, 707–708
Beta blockers, for hypertension
diabetogenic action of, 576–577
in chronic kidney disease, 708
in heart failure prevention, 671
in obesity, 741, 743
meta-analysis of, 535–536
Biomarkers
for hypertension, 536
for left ventricular hypertrophy, 643

Bisoprolol, for heart failure prevention, 671–672
Brachial pulse pressure, 611–612
Bradykinin receptor, AT-1 receptor interactions with, 562
Brain, reactive oxygen species in, 626–628
Brain natriuretic peptide
    in hypertensive heart disease, 668
    in obesity, 548
Bundle branch blocks, 546

C

Calcium channel blockers, for hypertension, 689, 742–743
    in cardiovascular disease prevention, 615
    in chronic kidney disease, 707–708
    in obesity, 741
    meta-analysis of, 535–536
Calpain-1, in arterial aging, 594
Candesartan in Heart Failure: Assessment of Reduction in Mortality and Morbidity
    study (CHARM), 576, 657, 671, 673
Captopril, for hypertension
    in chronic kidney disease, 700
    in heart failure prevention, 673
Captopril Nephropathy Trial, 703–704
Captopril Prevention Project, 575–576
Captopril renography, in renovascular hypertension, 728
Cardiac catheterization, in diastolic dysfunction, 654
Cardiac failure. See Heart failure.
Cardiac Insufficiency Bisoprolol Study (CIBIS), 672
Cardiometabolic syndrome
    angiotensin II-receptor blockers for, 575–576
    oxidative stress in, 572–575
    renin angiotensin aldosterone system in, 571
    sympathetic nervous system activation in, 570
Cardiomyocytes
    cytoskeletal proteins of, diastolic function and, 651
    hypertrophy of, in hypertensive heart disease, 638–639
    in remodeling, 639–641, 667
    obesity effects on, 735
Cardiotrophin-1, in cardiomyocyte hypertrophy, 642
Cardiovascular disease
    heart failure in. See Heart failure.
    hypertensive. See Hypertensive heart disease.
    in aging, **583–604**
    in obesity, 734–735
    J-curve controversy and, 544–545
    left ventricular hypertrophy in. See Left ventricular hypertrophy.
    prevention of, 555, 576
    risk for, 543, 547–548
        global assessment instrument for, 550–551
        preventive implications of, 554–555
        pulsatile hemodynamics and, 611–615

Cardiovascular Health Study, 666
Cardiovascular Outcomes for Renal Atherosclerotic Lesions, 717–718
Carvedilol, for hypertension
    in chronic kidney disease, 708
    in heart failure prevention, 671–672, 674
    in obesity, 743
Central nervous system, reactive oxygen species in, 626–628
Central pulse pressure, 613–614
Chlorthalidone, for hypertension
    in chronic kidney disease, 707
    in diastolic dysfunction, 658
    in heart failure prevention, 671
Circumventricular organ, reactive oxygen species effects on, 627
Clonidine, for hypertension, in obesity, 743
Cohort Study of Medication Adherence in Older Adults (CoSMO), **753–769**
Collagen fibers
    hypertension effects on, 650–651
    in aging arteries, 592
    in myocardial remodeling, 640–641
Compliance, assessment of, in diastolic dysfunction, 653–654
Computed tomography angiography, in renovascular hypertension, 729
Conduit Artery Function Evaluation (CAFE), 615
Contractility, in myocardial oxygen demand, 681–682
COOPERATE trial, 706
Coronary arteries, blood flow in, myocardial oxygen supply from, 682–683
Coronary flow reserve, in myocardial ischemia, 687
Coronary heart disease
    central pulse pressure and, 613–614
    electrocardiography in, 545–546
    myocardial ischemia in, 683–684
    risk for, 547
Cyclic mechanical forces, on arteries, 609
Cytochrome C, in cardiomyocyte apoptosis, 640
Cytokines, in extracellular matrix, 650–651
Cytoskeleton, hypertension effects on, 651

D

Diabetes mellitus
    angiotensin blockers in, 575–576
    nephropathy in, 699
Diabetes Reduction Assessment with Ramipril and Rosiglitazone Medication, 576
Diastolic dysfunction, heart failure in, **647–664**
Dietary Approaches to Stop Hypertension (DASH) diet, 703, 737–738
Dietary Intervention Study in Hypertension, 738
Diuretics, for hypertension, 742
    cardiovascular-renal damage due to, 535
    diabetogenic action of, 576–577
    in chronic kidney disease, 706–707
    in obesity, 741

Doppler ultrasonography
    in diastolic dysfunction, 654–655
    in renovascular hypertension, 727–728
Doxazosin, for hypertension
    in diastolic dysfunction, 658
    in obesity, 743

E

Echocardiography
    in diastolic dysfunction, 654, 656
    in hypertensive heart disease, 667–668
    in myocardial ischemia, 687
Effect of Losartan and Amlodipine on Left Ventricular Diastolic Function in Patients with Mild-to-Moderate Hypertension study, 659
Elastin, in aging arteries, 592
Elderly persons. *See* Older adults.
Electrocardiography, 545–546
    in myocardial ischemia, 686
    in obesity, 735
Enalapril
    for heart failure prevention, 671–672
    for hypertension, 689
End diastolic pressure, in diastolic dysfunction, 653–654
Endothelial cells
    dysfunction of
        diastolic dysfunction in, 651–652
        myocardial ischemia in, 685
        renovascular hypertension in, 721
    in arterial aging, 598–599
    reactive oxygen species produced in, 572
Endothelin, oxidative stress due to, 574–575
Endurance training, for diastolic dysfunction, 656
Epicardial arteries, myocardial oxygen supply from, 682–683
Epidermal growth factor receptor, AT-1 receptor interactions with, 562
Eplerenone Post-Acute Myocardial Infarction Heart Failure Efficacy and Survival Study (EPHESUS), 576, 673–674
European Working Party on High Blood Pressure in the Elderly trial, 611
Exercise
    for diastolic dysfunction, 656
    for obesity, 739
Exercise electrocardiography, in myocardial ischemia, 686
EXforge Aggressive Control of Hypertension to Evaluate Efficacy in Diastolic Dysfunction trial, 658
Extracellular matrix
    hypertension effects on, 650–652
    remodeling of, 608–609

F

Felodipine, for hypertension, 689, 744
Fibrillin defects, transforming growth factor excess and, 562–563

Fibromuscular dysplasia, of renal arteries, renovascular hypertension in, 719–721, 725–727
Fibrosis
    myocardial, 640–641
    perivascular, 685
Flow propagation velocity, in diastolic dysfunction, 655
Framingham Study, 541–555
Free fatty acids, in obesity, 736

G

Genetic factors
    in hypertension, 528–529
    in left ventricular hypertrophy, 641–642
Global risk assessment instrument, 549–552
Glomerular disease, in obesity, 735

H

Heart
    hypertension effects on, 529–530
    obesity effects on, 734–735
Heart disease. *See also* Cardiovascular disease; Heart failure; Left ventricular hypertrophy.
    hypertensive, **637–645**
Heart failure, **665–680**
    diagnosis of, 667–669
    diastolic dysfunction in, **647–664**
        assessment of, 653–656
        epidemiology of, 648
        pathophysiology of, 649–653
        physiology of, 648–649
        treatment of, 656–659
        with preserved ejection fraction, 647–659
    epidemiology of, 665–666
    in obesity, 735
    pathophysiology of, 666–667
    prevention of, 668, 670–671
    risk factors for, 666
    treatment of, 671–675
Heart Outcomes Prevention Evaluation (HOPE), 575, 657
Heart rate, in myocardial oxygen demand, 681–682
Hemodynamic effects, of obesity, 735–736
Hydrochlorothiazide, for hypertension, 742
    diabetogenic action of, 577
    in chronic kidney disease, 707
    in obesity, 742, 744
Hydrogen peroxide
    in hypertension, vasculature and, 628
    structure of, 621
Hydroxyl radical, structure of, 621
Hypertension
    arterial aging in, **583–604,** 607–608, 653, 656
    classification of, 549–550

Hypertension (*continued*)
    comorbid conditions with, 548
    diastolic dysfunction in, **647–664**
    epidemiology of, 650
    genetic factors in, 528–529
    heart disease in. *See* Heart disease.
    heart failure in, **647–680,** 735
    in chronic kidney disease, **697–715**
    large arteries and, **605–619**
    myocardial ischemia in, **681–695**
    obesity and. *See* Obesity.
    oxidative stress in, **621–635**
    pathophysiology of, **527–540**. *See also* Renin-angiotensin-aldosterone system.
    prevention of, 553–555
    progression to, 552–553
    renovascular, **717–732**
    risk factors for, **541–558**
    systolic. *See* Systolic hypertension.
    target organs in. *See* Heart; Kidney; Large arteries.
    treatment of
        global risk assessment for, 549–552
        in cardiovascular disease prevention, 614–615
        in diastolic dysfunction, 656–659
        in heart failure prevention, 670
        in myocardial ischemia, 688–690
        in target organ protection, **559–567**
        medication adherence in, **763–769**
        target blood pressure for, 689
    unresolved problems in, **527–540**
Hypertension in the Very Elderly Trial (HYVET), 671
Hypertension Obesity Sibutramine study (HOS), 744
Hypertensive heart disease, **637–645, 665–680**
    detection of, 641–642
    diagnosis of, 642–643, 667–669
    epidemiology of, 665–666
    pathophysiology of, 638–641, 666–667
    treatment of, 643–644, 670–675
Hypochlorous acid, structure of, 621

I

Indapamide, for hypertension, 615, 671
Inflammation, reactive oxygen species in, 629–630
Inflammatory cells, in aging arteries, 584–585
Insulin
    action of, in kidney, 570
    resistance to. *See also* Cardiometabolic syndrome.
        in obesity, 734–735
Integrins, in arterial wall stiffness, 610
Intima, of aging arteries, 584–585, 587
Intra-arterial angiography, in renovascular hypertension, 729
Intracrines, angiotensin II as, 563

Irbesartan, for hypertension, 742
Irbesartan in Diabetic Nephropathy Trial (IDNT), 700
Irbesartan in Heart Failure with Preserved Ejection Fraction (I-PRESERVE), 657
Isovolumetric ventricular relaxation, assessment of, in diastolic dysfunction, 653–656

J

J-curve controversy, 544–545

K

Kidney
    chronic disease of, hypertension in, **697–715**
        blood pressure goals for, 697–702
        epidemiology of, 697
        proteinuria in, 698–702
        pulse wave velocity in, 612–613
        treatment of, 614–615, 699–708
    hypertension effects on, 530–531
    obesity effects on, 735–736
    reactive oxygen species effects on, 624–626
    renal artery stenosis in, **717–732**
    sodium handling in, 570

L

Large arteries. *See also* Aorta.
    hemodynamics of, alterations for risk reduction, 614–615
    hypertension effects on, 530
    pulse pressure in
        cardiovascular disease risk and, 611–615
        diffusion, 609–611
        factors affecting, 606–609
    systolic blood pressure in, factors affecting, 606–609
Left Ventricular Dysfunction trial, 671
Left ventricular hypertrophy, 529–530, 545
    diagnosis of, 642–643
    early detection of, 641–642
    genetic factors in, 641–642
    heart failure in, 667–675
    in obesity, 735
    myocardial remodeling in, 652–653
    pathophysiology of, 541
    pulsatile-components index in, 611
    reference limits for, 669
    treatment of, 643–644, 671–676
Leptin
    elevated, sympathetic nervous system activation in, 570
    obesity and, 735–736
Lifestyle changes
    for heart failure prevention, 668, 670
    for hypertension, in chronic kidney disease, 703

Lifestyle (*continued*)
    for myocardial ischemia, 688–689
    for obesity, 736–739
Lipid peroxy radical, structure of, 621
Lisinopril, for hypertension, 658, 742
Losartan, for hypertension
    in chronic kidney disease, 700
    in diastolic dysfunction, 659
    in hypertensive heart disease, 643
Losartan Intervention For Endpoint Reduction in Hypertension Study (LIFE), 576,
    657, 670
LOX-1 receptor, 562

M

Magnetic resonance angiography, in renovascular hypertension, 728–729
Magnetic resonance imaging
    in left ventricular hypertrophy, 642
    in myocardial ischemia, 686–687
Marfan syndrome, vascular pathology in, 562–563
Matrix metalloproteinases, in arterial aging, 595
Medial hypertrophy, myocardial ischemia in, 684–685
Medication adherence, in older adults, **753–769**
Metabolic syndrome. *See* Cardiometabolic syndrome.
Metoprolol, for hypertension
    in chronic kidney disease, 700
    in heart failure prevention, 671–672, 674
    in obesity, 743
Metoprolol CR/XL Randomises Intervention Trial in Congestive Heart Failure
    (MERIT-HF), 672, 674
Microalbuminuria, in chronic kidney disease, 698–702
Micromanometer catheter, in diastolic dysfunction, 654
Mineralocorticoid receptor blockers, for cardiometabolic syndrome, 576
Mitochondrial respiratory chain, in reactive oxygen species production, 572–573
Modification of Diet in Renal Disease (MDRD) Study, 699, 701
Multiple Risk Factor Intervention Trial (MRFIT), 543
Myocardial contract echocardiography, in myocardial ischemia, 686
Myocardial infarction, unrecognized, 546–547
Myocardial ischemia, **691–695**
    asymptomatic, 684
    investigation of, 686–688
    mechanisms of, 683–685
    pathophysiology of, 681–683
    treatment of, 688–690
Myocardium
    fibrosis of, 640–641
    remodeling of, in hypertensive heart disease, 639–641

N

Natriuretic peptides, in obesity, 548
Nebivolol

for heart failure prevention, 671–672, 674
for hypertension, 689
    in chronic kidney disease, 708
    in obesity, 743
Necrosis, of cardiomyocytes, 639–641
Nicotinamide adenine dinucleotide phosphate oxidase complex
    in aging arteries, 589
    in reactive oxygen species production, 572–574, 622, 624–625, 627–630
Nifedipine, for hypertension, in chronic kidney disease, 707
Nitric oxide
    chemistry of, 621
    in aging arteries, 589
    in kidney, 625
Nitric oxide synthase
    action of, 622
    in kidney, 625–626
    in reactive oxygen species production, 572–573
Nitrogen dioxide, chemistry of, 621
Nitrosonium cation, chemistry of, 621
Nucleus tractus solitarii, reactive oxygen species effects on, 627

O

Obesity, **733–751**
    adipose tissue in, angiotensinogen in, 571
    epidemiology of, 733
    hypertension in, 531–532, 553
        cardiac effects of, 734–735
        hemodynamic effects of, 735–736
        mechanical effects of, 735–736
        renal effects of, 735–736
        treatment of, 736–744
        vascular adaptations in, 734–735
    leptin elevation in, 570
    natriuretic peptide levels in, 548
Obstructive sleep apnea, in obesity, 744
Older adults
    arterial aging in. See Arteries, aging of.
    diastolic dysfunction in, 647–664
    heart failure prevention in, 671
    hypertension prevalence in, 650
    medication adherence in, **753–769**
Oxidative stress. See also Reactive oxygen species.
    in insulin resistance, 572–575
Oxygen demand and supply, in myocardial ischemia, 681–683

P

Perindopril, for hypertension, 615
Perindopril in Elderly People with Chronic Heart Failure trial (PEP-CHF), 657

Perivascular fibrosis, myocardial ischemia in, 685
Peroxynitrate, in insulin resistance, 573
Peroxynitrite, structure of, 621
Positron emission tomography
    in left ventricular hypertrophy, 643
    in myocardial ischemia, 687
Prearterioles, myocardial oxygen supply from, 683
Precapillary arterioles, myocardial oxygen supply from, 683
Prehypertension, 543–544
Prorenin receptor, 560–561
Proteinuria, in chronic kidney disease, 698–702
Pulmonary venous flow Doppler studies, in diastolic dysfunction, 655
Pulsatile-components index, 611
Pulse pressure
    brachial, 611–612
    cardiovascular disease risk and, 611–615
    central, 613–614
    diffusion of, 609–611
    factors affecting, 606–609
    variation of, 609–611
    widened, 554–555
Pulse wave(s), in arterial aging, 591–592
Pulse wave velocity, in systolic hypertension, 605, 607–608, 612–613, 615
Pulsed-wave tissue Doppler imaging, in diastolic dysfunction, 655

R

Rac-1 protein, in hypertension, 627
Ramipril
    for cardiometabolic syndrome, 575–576
    for cardiovascular disease prevention, 575–576
    for diastolic dysfunction, 657
    for hypertension
        in chronic kidney disease, 700–701
        in obesity, 744
Ramipril Efficacy in Nephropathy (REIN) trial, 701
Randomized Aldacton Evaluation Study (RALES), 576, 673–674
Reactive nitrogen species, 621
Reactive oxygen species, **621–635**
    degradation of, 623
    functions of, 621–623
    in hypertension, 623–630
        central nervous system and, 626–628
        inflammation and, 629–630
        kidney and, 624–626
        vasculature and, 628
    in insulin resistance, 572–575
    pathogenicity of, 623
    types of, 621
REASON study, 615

Reduction of Endpoints in Non-insulin dependent diabetes mellitus with the Angiotensin II
    Antagonist Losartan (RENAAL), 700, 705–706
Renal arteries
    diagnostic evaluation of, 727–729
    revascularization of, 725–727
Renin inhibitors, for hypertension, in obesity, 741–742
Renin-angiotensin-aldosterone system, **569–582**
    AT-1 receptor in, 561–562
    blockade of. See Angiotensin-converting enzyme inhibitors; Angiotensin II-receptor
        blockers.
    chronic activation of, diastolic dysfunction in, 652
    description of, 571
    dysfunction of, vascular disease in, 559–560
    function of, 571
    in arterial aging, 592–597
    in insulin resistance, 574–575
    in reactive oxygen species generation, 572–575
    in sodium handling, 570
    intracrine, 563
    pathologic effects of, 571
    (pro)renin receptor in, 560–561
    sympathetic nervous system interactions with, 570
    transforming growth factor and, 562–563
Renography, captopril, in renovascular hypertension, 728
Renovascular hypertension, **717–732**
    clinical features of, 719–722
    diagnosis of, 727–729
    epidemiology of, 719–722
    pathophysiology of, 718–719
    treatment of, 722–727
Revascularization, for renovascular hypertension, 725–727
Risk factors and risk stratification, in hypertension, **541–558**
    antihypertensive guidelines and, 549–552
    cardiovascular hazards, 547
    electrocardiography in, 545–546
    global risk assessment, 549–552
    J-curve controversy in, 544–545
    left ventricular hypertrophy and. See Left ventricular hypertrophy.
    misconceptions in, 542–543
    predisposing, 552–553
    prehypertension category in, 543–544
    preventive implications of, 552–553
    unrecognized myocardial infarction and, 546–547
Rosiglitazone, for cardiometabolic syndrome, 576

S

Salt intake, hypertension and, 532–535
SERCA2a receptor, in diastolic function, 651
Serine kinases, in oxidative stress, 575

Shear stress, cyclic, on arteries, 609
Sibutramine, for obesity, 744
Single-photon emission computed tomography
    in left ventricular hypertrophy, 643
    in myocardial ischemia, 687
Sleep apnea, obstructive, in obesity, 744
Smoking, hypertension and, 531–532
Sodium
    excretion of, renovascular hypertension and, 721–722
    restriction of
        for hypertension, in chronic kidney disease, 703
        in hypertension, 738–739
    retention of, in obesity, 735–736
Speckle tracking technology, in diastolic dysfunction, 656
Spironolactone, for hypertension, 689
    in cardiometabolic syndrome, 576
    in diastolic dysfunction, 652
    in heart failure prevention, 673–675
Stents, renal artery, 727
Stiffness, in arterial aging, 591–592, 599, 609–611, 653, 656
Stress echocardiography, in myocardial ischemia, 687
Stress electrocardiography, in myocardial ischemia, 686
Stroke, risk for, 547, 549
Strong Heart Study, 648, 666
Studies of Left Ventricular Dysfunction (SOLVD), 576, 672
Study of the Effects of Nebivolol Intervention on Outcomes and Hospitalization in
    Seniors with Heart Failure study (SENIORS), 672, 674
Subfornical organ, reactive oxygen species effects on, 627
Superoxide
    in hypertension
        in kidney, 625–626
        vasculature and, 628
    in insulin resistance, 572–575
    structure of, 621
Superoxide dismutase
    action of, 623
    blood pressure reduction due to, 573–574
    in aging arteries, 589
    in hypertension, 623, 627
Survival and Ventricular Enlargement (SAVE) trial, 671–672
Sympathetic nervous system, activation of, in insulin resistance, 570
Syst-China trial, 611
Syst-Eur trial, 611
Systolic blood pressure, factors affecting, 606–609
Systolic dysfunction, 667
Systolic hypertension
    brachial pulse pressure in, 611–612
    cardiovascular disease prevention in, 614–615
    isolated, 544–545
        aging and, 598
        treatment guidelines for, 554–555

pulse wave reflections in, 607–608
    treatment of, 656–657
Systolic Hypertension in Europe trial, 545
Systolic Hypertension in the Elderly Program (SHEP), 544–545

T

T lymphocytes, in atherosclerosis, 629–630
Target organs. See Cardiovascular disease; Heart; Kidney; Large arteries.
Telmisartan, for hypertension, in obesity, 742
Torsemide, for hypertension, 707
Trandolapril, for hypertension, 689, 742, 744
Trandolapril Cardiac Evaluation trial (TRACE), 671
Transforming growth factor
    angiotensin II interactions with, 562–563
    in arterial aging, 595–596
    obesity and, 736
Treatment of Obese Patients With Hypertension Study Group, 742
Treatment of Preserved Systolic Function Heart Failure with an Aldosterone Antagonist
    trial (TOPCAT), 658–659
Trial of Hypertension Prevention (TOPH), 534, 738
Trial of Nonpharmacological Interventions in the Elderly (TONE), 738
Tubuloglomerular feedback, in hypertension, 625

U

Ultrasonography
    in diastolic dysfunction, 654–655
    in left ventricular hypertrophy, 642
    in renovascular hypertension, 727–728
United States Carvedilol Heart Failure Study, 672, 674

V

Valsartan Heart Failure Trial, 671, 673
Valsartan in Acute Myocardial Infarction trial (VALIANT), 671
Valsartan in Diastolic Dysfunction trial (VALIDD), 649–650, 657–658
Vascular smooth muscle cells
    cyclic stress on, 609
    in aging arteries, 584–585, 608–609
    reactive oxygen species produced in, 572
Ventral lateral medulla, reactive oxygen species effects on, 627
Ventricle(s), left
    coupling with aging arteries, 599–600
    filling pressure measurement, 654–656
    hypertrophy of. See Left ventricular hypertrophy.
    stiffness of, 653

Verapamil, for hypertension, 689
   in chronic kidney disease, 708
   in obesity, 742, 744

W

Wall tension, in myocardial oxygen demand, 681–682
Weight loss, for obesity, 736–740, 744

X

Xanthine oxidase, in reactive oxygen species production, 572–573, 622

Moving?

Make sure your subscription moves with you!

To notify us of your new address, find your **Clinics Account Number** (located on your mailing label above your name), and contact customer service at:

E-mail: elspcs@elsevier.com

800-654-2452 (subscribers in the U.S. & Canada)
314-453-7041 (subscribers outside of the U.S. & Canada)

Fax number: 314-523-5170

Elsevier Periodicals Customer Service
11830 Westline Industrial Drive
St. Louis, MO 63146

*To ensure uninterrupted delivery of your subscription, please notify us at least 4 weeks in advance of move.